Diana J. Wood

Medical Unit
Royal London Hospital
London E1 1BB.

Polycystic Ovary Syndrome

CURRENT ISSUES IN ENDOCRINOLOGY AND METABOLISM

Series Editor

JEROME M. HERSHMAN MD
Chief, Endocrinology Section,
Wadsworth VA Medical Center, Los Angeles, California;
Professor of Medicine, University of California, Los Angeles

Previous volumes in the series

Graves' Ophthalmopathy
JACK R. WALL AND JACQUES HOW

Molecular and Clinical Advances in Pituitary Disorders
SHLOMO MELMED AND RICHARD J. ROBBINS

Thyroid Hormone Metabolism: Regulation and Clinical Implications
SING-YUNG WU

CURRENT ISSUES IN ENDOCRINOLOGY AND METABOLISM

Polycystic Ovary Syndrome

Edited by

ANDREA DUNAIF MD
Department of Medicine, Division of Endocrinology
Mount Sinai Medical Center
New York

JAMES R. GIVENS MD
Department of Medicine
University of Tennessee
Memphis, Tennessee

FLORENCE P. HASELTINE PhD, MD
Center for Population Research
Bethesda, Maryland

GEORGE R. MERRIAM MD
Developmental Endocrinology Branch
National Institute of Child Health and Human Development
Bethesda, Maryland

BOSTON

BLACKWELL SCIENTIFIC PUBLICATIONS

OXFORD LONDON EDINBURGH

MELBOURNE PARIS BERLIN VIENNA

To our spouses, who have tolerated our interest and our work. We do not know how much androgens influenced either.

Editorial offices:
3 Cambridge Center, Cambridge
Massachusetts 02142, USA
Osney Mead, Oxford OX2 0EL, England
25 John Street, London WC1N 2BL
England
23 Ainslie Place, Edinburgh EH3 6AJ
Scotland
54 University Street, Carlton
Victoria 3053, Australia

Other Editorial offices:
Arnette SA
2, rue Casimir-Delavigne
75006 Paris
France

Blackwell Wissenschaft
Meinekestrasse 4
D-1000 Berlin 15
Germany

Blackwell MZV
Feldgasse 13
A-1238 Wien
Austria

First published 1992

Set by Excel Typesetters Ltd., Hong Kong
Printed and bound in the United States of America by BookCrafters, Chelsea, Michigan

92 93 94 95 5 4 3 2 1

DISTRIBUTORS

USA and Canada
Mosby-Year Book, Inc.
11830 Westline Industrial Drive
St Louis, Missouri 63146
(*Orders*: Tel: 800 633–6699)

Australia
Blackwell Scientific Publications
(Australia) Pty Ltd
54 University Street
Carlton, Victoria 3053
(*Orders*: Tel: 03 347 0300)

Outside North America and Australia
Marston Book Services Ltd
PO Box 87
Oxford OX2 0DT
(*Orders*: Tel: 0865 791155
Fax: 0865 791927
Telex: 837515)

Library of Congress
Cataloging-in-Publication Data

Polycystic ovary syndrome/
edited by Andrea Dunaif *et al.*
p. cm.—(Current issues in endocrinology and metabolism)
Includes bibliographical references and index.
ISBN 0-86542-142-0
1. Stein–Leventhal syndrome.
I. Dunaif, Andrea.
II. Series.
[DNLM: 1. Polycystic Ovary Syndrome.
WP 320 P7825]
RG480. S7P66 1991
618.1–dc20
DNLM/DLC
for Library of Congress

Contents

Section 6: Growth Factors

Section 7: Insulin

Section 8: Consequences and Treatment of Polycystic Ovary Syndrome

Section 9: Diagnostic Criteria: Towards a Rational Approach

List of Contributors

DOMENICO A. ACCILI MD *Diabetes Branch, National Institute of Diabetes and Digestive and Kidney Diseases, National Institutes of Health, Bethesda, MD 20892*

ELI Y. ADASHI MD *Division of Reproductive Endocrinology, Department of Obstetrics and Gynecology, University of Maryland School of Medicine, Baltimore, MD 21201*

BARRY D. ALBERTSON PhD *Division of Endocrinology, Oregon Health Sciences University, Portland, OR 97201*

ROBERT L. BARBIERI MD *Department of Obstetrics and Gynecology, Health Sciences Center, State University of New York at Stony Brook, Stony Brook, NY 11794*

RANDALL B. BARNES MD *Department of Obstetrics and Gynecology, University of Chicago, Pritzker School of Medicine, Chicago, IL 60637*

WILLIAM G. BLACKARD MD *Division of Endocrinology and Metabolism, Medical College of Virginia, Richmond, VA 23298*

KATRYNA BOGOVICH PhD *University of South Carolina School of Medicine, Columbia, SC 29208*

DEBORAH F. BRIGELL MD *Department of Medicine, University of Chicago, Pritzker School of Medicine, Chicago, IL 60637*

CYNTHIA K. BUFFINGTON PhD *Departments of Medicine and Biochemistry, University of Tennessee at Memphis, Memphis, TN 38163*

ALESSANDRO CAMA MD *Diabetes Branch, National Institute of Diabetes and Digestive and Kidney Diseases, National Institutes of Health, Bethesda, MD 20892*

DONALD W. CHANDLER PhD *Endocrine Sciences, Tarzana, CA 91356*

R. JEFFREY CHANG MD *Division of Reproductive Biology and Medicine, Department of Obstetrics and Gynecology, University of California at Davis Medical Center, Sacramento, CA 95816*

JOHN N. CLORE MD *Division of Endocrinology and Metabolism, Medical College of Virginia, Richmond, VA 23298*

JEFFREY R. CRAGUN MD *Division of Reproductive Biology and Medicine, Department of Obstetrics and Gynecology, University of California at Davis Medical Center, Sacramento, CA 95816*

WILLIAM F. CROWLEY Jr MD *Reproductive Endocrine Unit, Department of Medicine, Massachusetts General Hospital, Boston, MA 02114*

SEAN K. CUNNINGHAM PhD, MSc *Department of Endocrinology, St Vincent's Hospital, Elm Park, Dublin 4, Ireland*

GORDON B. CUTLER Jr MD *Developmental Endocrinology Branch, National Institute of Child Health and Human Development, National Institutes of Health, Bethesda, MD 20892*

MICHELLE DEMETER BA, *Departments of Biochemistry and Obstetrics and Gynecology, University of Texas Southwestern Medical Center at Dallas, Dallas, TX 75235*

ANDREA DUNAIF MD *Department of Medicine, Division of Endocrinology, Mount Sinai Medical Center, New York, NY 10029*

ANKE A. EHRHARDT PhD *Psychiatric Institute, Children's Division, Columbia University College of Physicians and Surgeons, New York, NY 10032*

DAVID A. EHRMANN MD *Department of Medicine, University of Chicago, Pritzker School of Medicine, Chicago, IL 60637*

GREGORY F. ERICKSON PhD *Department of Reproductive Medicine, University of California, San Diego, La Jolla, CA 92093*

MARCO FILICORI MD *Center for Chronobiology of Reproduction and Reproductive Medicine Unit, University of Bologna, Bologna, Italy*

CARLO FLAMIGNI MD *Center for Chronobiology of Reproduction and Reproductive Medicine Unit, University of Bologna, Bologna, Italy*

STEPHEN FRANKS MD *Department of Obstetrics and Gynaecology, University of London, St Mary's Hospital Medical School, London W2 1PG, UK*

CATHERINE FRAPIER MD *Diabetes Branch, National Institute of Diabetes and Digestive and Kidney Diseases, National Institutes of Health, Bethesda, MD 20892*

JAMES R. GIVENS MD *Department of Medicine, University of Tennessee at Memphis, Memphis, TN 38163*

LINDA C. GIUDICE PhD, MD *Department of Gynecology/Obstetrics and Department of Pediatrics, Stanford University School of Medicine, Stanford, CA 94305*

JANET E. HALL MD *Reproductive Endocrine Unit, Department of Medicine, Massachusetts General Hospital, Boston, MA 02114*

FLORENCE P. HASELTINE PhD, MD *Center for Population Research, National Institute of Child Health and Human Development, Rockville, MD 20892*

ELEUTERIO R. HERNANDEZ MD, PhD *Division of Reproductive Endocrinology, Department of Obstetrics and Gynecology, University of Maryland School of Medicine, Baltimore, MD 21201*

ARYE HURWITZ MD *Division of Reproductive Endocrinology, Department of Obstetrics and Gynecology, University of Maryland School of Medicine, Baltimore, MD 21201*

EIICHI IMANO MD *Diabetes Branch, National Institute of Diabetes and Digestive and Kidney Diseases, National Institutes of Health, Bethesda, MD 20892*

HIROSHI INOUYE MD *Departments of Medicine and Biochemistry and Clinical Research Center, University of Tennessee at Memphis, Memphis, TN 38163*

HIROKO KADOWAKI MD *Diabetes Branch, National Institute of Diabetes and Digestive and Kidney Diseases, National Institutes of Health, Bethesda, MD 20892*

TAKASHI KADOWAKI MD *Diabetes Branch, National Institute of Diabetes and Digestive and Kidney Diseases, National Institutes of Health, Bethesda, MD 20892*

AHMED KISSEBAH MD, PhD *Department of Medicine, Medical College of Wisconsin, Froedtert Memorial Lutheran Hospital, Milwaukee, WI 53226*

ABBAS E. KITABCHI PhD, MD *Department of Medicine, Division of Endocrinology and Metabolism, University of Tennessee at Memphis, Memphis, TN 38163*

MARKUS LAUBER PhD *Departments of Biochemistry and Obstetrics and Gynecology, University of Texas Southwestern Medical Center at Dallas, Dallas, TX 75235*

DEREK LEROITH MD, PhD *Diabetes Branch, National Institute of Diabetes and Digestive and Kidney Diseases, National Institutes of Health, Bethesda, MD 20892*

RACHEL LEVY-TOLEDANO MD *Diabetes Branch, National Institute of Diabetes and Digestive and Kidney Diseases, National Institutes of Health, Bethesda, MD 20892*

ROGERIO A. LOBO MD *Department of Obstetrics and Gynecology, Division of Reproductive Endocrinology and Infertility, University of Southern California School of Medicine, Los Angeles, CA 90033*

D. LYNN LORIAUX MD, PhD *Division of Endocrinology, Oregon Health Sciences University, Portland, OR 97201*

KATHRYN A. MARTIN MD *Reproductive Endocrine Unit, Department of Medicine, Massachusetts General Hospital, Boston, MA 02114*

JAN M. MCALLISTER PhD *Departments of Biochemistry and Obstetrics and Gynecology, University of Texas Southwestern Medical Center at Dallas, Dallas, TX 75235*

T. JOSEPH MCKENNA MD, FRCPI, FRCP, FACP *Department of Endocrinology, St Vincent's Hospital, Elm Park, Dublin 4, Ireland*

GEORGE R. MERRIAM MD *Developmental Endocrinology Branch, National Institute of Child Health and Human Development, Bethesda, MD 20892*

MANUBAI NAGAMANI MD *Department of Obstetrics and Gynaecology, University of Texas Medical Branch, Galveston, TX 77550*

JOHN E. NESTLER MD *Division of Endocrinology and Metabolism, Medical College of Virginia, Richmond, VA 23298*

MARIA I. NEW MD *Department of Pediatrics, New York Hospital Cornell Medical Center, New York, NY 10021*

CAROL E. RESNICK *Division of Reproductive Endocrinology, Department of Obstetrics and Gynecology, University of Maryland School of Medicine, Baltimore, MD 21201*

CHARLES T. ROBERTS PhD *National Institute of Diabetes and Digestive and Kidney Diseases, National Institutes of Health, Bethesda, MD 20892*

RON G. ROSENFELD MD *Division of Pediatric Endocrinology, Stanford University*

EVAN R. SIMPSON PhD *Departments of Biochemistry and Obstetrics and Gynecology, Cecil H. and Ida Green Center for Reproductive Biology Sciences, University of Texas Southwestern Medical Center at Dallas, Dallas, TX 75235*

EVAN R. SIMPSON PhD *Departments of Biochemistry and Obstetrics and Gynecology, University of Texas Southwestern Medical Center at Dallas, Dallas, TX 75235*

JOE LEIGH SIMPSON MD *Department of Obstetrics and Gynecology, University of Tennessee at Memphis, Memphis, TN 38163*

CHARLES A. STUART MD *Department of Internal Medicine, University of Texas Medical Branch, Galveston, TX 77550*

ANN E. TAYLOR, MD *Reproductive Endocrine Unit, Department of Medicine, Massachusetts General Hospital, Boston, MA 02114*

SIMEON I. TAYLOR MD, PhD *Diabetes Branch, National Institute of Diabetes and Digestive and Kidney Diseases, National Institutes of Health, Bethesda, MD 20892*

MICHAEL R. WATERMAN PhD *Departments of Biochemistry and Obstetrics and Gynecology, University of Texas Southwestern Medical Center at Dallas, Dallas, TX 75235*

ROBERT A. WILD MD *Department of Obstetrics and Gynecology, University of Oklahoma, Oklahoma City, OK 73190*

JOANNA K. ZAWADZKI MD *Department of Medicine, Division of Endocrinology, Georgetown University Hospital, Washington, DC 20007*

Preface

Although it has been more than 50 years since Stein and Leventhal identified the symptom complex of hirsutism, menstrual dysfunction and obesity associated with the pathologic finding of enlarged cystic ovaries, the etiology of the polycystic ovary syndrome (PCO) remains unknown. Indeed, even standardized diagnostic criteria for PCO have not been established and there are as many definitions of PCO as investigators working in the field. Thus PCO has been to endocrinologists what pornography is to judges: we do not know how to define it but we know it when we see it.

This volume is the result of the NIH–NICHD Conference on PCO in April 1990 which was organized with the goals of: synthesizing current research in the field; exploring areas of promise for future investigation; and developing diagnostic criteria for the syndrome.

We believe that this volume will demonstrate that the first two goals were amply accomplished. Alas, we achieved little order out of chaos in the development of diagnostic criteria. However, the areas of controversy have been brought into sharper focus and a mechanism for achieving consensus is presented in the final chapter.

The book is divided into nine major sections and the chapters in the sections were contributed by the speakers at the conference. Since a major part of the conference was open discussion among the participants, this is summarized in overview chapters where appropriate.

The chapters in this volume address five main areas. First, an overview of important topics relating to PCO, such as the history of the syndrome (Givens and Wild), ovarian morphology (Franks) and function (Erickson), hypothalamic–pituitary derangements (Filicori and Flamigni), adrenal function (McKenna) and animal models (Bogovich). Second, fields that may contribute to the clarification of the etiologies of

PCO are reviewed. These include growth factor physiology (Adashi *et al.* and Rosenfeld *et al.*), adrenarche (Albertson *et al.*), a population genetics approach to PCO (Simpson), and the molecular genetics of steroid enzymes (Simpson *et al.*), nonclassical congenital adrenal hyperplasia (New) and syndromes of extreme insulin resistance (Taylor *et al.*). Third, hypotheses for the pathogenesis of PCO are presented. Cogent arguments are made for primary hypothalamic–pituitary abnormalities (Hall *et al.*), ovarian and adrenal steroidogenic abnormalities (Rosenfield) and insulin resistance (Nestler *et al.*, Barbieri) as causes of PCO.

Complications (Lobo) and treatment (Chang) of PCO are reviewed. Particular attention is paid to the newly recognized and important metabolic consequences of the disorder (Wild, Kitabchi, Dunaif, Kissebah). In addition, the potential psychological consequences of hyperandrogenism and its treatment are discussed (Erhardt).

Finally, the round table discussion of possible diagnostic criteria is summarized by Zawadzki and Dunaif. An overview of the development of diagnostic criteria for other heterogeneous syndromes such as non-insulin-dependent diabetes mellitus and rheumatoid diseases is presented as a model for the development of diagnostic criteria for PCO. Although it is evident from the discussion that a consensus on the diagnosis of PCO was not achieved, there was general agreement on three major criteria for the syndrome: hyperandrogenism, chronic anovulation and the absence of secondary causes of PCO such as non-classical adrenal hyperplasia or androgen sensitive neoplasms. Further work will be needed to refine those criteria and to address the utility of ovarian ultrasonography as well as suppression and stimulation testing with dexamethasone and gonadotropin-releasing hormone analogs, respectively.

We believe that the progress, diversity and controversy in this field are addressed in this volume. Further, it is evident from this volume that clarifying the pathogenesis of PCO will elucidate not only a number of important areas of reproductive physiology but also provide insight into the association between gonadal function and carbohydrate metabolism.

Acknowledgments

We are deeply grateful to Ms Lisa Gawley and Margie Perikles for the outstanding assistance they provided in organizing the PCO Conference and in preparing the manuscript.

Abbreviations

17-hydroxylase	17α-hydroxylase
17-lyase	17, 20-lyase
17-PROG/17-OHP	17-hydroxyprogesterone
3β-HSD	3β-hydroxysteroid dehydrogenase
α-MSH	α-melanocyte-stimulating hormone
ACTH	Adrenocorticotropic hormone
AD	Androstenedione
AN	Acanthosis nigricans
apo-B	Apolipoprotein B
BBT	Basal body temperature
Bcr	Bromocriptine
CAH	Congenital adrenal hyperplasia
cAMP	Cyclic adenosine monophosphate
CRF	Corticotropin-releasing factor
CPA	Cyproterone acetate
DA	Dopamine
DES	Diethylstilbestrol
dex, DEX	Dexamethasone
DHA/DHEA	Dehydroepiandrosterone
DHAS/DHEAS	Dehydroepiandrosterone sulfate
DHT	Dihydrotestosterone
E_2/E2	Estradiol
EFP	Early follicular phase
EGF	Epidermal growth factor
FAS	Free α-subunit
FFA	Free fatty acid
FGF	Fibroblast growth factor
FSH	Follicle-stimulating hormone

GnRH	Gonadotropin-releasing hormone
GnRHa	Long-acting gonadotropin-releasing hormone analog
HCA	Hyperandrogenic chronic anovulation
hCG	Human chorionic gonadotropin
HDL	High-density lipoprotein
HLA	Human leukocyte antigens
I/G	Insulin/glucose
IGF	Insulin-like growth factor
IGFBP	Insulin-like growth factor-binding protein
IH	Idiopathic hirsutism
LDL	Low-density lipoprotein
LFP	Late follicular phase
LH	Luteinizing hormone
LHRH	Luteinizing hormone-releasing hormone
LPD	Luteal phase deficiency
LPH	Lipotropic hormone
LPL	Lipoprotein lipase
MCR	Metabolic clearance rate
MFP	Midfollicular phase
NC21OHD	Nonclassical 21-hydroxylase deficiency
NE	Norepinephrine
NIDDM	Non-insulin-dependent diabetes mellitus
$P\text{-}450_{scc}$	Side-chain cleavage cytochrome P-450
$P\text{-}450_{17\alpha}$	17α-hydroxylase cytochrome P-450
$P\text{-}450_{arom}$	Aromatase cytochrome P-450
PCO	Polycystic ovary syndrome
PDH	Pyruvate dehydrogenase
PEG	Polyethylene glycol
POMC	Pro-opiomelanocortin
PR	Production rates
PRL	Prolactin
PROG	Progesterone
RFLP	Restriction fragment length polymorphism
SHBG	Sex hormone-binding globulin
T	Testosterone
TG	Triglycerides
TGF	Transforming growth factor
TIC	Theca interstitial cells
TRH	Thyrotrophin-releasing hormone
TSH	Thyroid-stimulating hormone
VLDL	Very-low-density lipoprotein
WHR	Waist-to-hip ratio

DISCLAIMER: The indications and dosages of all drugs in this book have been recommended in the medical literature and conform to the practices of the general medical community. The medications described do not necessarily have specific approval by the Food and Drug Administration for use in the diseases and dosages for which they are recommended. The package insert for each drug should be consulted for use and dosage as approved by the FDA. Because standards for usage change, it is advisable to keep abreast of revised recommendations, particularly those concerning new drugs.

Section 1
History and Clinical Features

Chapter 1
Historical Overview of the Polycystic Ovary

JAMES R. GIVENS & ROBERT A. WILD

It was inconceivable to clinicians and investigators, as late as the nineteenth century, that the ovary could be a source of androgens causing hirsutism and infertility. Consequently, male hormones were considered to be the exclusive product of the adrenals. However, careful studies using grafting procedures on castrated animals identified the ovary as a source of androgens [1,2]. Cystic degeneration of human ovaries was described in the middle of the nineteenth century and removal of both ovaries or ovarian wedge resection was performed on a limited number of women by the turn of the century [3].

The Stein–Leventhal syndrome

Stein and Leventhal published their initial report in 1935 in which they called attention to women with amenorrhea, hirsutism and enlarged polycystic ovaries [4]. Previous reports had emphasized menometrorrhagia in association with microcystic disease. Stein and Leventhal performed ovarian wedge resection as a biopsy and found that reproductive function was restored. Following the initial report, Stein and Leventhal published their accumulated experience with the ovarian wedge resection at 5-year intervals [4–10]. They were primarily interested in the factors that influence the therapeutic effectiveness of ovarian wedge resection. The Stein–Leventhal syndrome consists of "secondary amenorrhea, a male type of hirsutism, sterility, hypoplasia of the uterus, and bilaterally enlarged ovaries" (Fig. 1.1) [4]. Excluded from the syndrome were: women with cyclic menses, normal-sized ovaries, elevated urinary 17-ketosteroids, adrenal virilism and stromal thecosis. The Stein–Leventhal syndrome is a rare disorder; Stein

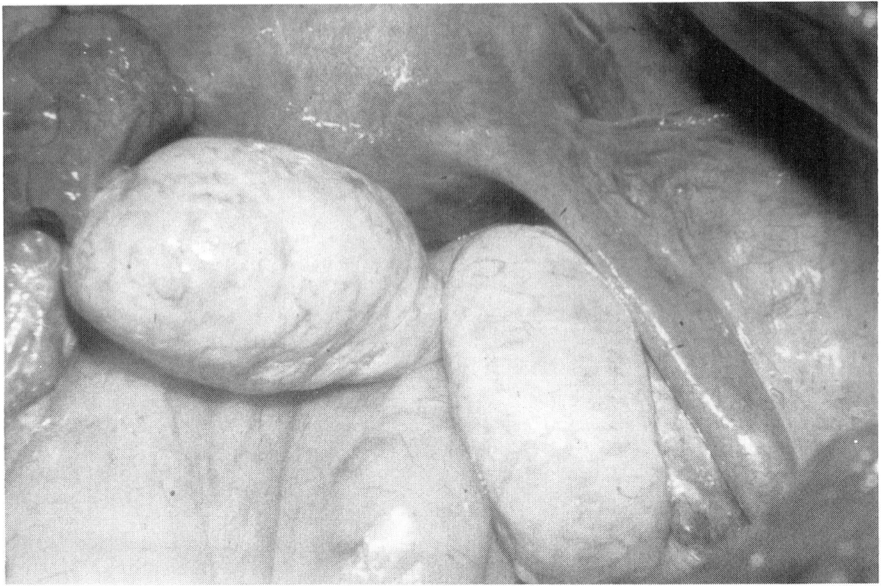

Fig. 1.1 Enlarged, sclerocystic ovaries; a nonspecific finding in the various causes of androgenic ovaries. They are a sign, not a specific diagnosis.

personally treated only 90 affected women in 29 years with a pregnancy rate after wedge resection of 88% [10].

The wide variability of the clinical and histologic findings among patients, which resulted in the inability to clearly identify any consistent characteristic features of the syndrome, formed the basis for doubts concerning its existence. For example, Roberts and Haines [11], in an article published in 1960 entitled "Is there a Stein–Leventhal syndrome?", reported typical ovarian histologic findings in the absence of symptoms. Roberts and Haines also did not observe hyperplasia of the theca interna in a single case and a corpus luteum was not uncommonly found [11]. Leventhal had noted that these two findings were the most frequently observed in the syndrome.

On the basis of these data, Roberts and Haines [11] reasoned that it is difficult to believe that there is a definite entity as the Stein–Leventhal syndrome. Goldzieher and Axelrod [12], in their classic paper published in 1963, came to the same conclusion, based on the analysis of 1097 published cases in the world literature showing a wide variation of signs and symptoms associated with sclerocystic ovaries. For example, the incidence of infertility ranged from 35 to 77%, with an average of 74%. The most common complaint recorded was hirsutism (mean 69%), also with wide variation (17–83%).

It must be emphasized that the inclusion and exclusion criteria of the Stein–Leventhal syndrome were for the purpose of selecting those women who would benefit from ovarian wedge resection [4–10]. It was not their intention to define the limits of the disorder. The excellent results of wedge resection experienced by Stein and Leventhal have not been duplicated, particularly in regard to reversing the infertility. According to Goldzieher and Axelrod [12], 63% of 640 women reported in the world literature with polycystic ovaries who had ovarian wedge resection became pregnant after the procedure.

The hyperthecosis syndrome

Culiner and Shippel [13], in 1949, applied the term hyperthecosis ovarii to a subgroup of women with polycystic ovaries who failed to respond to ovarian wedge resection and whose ovaries were characterized by nests of theca cells out in the stroma away from follicles (Fig. 1.2). Clinically, they were masculinized, had a high incidence of diabetes and hypertension, and had a familial aggregation suggesting genetic transmission.

The Stein–Leventhal syndrome and the hyperthecosis syndrome ovaries each have hyperplasia of the theca interna lining the atretic follicles (Fig. 1.3). The number of atretic cysts, however, is greater in the hyperthecosis syndrome, and thus the number of theca cells secreting androstenedione and testosterone far outnumber those in the Stein–Leventhal ovary, which accounts for the masculinization and other features of the hyperthecosis syndrome.

A major question, which remains unanswered, is whether the Stein–Leventhal syndrome and the hyperthecosis syndrome are part of the continuum of a single disorder or whether they are two separate disorders with different degrees of severity. There is a continuum of the relative frequency of follicular vs. atretic cysts along with the degree of stroma thecosis. The Stein–Leventhal syndrome ovary has large numbers of follicular cysts, a small number of atretic cysts and minimal stroma involvement. The hyperthecosis syndrome ovary has large numbers of atretic cysts, only a few follicular cysts, along with marked stromal hyperplasia. There is paucity of ova in the hyperthecotic ovary due at least in part to the massive atresia rate.

There is a broad spectrum of clinical features of women with the polycystic ovary syndrome. The spectrum extends from women with no complaints to the other extreme of masculinization in the hyperthecosis

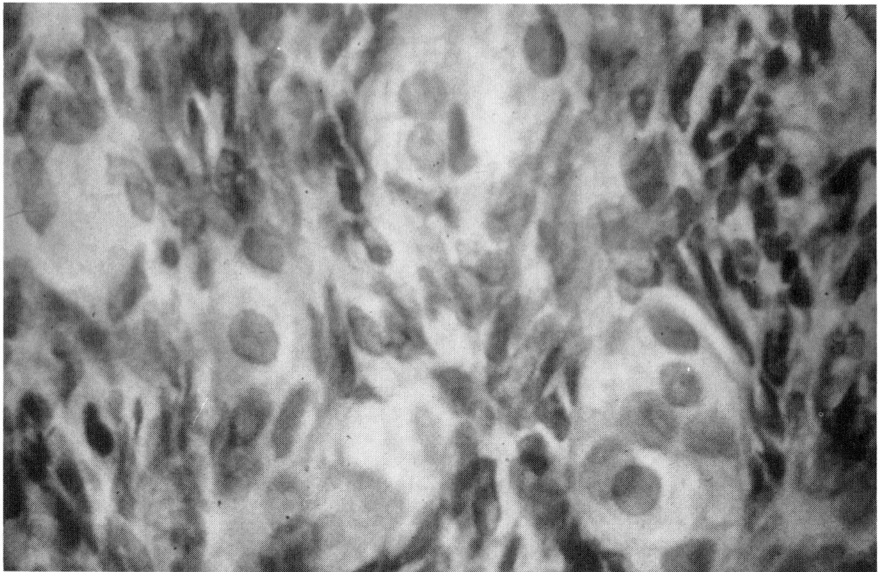

Fig. 1.2 A cluster of luteinized ovarian stroma cells not associated with a follicle observed in hyperthecosis.

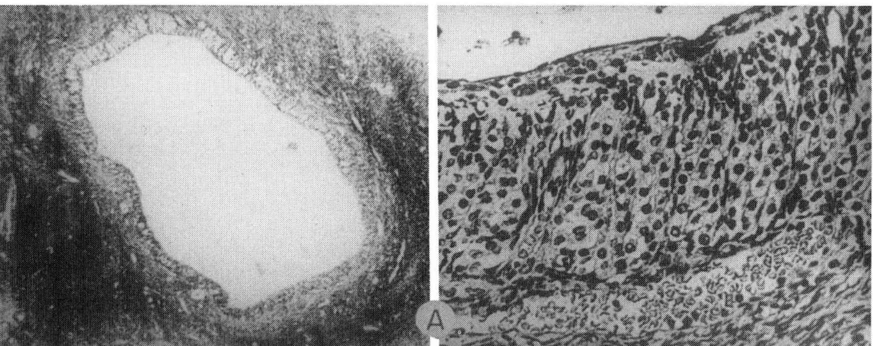

Fig. 1.3 An atretic follicle with a hyperplastic theca interna commonly observed in increased numbers in androgenic ovaries. (Used with permission. Givens JR *et al.* Am J Obstet Gynecol 110: 959–72, 1971.)

syndrome. The Stein–Leventhal syndrome occupies a position intermediate between these two extremes.

The hyperthecosis syndrome is associated with a high incidence of diabetes mellitus, obesity, insulin resistance, acanthosis nigricans, hyper-

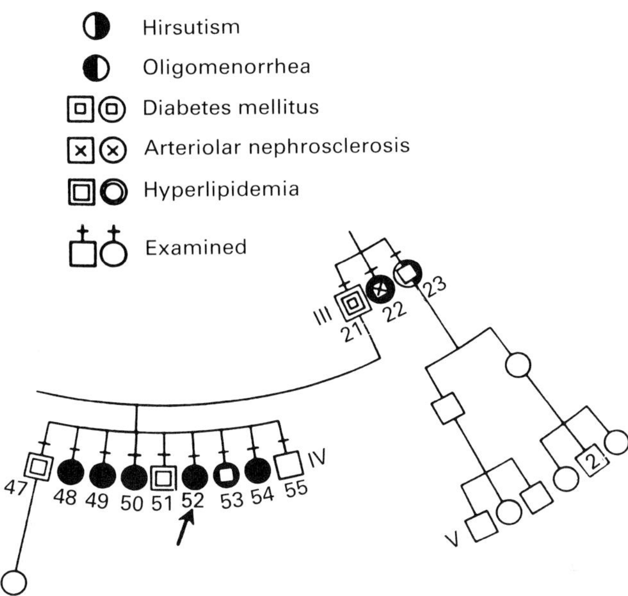

Fig. 1.4 Two sibships of a family with a high incidence of acanthosis nigricans, hyperthecosis and lipid and carbohydrate abnormalities. (Used with permission. Givens JR *et al.* Am J Obstet Gynecol 110: 959–72, 1971.)

tension and abnormal lipids [14]. Illustrated in Fig. 1.4 is the pedigree of two sibships of a black family with hyperthecosis, documenting the high frequency of amenorrhea and hirsutism. All six female siblings were affected as evidenced clinically and by laboratory data of elevated serum levels of testosterone and androstenedione. Their two paternal aunts were also affected. The relationship of the diabetes mellitus, hypertension, arteriolar nephrosclerosis, and hyperlipidemia, which is present in both males and females, is not known. This family was studied 10 years before there was any knowledge of a relationship between insulin resistance and polycystic ovaries. We have recently restudied two of the male members of this family who have acanthosis nigricans and their fasting insulin levels were 10 times normal. These interesting males are described in greater detail in Chapter 26. A total of five generations of this family were studied and the diagnosis of hyperthecosis was made on histologic findings in ovaries obtained at autopsy or surgery.

Until recently, we considered that hyperthecosis and the Stein–Leventhal syndrome represented different degrees of severity of the same disorder. However, the complex and varied presentation of hyperthecosis compared to the Stein–Leventhal syndrome suggests that they are different disorders.

In summary, considerable progress has been made in describing the anatomical changes in the ovary, as well as the associated hormonal changes in women with polycystic ovaries. A major obstacle to an understanding of the pathogenesis of polycystic ovaries is the failure to appreciate the heterogeneity of the associated disorders. Another hindrance, which has narrowed the concept and therefore falsely underestimated its incidence, has been the misapplication of the inclusion and exclusion criteria of Stein and Leventhal for the wedge resection of the ovaries to the diagnosis of global polycystic ovaries. Their rigid criteria, when erroneously applied to the general diagnosis, severely underestimate the breadth of the phenotypic spectrum.

The major diagnostic criterion that distinguishes the Stein–Leventhal syndrome from the hyperthecosis syndrome is the presence of luteinized theca cells distributed throughout the stroma in the latter condition (Fig. 1.2). Because this diagnosis requires ovarian tissue, a relatively small number of patients have been assigned a diagnosis of hyperthecosis syndrome.

The eponym, Stein–Leventhal syndrome, no longer serves a useful purpose to either investigators or clinicians. It is now clear that a number of specific disorders can induce polycystic ovaries. The presence of multiple cysts in the ovary does not reflect a specific diagnostic entity. Thus, multicystic ovaries are a sign, and not a diagnosis [15].

Future investigative effort should be aimed at developing a strategy that would permit identification of those women whose polycystic ovaries are due to a proximate defect primary in the ovary vs. those that have an extraovarian cause inducing arrest or dysrhythmia of folliculogenesis as a secondary phenomenon. The use of the terms Stein–Leventhal syndrome and hyperthecosis syndrome should be discontinued and replaced with primary and secondary ovarian hyperandrogenism. The nosology should have a pathophysiologic basis rather than a histopathologic one (Table 1.1).

Polycystic ovaries and primary ovarian hyperandrogenism

Steroidogenic enzyme deficiency

OVARIAN 17-KETOSTEROID REDUCTASE DEFICIENCY

Pang *et al.* [16] in 1987 reported deficiency of the enzyme 17-ketosteroid reductase, which converts androstenedione to testosterone and estrone

Table 1.1 Nosology of polycystic ovaries based on pathophysiology.

Polycystic ovaries and primary ovarian hyperandrogenism
Steroidogenic enzyme deficiency
  Ovarian 17-ketosteroid reductase deficiency
  Ovarian 3β-hydroxysteroid dehydrogenase Δ^{5-4} isomerase
Dysrhythmia or arrest of folliculogenesis: a hypothesis
Androgen-secreting ovarian tumors

Polycystic ovaries and secondary ovarian hyperandrogenism
CNS dysfunction
  Decreased dopamine
  Abnormal opiate metabolism
Adrenal hyperandrogenism
  Steroidogenic enzyme deficiency
  Hyperresponsiveness to ACTH
  Precocious adrenarche
  Androgen-secreting tumors
Hyperinsulinemia
  Insulin resistance
    Kahn A syndrome
    Kahn B syndrome
    Kahn C syndrome
  Abnormal gene products
    Abnormal insulins
    Abnormal proinsulin
    Abnormal insulin receptor
  Obesity
A model for the genetic basis of polycystic ovary syndrome with environmental cofactors

to estradiol. These patients have high levels of androstenedione and estrone associated with polycystic ovaries. The elevated testosterone level is due primarily to the peripheral conversion of androstenedione to testosterone. It is not clear whether the elevated estrone is responsible for the enlarged polycystic ovaries through the positive feedback on the release of gonadotropin-releasing hormone (GnRH) and luteinizing hormone (LH).

3β-HYDROXYSTEROID DEHYDROGENASE, Δ^{5-4} ISOMERASE DEFICIENCY

This is primary ovarian deficiency of the steroidogenic enzyme 3β-hydroxysteroid dehydrogenase, Δ^{5-4} isomerase, which converts the Δ^5 to Δ^4 compounds, including dehydroepiandrosterone to androstenedione [17]. This enzyme system is also deficient in the adrenals, but not in the peripheral tissues. The elevated testosterone level reflects the increased amount of the substrate androstenedione being converted to testosterone in the peripheral tissues, where the activity of the enzyme system remains intact.

A mild defect in this system is not uncommon among young hirsute women. The enzymatic block results in the accumulation of dehydroepiandrosterone. Our observation that hirsute females with this enzyme defect do not have insulin resistance, even when obese, caused us to look at dehydroepiandrosterone as a possible modulator of hormone action of insulin. Preliminary data suggest that dehydroepiandrosterone does enhance tissue sensitivity to insulin [18].

Dysrhythmia or arrest of folliculogenesis: a hypothesis

The integrity of the developing ovarian follicle requires intact and functioning interchanging control mechanisms between the oocyte and the surrounding follicular cells. For example, an oocyte maturation inhibitor produced by the granulosa cells is essential for maintaining a viable oocyte suspended in prophase, and a luteinization inhibitor prevents luteinization of the follicular cells. A defect in either of these factors, or some other intraovarian controlling influence, such as growth factors, could lead to increased atresia of the follicles producing increased numbers of atretic follicles with theca cell hyperplasia, decreased numbers of granulosa cells causing decreased estrogen production, and increased androgen production. Paucity of oocytes and increased numbers of atretic follicles are observed in hyperthecosis, which could result from a defective intrafollicular control mechanism. In support of this concept, lipoid degeneration of ova has been observed as an early sign of follicular atresia suggesting a defect involving the integrity of the control mechanism for normal folliculogenesis.

Increased follicular atresia may be related to deficient function of the granulosa cells. In this regard, it is of interest that Ohno, in reviewing the material of Singh and Carr, was of the opinion that the reason for the increased atresia rate in 45, X fetuses was the paucity of progranulosa cells with which the ovum must align in order to survive. The apparent involvement of the heterochromatic X-chromosome in the control of atresia, as evidenced by the increased atresia rate in gonadal dysgenesis, raises the possibility that a similar though less severe genetic defect exists in some cases of polycystic ovarian disease causing increased follicular atresia with theca cell hyperplasia. Increased numbers of degenerative ova are present in some ovaries with hyperthecosis. Using *in vitro* culture technique, a higher degenerative rate of ova from polycystic ovaries has been noted. Dermatoglyphic data also suggest X-linked transmission of polycystic ovaries [15].

Androgen-secreting ovarian tumors

Stromal tumors, such as luteomas, occur with polycystic ovaries [19]. A patient with polycystic ovaries and a stromal luteoma is described in detail in the section on hyperinsulinemia.

Polycystic ovaries and secondary ovarian hyperandrogenism

CNS dysfunction

A major landmark in the progress toward understanding the pathophysiology of polycystic ovaries was the report of Keettel and associates [20] that 10 of 11 women with the Stein–Leventhal syndrome had increased amounts of LH in their urine. Subsequent investigation revealed erratic bursts of LH indicating a disordered secretion of gonadotropins [21]. Plasma assays confirmed the finding of an elevated LH to follicle-stimulating hormone (FSH) ratio in the Stein–Leventhal syndrome [22,23]. Further insight into the abnormal physiology of the disorder occurred when the hyperandrogenism was shown to be LH dependent [24]. This was a significant observation because it formed the basis for the medical therapy of hyperandrogenism by suppressing LH with an oral contraceptive [24].

The observation that some women with polycystic ovaries have consistently normal LH levels was disturbing in view of the above findings. A study was undertaken to see if there were differences in the responses to dynamic testing of the hypothalamus–pituitary axis in women with polycystic ovaries who had elevated vs. normal LH [25]. The majority of those in the normal LH group had hyperthecosis and those who had LH above normal had Stein–Leventhal syndrome. The effect on LH levels of dexamethasone alone followed by dexamethasone plus ethinyl estradiol was determined. This study showed that women with normal LH did not have an LH response to dexamethasone plus ethinyl estradiol. On the other hand, those with elevated LH had a marked LH response to dexamethasone plus ethinyl estradiol. These data identify one of the differences of the two subgroups of polycystic ovaries. Future research should carefully titrate the relative sensitivity of the hypothalamus–pituitary axis to the feedback effect of variable estrogen blood levels in polycystic ovary subgroups with elevated vs. normal LH. At the time of the above study, the effect of insulin on the hypothalamus–pituitary–ovarian axis was not known. The marked hyperinsulinemia of hyperthecosis could enhance the LH effects on the theca and stroma thereby producing marked hyperandrogenemia, which suppresses the estrogenic positive feedback mechanism controlling LH secretion. Alternatively, high levels of insulin could directly enhance or suppress the estrogenic positive feedback mechanism in polycystic ovaries–acanthosis nigricans.

DECREASED DOPAMINE

Destructive lesions of the CNS can produce decreased dopamine tone and increased LH secretion [26]. The mechanism for the increased LH in women with polycystic ovaries may be a reduction in the inhibitory influence of dopamine on GnRH secretion [27].

ABNORMAL OPIATE METABOLISM

Opioids also participate in the control of GnRH secretion. β-Endorphin levels are elevated in women with polycystic ovaries [28]. β-Endorphin suppresses LH in normal women, but has been reported not to in women with polycystic ovaries [29–32]. This may represent uncoupling of the opioid influence on GnRH secretion.

Adrenal hyperandrogenism

STEROIDOGENIC ENZYME DEFICIENCY

Congenital adrenal hyperplasia (classical and nonclassical) may be associated with enlarged, polycystic ovaries. However, enlarged cystic ovaries are not always present in 21- or 11β-hydroxylase deficiency. Hyperresponsiveness of androstenedione to adrenocorticotropic hormone (ACTH) occurs in 50% of the women with polycystic ovaries without deficiency of a steroidogenic enzyme. Some of these women are obese, which is associated with adrenal hyperandrogenism.

HYPERRESPONSIVENESS TO ACTH

Because obesity commonly accompanies polycystic ovaries, the response of androstenedione and dehydroepiandrosterone to physiologic doses of ACTH was tested in women who were obese but were nonhirsute and eumenorrheic. Hyperresponsiveness of androstenedione and dehydroepiandrosterone was demonstrated, indicating obesity is at least one cause of adrenal hyperandrogenism in polycystic ovaries.

Further confirmation of adrenal hyperandrogenism in obesity was obtained by determining the metabolic clearance rates and production rates for androstenedione and dehydroepiandrosterone [33]. Both are increased in simple obesity. The fact that the serum levels of androstenedione and dehydroepiandrosterone were not different from normal is of particular interest because it means the production rate of the steroids is increased to the same magnitude as the metabolic clearance rate and are coupled through insulin [34] (see Chapter 24).

PRECOCIOUS ADRENARCHE

Other data supporting the concept that adrenal androgen excess is involved in the pathogenesis of polycystic ovaries is the observation that precocious adrenarche may occur prior to developing the full picture of polycystic ovaries. Yen [22] has suggested that polycystic ovaries may be induced by an exaggerated adrenarche with increased adrenal androgen levels. Yen has proposed that adrenal androgen excess may herald the development of polycystic ovaries through positive feedback of non-cyclic estrogen levels causing dysrhythmia of folliculogenesis and other characteristics of polycystic ovaries (Fig. 1.3).

ANDROGEN-SECRETING TUMORS

Androgen-secreting tumors may induce cystic ovaries.

Hyperinsulinemia

INSULIN RESISTANCE

The first suggestion that insulin might be involved in polycystic ovaries came from the studies on a 16-year-old black female whom we saw in consultation because of amenorrhea and acanthosis nigricans [19] (Fig. 1.5). Serum androstenedione was massively elevated at 3000–5000 ng/dl, both ovaries were enlarged, growth hormone and insulin were increased and insulin rose five times normal on a glucose tolerance test. She was tall, had acral enlargement and acromegaloid facial features. Cushing's syndrome and acromegaly were ruled out by appropriate tests. A stromal luteoma was removed from an ovary and there was almost complete clearing of the acanthosis nigricans postsurgery while on oral contraceptive pill ovarian suppression.

George Burghen [35] had performed the original insulin assays on this index case, and assayed insulin levels in a group of women with polycystic ovaries to compare the levels to those with simple obesity.

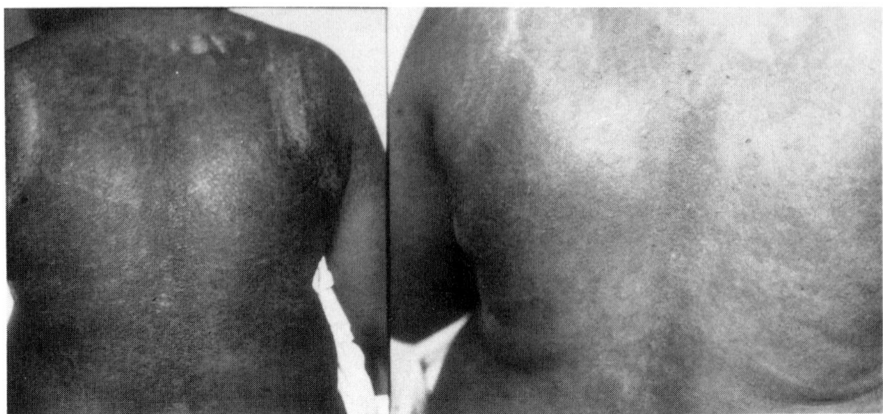

Fig. 1.5 Acanthosis nigricans before and after removal of an androstenedione secreting ovarian tumor and pituitary–ovarian suppression. (Used with permission. Givens JR *et al.* J Clin Endocrinol Metab 38: 347–55, 1974.)

A highly significant positive correlation was observed between serum androstenedione and testosterone across a broad range of circulating insulin in simple obesity and in obese women with polycystic ovaries. Numerous investigators have confirmed and extended these data.

Kahn A syndrome, Kahn B syndrome, Kahn C syndrome

The seminal observations of Kahn [36,37] on ovarian hyperandrogenism in association with various causes of insulin resistance and the description of polycystic ovaries–acanthosis nigricans by Barbieri, Makris and Ryan [38] are important landmarks in the evolution of the concept of polycystic ovaries.

ABNORMAL GENE PRODUCTS

The following abnormal gene products are associated with hyperinsulinemia: abnormal insulins, abnormal proinsulin, and abnormal insulin receptors [39] (see Chapter 20).

OBESITY

In normals and in simple obesity, insulin is significantly positively correlated with the metabolic clearance rate and production rate of dehydroepiandrosterone, and the magnitude of the correlation coefficients is identical. These data suggest that in normal women insulin enhances the response of the production rate of dehydroepiandrosterone to ACTH and increases the metabolic clearance rate of dehydroepiandrosterone to the same degree. These relationships are not present in polycystic ovaries–acanthosis nigricans because when the insulin is above 40 μU/ml the production rate of dehydroepiandrosterone is negatively correlated with insulin. Thus, the insulin level determines the nature of the interaction between dehydroepiandrosterone and insulin (see Chapters 22–24). In the face of excess insulin, with insulin levels above 40 μU/ml, dehydroepiandrosterone production rate is decreased. On the other hand, when the insulin is below 40 μU/ml, insulin stimulates dehydroepiandrosterone production.

There is hyperresponsiveness of dehydroepiandrosterone and androstenedione to physiologic amounts of ACTH in women with simple obesity who are nonhirsute and eumenorrheic [40]. There is a significant positive correlation between the insulin level and the degree of hyperresponsiveness of the steroids to ACTH, which suggests that insulin enhances the androgen–ACTH interaction. These data suggest that insulin modulates both LH and ACTH action and likely serves a pivotal role in the interaction of the adrenals and the ovaries [40].

A model for the genetic basis of polycystic ovaries with environmental cofactors

Microcystic degeneration of the ovaries or polycystic ovaries, associated with infertility, were recorded in dairy cattle over 150 years ago. The term nymphomania is a synonym for cystic degeneration of the ovaries in the veterinary literature. The clinical features of the disorder include bull-like behavior, such as low-pitch bellowing, digging with horns and feet and bullying cows [41,42]. They have a masculine appearance with thickening of the head and neck. Relaxation of the pelvic ligaments results in raising of the tailhead. Most are sterile due to anovulation and constant estrus. This constellation of signs and symptoms does not reflect a single disorder; it is the expression of several subgroups including adrenal virilism and varying degrees of a mixture of ovarian hyperestrogenism and of hyperandrogenism. Nymphomania has been induced experimentally by the administration of androgen or estrogen. In some pure dairy breeds there is apparent genetic transmission, which is associated with increased food intake, early maturity and high milk production. Nymphomania is rare in beef cattle and is uncommon in the ordinary grazing dairy cow. It occurs predominantly in highly-fed, purebred dairy cows and the severity is positively correlated with the magnitude of milk production. The onset of nymphomania occurs usually after the second or third calving. The frequency of occurrence is directly correlated with the intensity of feeding and the efficiency of milk production by the cow. The expression of nymphomania in dairy cows apparently requires a coupling of environmental factors, such as increased food intake especially protein, along with a genetic propensity. Hyperprolactinemia, obesity, and dietary factors are also apparently important in the expression of polycystic ovaries in some humans [41,42].

References

1 Deanesly R. The androgenic activity of ovarian grafts in castrated male rats. Proc R Soc Lond B 1938; 126:122–35.
2 Hill HT. Ovaries secrete male hormone: I. Restoration of the castrate type of seminal vesicle and prostate glands to normal by grafts of ovaries in mice. Endocrinology 1937; 21:495–502.
3 Greenblatt RB. The polycystic ovary syndrome of Stein–Leventhal. In: Greenblatt RB, ed. The Hirsute Female. Springfield, IL: Charles C. Thomas, 1963, pp. 149–78.
4 Stein IF, Leventhal ML. Amenorrhea associated with bilateral polycystic ovaries. Am J Obstet Gynecol 1935; 29:181–91.
5 Stein IF. The management of bilateral polycystic ovaries. Fertil Steril 1955; 6:189–205.
6 Stein IF. Duration of fertility following ovarian wedge resection—Stein–Leventhal syndrome. West J Surg 1964; 72:237–42.
7 Stein IF. Multiple pregnancy following wedge resection in the Stein–Leventhal syndrome. Int J Fertil 1964; 9:343–50.
8 Stein IF, Cohen MR, Elson R. Results of bilateral ovarian wedge resection in 47 cases of sterility. Am J Obstet Gynecol 1949; 58:267–74.
9 Stein IF, Cohen MR. Surgical treatment of bilateral polycystic ovaries—amenorrhea and sterility. Am J Obstet Gynecol 1939; 38:465–80.
10 Leventhal ML. Functional and morphologic studies of the ovaries and suprarenal glands in the Stein–Leventhal syndrome. Am J Obstet Gynecol 1962; 84:154–64.
11 Roberts DW, Haines M. Is there a Stein–Leventhal syndrome? Br Med J 1960; 1: 1709–11.
12 Goldzieher JW, Axelrod LR. Clinical and biochemical features of polycystic ovarian disease. Fertil Steril 1963; 14:631–53.
13 Culiner A, Shippel S. Virilism and theca cell hyperplasia of the ovary syndrome. J Obstet Gynaecol Br Comm 1949; 56:439–45.
14 Givens JR, Wiser WL, Coleman SA, *et al.* Familial ovarian hyperthecosis: a study of two families. Am J Obstet Gynecol 1971; 110:959–72.
15 Givens JR. Polycystic ovaries—a sign, not a diagnosis. Semin Reprod Endocrinol 1984; 2:271–80.
16 Pang S, Softness B, Sweeney WJ, New MI. Hirsutism, polycystic ovarian disease, and ovarian 17-ketosteroid reductase deficiency. N Engl J Med 1987; 316:1295–301.
17 Axelrod LR, Goldzieher JW, Ross SD. Concurrent 3β-hydroxysteroid dehydrogenase deficiency in adrenal and sclerocystic ovary. Acta Endocrinol 1965; 48:392–412.
18 Buffington CK, Givens JR, Kitabchi AE. Opposing actions of dehydroepiandrosterone and testosterone on insulin sensitivity in activated T-lymphocytes of hyperandrogenic females. Diabetes 1991; 40:693–700.
19 Givens JR, Kerber IJ, Wiser WL, Andersen RN, Coleman SA, Fish SA. Remission of acanthosis nigricans associated with polycystic ovarian disease and a stromal luteoma. J Clin Endocrinol Metab 1974; 38:347–55.

20 Keettel WC, Bradbury JT, Stoddard FJ. Observations on the PCO syndrome. Am J Obstet Gynecol 1957; 73:954–65.
21 McArthur JW, Ingersall FM, Worcester J. The urinary excretion of interstitial cell and follicle-stimulating hormone activity by women with diseases of the reproductive system. J Clin Endocrinol 1958; 18:1202–15.
22 Yen SS, Chaney C, Judd HL. Functional aberrations of the hypothalamic–pituitary system in polycystic ovary syndrome: a consideration of the pathogenesis. In: James VHT, Serio M, Giusti G, eds. The Endocrine Function of the Human Ovary. New York: Academic Press, 1976. pp. 373–85.
23 Yen SS, Vela P, Rankin J. Inappropriate secretion of follicle-stimulating hormone and luteinizing hormone in polycystic ovarian disease. J Clin Endocrinol Metab 1970; 30:435–42.
24 Givens JR, Andersen RN, Wiser WL, Fish SA. Dynamics of suppression and recovery of plasma FSH, LH, androstenedione and testosterone in polycystic ovarian disease using an oral contraceptive. J Clin Endocrinol Metab 1974; 38:727–35.
25 Givens JR, Andersen RN, Umstot ES, *et al.* Clinical findings and hormonal responses in patients with polycystic ovarian disease with normal versus elevated LH levels. Obstet Gynecol 1976; 47:388–94.
26 Bartuska DG, Eskin BA, Smith EM, *et al.* Brain damage, hypertrichosis, and polycystic ovaries. Am J Obstet Gynecol 1967; 99:387–9.
27 Quigley ME, Rakoff JS, Yen SS. Increased luteinizing hormone sensitivity to dopamine inhibition in polycystic ovary syndrome. J Clin Endocrinol Metab 1981; 52:231–4.
28 Givens JR, Wiedemann E, Andersen RN, Kitabchi AE. β-Endorphin and β-lipotropin plasma levels in hirsute women: correlation with body weight. J Clin Endocrinol Metab 1980; 50:975–6.
29 Quigley ME, Yen SS. The role of endogenous opiates on LH secretion during the menstrual cycle. J Clin Endocrinol Metab 1980; 51:179–81.
30 Cumming DC, Reid RL, Quigley ME, Rebar RW, Yen SS. Evidence for decreased endogenous dopamine and opioid inhibitory influences on LH secretion in polycystic ovary syndrome. Clin Endocrinol 1984; 20:643.
31 Reid RL, Hoff JD, Yen SS, Li CH. Effects of exogenous β-endorphin on pituitary hormone secretion and its disappearance rate in normal human subjects. J Clin Endocrinol Metab 1981; 52:1179–84.
32 Broster LR. Eight years' experience with adrenal gland. Arch Surg 1937; 34:761–91.
33 Kurtz BR, Givens JR, Komindr S, *et al.* Maintenance of normal circulating levels of Δ^4-androstenedione and dehydroepiandrosterone in simple obesity despite increased metabolic clearance rates: evidence for a servo-control mechanism. J Clin Endocrinol Metab 1987; 64:1261–7.
34 Farah MJ, Givens JR, Kitabchi AC. Bimodal correlation between the circulating insulin level and the production rate of dehydroepiandrosterone: positive correlation in controls and negative correlation in the polycystic ovary syndrome with acanthosis nigricans. J Clin Endocrinol Metab 1990; 70:1075–81.
35 Burghen GA, Givens JR, Kitabchi AE. Correlation of hyperandrogenism with hyperinsulinism in polycystic ovarian disease. J Clin Endocrinol Metab 1980; 50:113–16.
36 Kahn CR, Flier JS, Bar RS, *et al.* The syndromes of insulin resistance and acanthosis nigricans. Insulin-receptor disorders in man. N Engl J Med 1976; 294:739–45.
37 Kahn CR, Podskainy JM. Demonstration of a primary (?genetic) defect in insulin receptors in fibroblasts from a patient with the syndrome of insulin resistance and acanthosis nigricans type A. J Clin Endocrinol Metab 1980; 50:1139–41.
38 Barbieri Rl, Makris A, Ryan KJ. Effects of insulin on steroidogenesis in cultured porcine ovarian theca. Fertil Steril 1983; 40:237–41.
39 Tager HS. Insulin gene mutations and abnormal products of the human insulin gene.

In: Cohen MP, Foa PP, eds. Hormone Resistance and Other Endocrine Paradoxes. New York: Springer-Verlag, 1987. pp. 35–61.

40 Komindr S, Kurtz BR, Stevens MD, Karas JG, Bittle JB, Givens JR. Relative sensitivity and responsivity of serum cortisol and two adrenal androgens to δ-adrenocorticotropin-(1–24) in normal and obese, nonhirsute, eumenorrheic women. J Clin Endocrinol Metab 1986; 63:860–4.

41 Williams WL, Williams WW. Nymphomania of the cow. North Am Vet 1923; 4:232–41.

42 Dawson FL. Bovine cystic ovarian disease—a review of recent progress. Br Vet J 1951; 113:112–33.

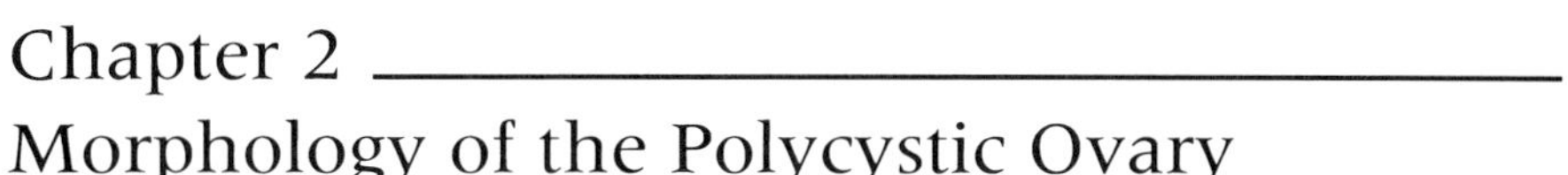

Chapter 2
Morphology of the Polycystic Ovary

STEPHEN FRANKS

Pelvic ultrasound provides a noninvasive technique for visualization of the ovaries and has led to a reappraisal of the definition, diagnosis, and prevalence of polycystic ovaries in women with hyperandrogenemia and anovulation. The histologic features of the polycystic ovary are reviewed and this is followed by a discussion of the role of ultrasound imaging of the ovaries in the investigation and management of women with polycystic ovary syndrome (PCO).

Histologic features of the polycystic ovary

There have been numerous studies documenting the morphology of the polycystic ovary [1–8] but few have made a concerted attempt to quantitate the histologic features that distinguish the polycystic from the normal ovary. However, Hughesdon [9] used both a descriptive and quantitative approach to the analysis of ovarian tissue obtained after a full-thickness, transverse wedge resection. A summary of his findings in 34 polycystic ovaries, compared with those in 30 normal ovaries, is given in Table 2.1 and depicted in Fig. 2.1. The polycystic ovaries were typically larger than normal, although normal-sized ovaries with all the other characteristic histologic features of polycystic ovaries were observed in his series. An important feature of the polycystic ovary was that although the average number of primordial follicles was the same as in the normal ovary, the number of ripening and atretic follicles was doubled. Thus, all stages of folliculogenesis are found with increased frequency in the polycystic ovary (Table 2.2) but the proportions of immature, mature, and atretic follicles are similar to those observed in the normal ovary.

There is a tendency for the tunica to be increased in size and to

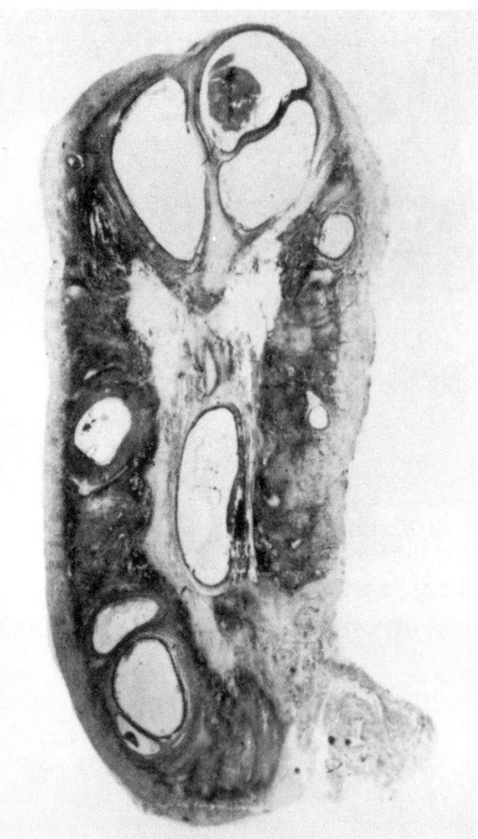

Fig. 2.1 Section of a polycystic ovary. Note thick tunica, numerous cystic follicles and thickened cortical and subcortical stroma. (From Hughesdon [9], with permission.)

Table 2.1 Histologic features of the polycystic ovary as compared with those of the normal ovary. (Adapted from Hughesdon [9].)

Increased volume (2× cross-sectional area)
Same number of primordial follicles
Double the number of ripening and atretic follicles
Increased and more collagenized tunica
Slight increase in cortical stromal thickness
Greatly increased (5×) amount of subcortical stroma with increased vascularity and innervation
Frequent occurrence of nests of hilar cells

contain many collagen fibers. There is a slight increase in the thickness of the cortical stroma but the subcortical stroma is greatly increased in amount with the appearance of many small blood vessels and nerves, in particular, in the hilar region. Small nests of hilar cells (which, under

Table 2.2 Ovarian cross-sectional area and follicle count in polycystic and control ovaries. (Adapted, with permission, from Hughesdon [9].)

	Size (cm^2)	pf	Follicle count 1°	2°	3°
PCO	9.8	81	3.7	1.4	12.4
Normal	5.0	80	1.8	0.7	5.2

pf, primordial follicles; follicle count refers to the average number per section.

the electron microscope, have features of steroid-secreting cells) are also commonly found in the polycystic ovary [10].

The increased amount of stroma that is so characteristic of the polycystic ovary appears to be derived primarily from atretic follicles. During atresia, there is a striking hypertrophy of the theca cells [10], which then disperse into the interstitial tissue, often accumulating around small blood vessels [9]. It is the increased population of atretic follicles that accounts for the previously described "theca cell hyperplasia" but it is important to realize that such hyperplasia is probably a normal function of atresia itself rather than an abnormality that affects developing follicles in the polycystic ovary. Primary mesenchymal hyperplasia may also contribute to the increase in the amount of the stroma [9] but it appears to play a lesser role in the genesis of the polycystic ovary than that of the theca-derived cells.

It remains unclear whether the increased production of androgens from the polycystic ovary is simply a feature of the increased number of (luteinizing hormone (LH)-responsive) theca-interstitial cells or whether the cells themselves are qualitatively different in their steroidogenic capacity from those in the normal ovary (Fig. 2.2).

Ultrasound diagnosis of polycystic ovaries

The increased number of follicles and, in particular, of the medium-sized to large antral follicles (2–10 mm in diameter) can be readily visualized using high-resolution ultrasound scanning (Figs 2.3 and 2.4). Ultrasound will also demonstrate the increased stroma, which typifies the polycystic ovary [11–14]. The basis for the diagnosis (using the transabdominal route of scanning) is the finding of 10 or more follicles in one plane, together with an increased amount of stroma [13]. Identification of an increased amount of stroma is relatively straightforward when the overall ovarian volume is greater than 9 ml (i.e. 2 SD above the mean

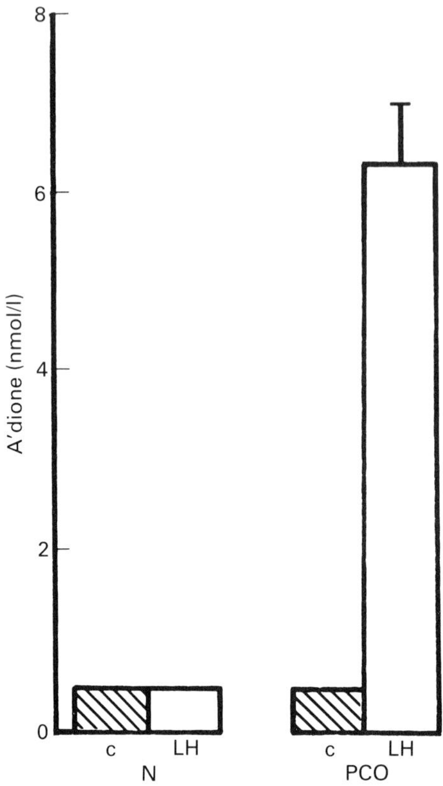

Fig. 2.2 Androstenedione (A'dione) concentrations in conditioned media from incubations of stromal tissue obtained from normal (N) or polycystic ovaries (PCO). Note stimulation of A'dione secretion in the presence of LH in stroma from PCO only. C = control incubation without LH.

for 114 normal ovaries [15]) but is more difficult to assess if the ovary is of normal volume. The appearance then has to be differentiated from that of the so-called multifollicular ovary [11] (Fig. 2.5). The multifollicular ovary is observed during normal puberty and in women with mild or partially recovered hypothalamic amenorrhea related to weight loss and is associated with a slowing of pulses of LH [16]. In such cases, the ovary is normal in size or slightly increased in volume and there is an increased number of follicles. However, the amount of the stroma is not increased and the ovary can be distinguished quite clearly from the normal-sized polycystic ovary.

Transvaginal ultrasonography allows the definition of a larger number of small follicles than does transabdominal scanning, even in the normal ovary. The criteria for the diagnosis of polycystic ovaries described above may need to be revised for the assessment of polycystic ovaries by vaginal ultrasonography.

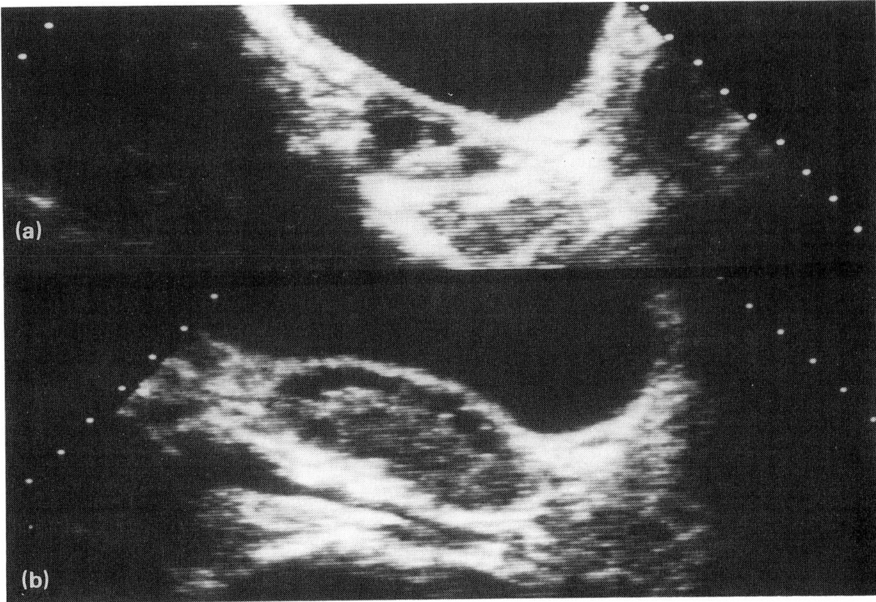

Fig. 2.3 Sagittal ultrasound scans of (a) a normal ovary in the midfollicular phase of the menstrual cycle and (b) an enlarged polycystic ovary in an anovulatory woman. Pictures courtesy of Miss J. Adams and published with permission from *Clinical Endocrinology* [15].

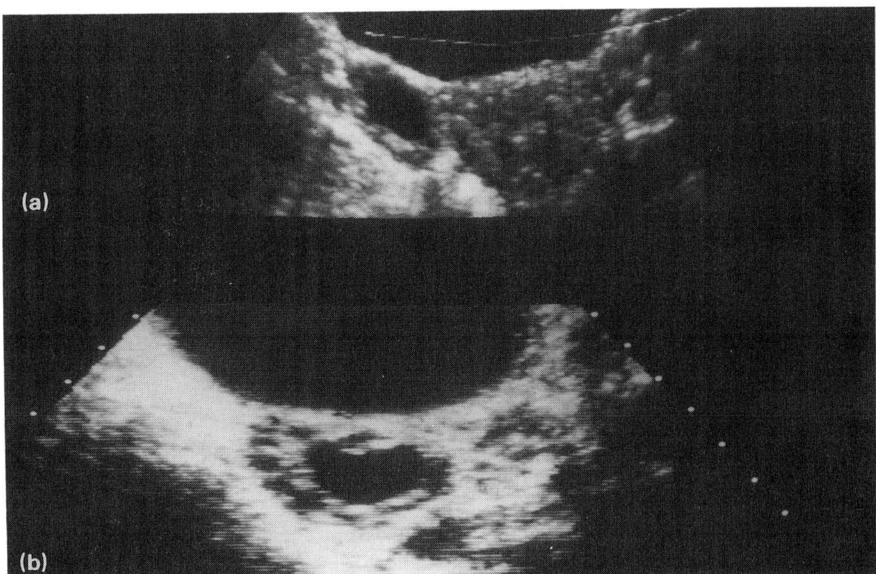

Fig. 2.4 Sagittal ultrasound scans of (a) a normal ovary in the late follicular phase, showing a pre-ovulatory follicle, and (b) a polycystic ovary at a similar stage of the cycle in a woman with hirsutism and regular ovulatory cycles. Pictures courtesy of Miss J. Adams and published with permission from *Clinical Endocrinology* [15].

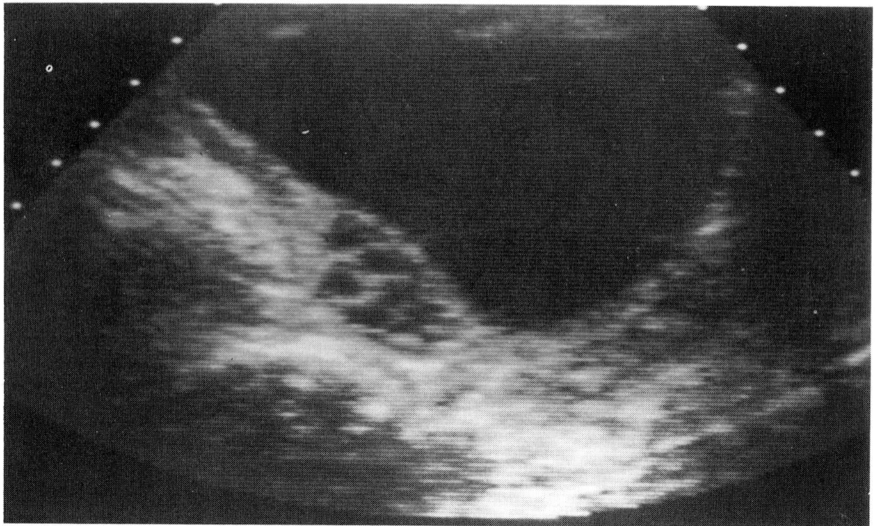

Fig. 2.5 A multifollicular ovary in a woman with weight loss-related amenorrhea. The ovary is of normal size and is filled with follicles but, in contrast to a polycystic ovary, with no increase in stroma. Picture courtesy of Miss J. Adams and published with permission from *Clinical Endocrinology* [15].

Correlation of ultrasound with histology

It is important, when possible, to corroborate the findings on ultrasound by those obtained by histologic analysis. In a recent study, Saxton *et al.* [17] showed an excellent correlation between the morphologic appearance as observed on ultrasound and that seen by histologic analysis. These observations lend weight to the assertion that ultrasound can be used reliably for the diagnosis of polycystic ovaries.

Prevalence of polycystic ovaries in anovulatory, hirsute, and normal subjects

The prevalence of polycystic ovaries was assessed in a population of patients at a gynecologic endocrine clinic presenting with menstrual disturbances, hirsutism or both [14,17]. The prevalence of polycystic ovaries in the various groups of women is summarized in Table 2.3. The vast majority of women with oligomenorrhea were found to have polycystic ovaries on ultrasound but, more surprisingly, those with regular ovulatory cycles who presented with hirsutism also had a high prevalence of polycystic ovaries.

The appearance of polycystic ovaries in women with regular

Table 2.3 Prevalence of PCO on ultrasound in women with anovulation and/or hirsutism.

			Hormone concentrations in women with PCO	
Presenting symptom	No.	Prevalence of PCO (%)	LH (U/l) median (range)	Testosterone (nmol/l) mean (SD)
Secondary amenorrhea	100	32	16.0 (4.8–29)	3.1 (1.1)
Oligomenorrhea	75	87	13.9 (4.0–42)	3.3 (1.2)
Hirsutism (regular cycle)	46	87	9.9 (5.0–15)	2.6 (0.9)
Normal controls	60	—	5.3 (2.0–14)	1.7 (0.4)

Hormone concentrations in women with PCO are compared with those at the early to midfollicular phase in subjects with normal ovaries and ovulatory cycles. Levels of LH were compared by the Mann–Whitney U test and those of testosterone by Student's test. Levels of both LH and testosterone in each group of women with PCO were significantly higher ($P < 0.01$) than those in normal controls [15].

ovulatory cycles was an important finding since it suggests that the polycystic ovary represents a primary ovarian abnormality rather than the response of the ovary to chronic anovulation [17].

The endocrine evaluation of these three groups of women revealed that serum concentrations of LH were significantly elevated as compared with normal levels in all three groups but that the levels in women with regular cycles and hirsutism were intermediate between those of normal subjects and those of women with anovulatory cycles (Table 2.3). A similar pattern was seen in serum levels of testosterone. These endocrine features support the ultrasound diagnosis of polycystic ovaries. Subsequent results from a much larger series of subjects, in whom the primary diagnosis of polycystic ovary syndrome was made on ultrasound, have confirmed these initial endocrine findings [17].

Because of the high prevalence of polycystic ovaries in our population of patients, we decided to examine a large group of volunteers from the normal population. All these women considered themselves to be normal and had not presented to a physician for treatment of menstrual disturbance or symptoms of hyperandrogenemia. We found that 22% of 257 women who presented for ultrasound scans had polycystic ovaries [18]. There was a strong correlation between the cycle history and the appearance of the ovaries (Table 2.4), such that the majority of women in the normal population who had polycystic ovaries had slightly irregular cycles. Furthermore, although the mean and median serum concentrations of LH in women with polycystic ovaries

Table 2.4 Correlation of the appearance of ovaries on ultrasound with menstrual history in the normal population.

	Menses	
Ultrasound appearance	Regular	Irregular
Normal ovaries	115	1
Polycystic ovaries	8*	24

*6 of 8 women with PCO and regular cycles were hirsute [15,18].

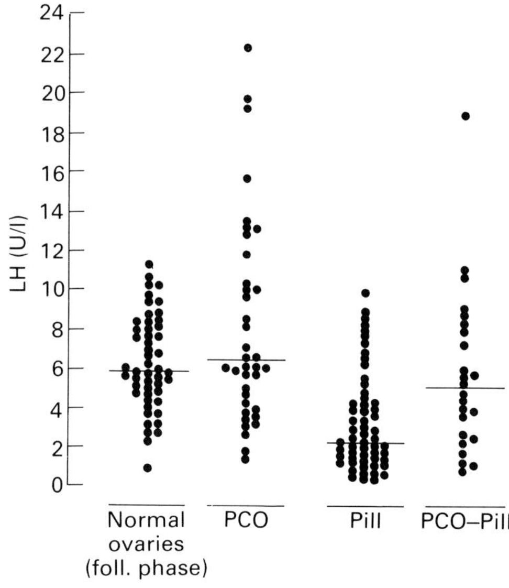

Fig. 2.6 Serum LH concentrations in the normal population, grouped according to ovarian morphology on ultrasound and to whether or not subjects were taking the oral contraceptive. Note preponderance of elevated LH values even in this asymptomatic group of subjects with PCO. From Polson *et al.* [18], with permission.

were no different from those in women with normal ovaries, there was a difference in the distribution of concentrations of LH such that there was a preponderance of higher levels in the case of women with polycystic ovaries [18] (Fig. 2.6).

Significance of the polycystic ovary on ultrasound

The evidence suggests that the ovarian phenotype of the polycystic ovary is extremely common, and other studies have suggested that it is genetic in origin [19,20]. It is clear that women with PCO exhibit a wide spectrum of clinical and biochemical features. The explanation for this heterogeneity remains uncertain. It is possible that there are a number of discrete syndromes associated with PCO and, indeed, it seems that there is more than one cause of PCO. However, an alternative view (favored by this author) is that there is one major underlying cause, ovarian in origin, which is associated with variable clinical and biochemical expression. Development of PCO probably depends on the interaction of other genetic and environmental factors (e.g. insulin resistance with or without obesity) that affect the clinical and biochemical presentation of the disorder [17,18,21].

Despite the apparent heterogeneity, there is more that unites women with the appearance of polycystic ovaries on ultrasound than divides them. This statement is supported by the observations, detailed above, that women in the normal population who have PCO are much more likely to have irregular menstrual cycles than women with non-polycystic ovaries and that the patterns of secretion of LH in the two groups are different (Table 2.4; Fig. 2.6).

Even the "incidental" finding of a polycystic picture on ultrasound in women with regular cycles and tubal disease who are being considered for *in vitro* fertilization may be clinically significant; such patients are more likely to produce multiple follicles during superovulation and may have higher than normal serum concentrations of androgens (as well as estrogens) in response to exogenous gonadotropins (A. Rutherford, R.M. Winston, R. Margara & S. Franks, unpublished data).

In summary, the morphology of the polycystic ovary is characterized by an increase in the number of developing and atretic follicles and a substantial increase in the amount of subcortical stroma compared with the normal ovary. These features can be identified by pelvic ultrasound and are present at high frequency not only in anovulatory women (with or without hirsutism) but also in subjects with hirsutism who have regular ovulatory cycles. The heterogeneity of clinical and biochemical features in women with PCO may be related to interactions with other, extraovarian factors that influence the production, transport or action of androgens.

References

1 Allen WM, Woolf RB. Medullary resection of the ovaries in the Stein–Leventhal syndrome. Am J Obstet Gynecol 1959; 77:826–34.

2 Goldzieher JW, Green JA. The polycystic ovary. I. Clinical and histologic features. J Clin Endocrinol Metab 1962; 22:325–38.

3 Green JA, Goldzieher JW. The polycystic ovary. IV. Light and electron microscopic studies. Am J Obstet Gynecol 1965; 91:173–81.

4 Ingersoll FM, McDermott WV. Bilateral polycystic ovaries, Stein–Leventhal syndrome. Am J Obstet Gynecol 1950; 60:117–25.
5 Leventhal ML. The Stein–Leventhal syndrome. Am J Obstet Gynecol 1958; 76: 825–38.
6 Plate WP. The pathologic anatomy of the Stein–Leventhal syndrome. Fertil Steril 1958; 9:545–54.
7 Shippel S. The ovarian theca cell. IV. The hyperthecosis syndrome. J Obstet Gynaecol Br Emp 1955; 62:321–53.
8 Westman A. The histology and structure of the ovary in cases of virilism. Acta Obstet Gynecol Scand 1955; 34:92–104.
9 Hughesdon PE. Morphology and morphogenesis of the Stein–Leventhal ovary and of so-called "hyperthecosis." Obstet Gynecol Surv 1982; 37:59–77.
10 Erickson GF, Magoffin DA, Dyer CA, Hofeditz C. The ovarian androgen-producing cells: a review of structure/function relationships. Endocr Rev 1985; 6:371–99.
11 Swanson M, Sauerbrei EE, Cooperberg PL. Medical implications of ultrasonically detected polycystic ovaries. J Clin Ultrasound 1981; 9:219–22.
12 Parisi L, Tramonti M, Casciano S, Zurli A, Gazzarrini Q. The role of ultrasound in the study of polycystic ovarian disease. J Clin Ultrasound 1982; 10:167–72.
13 Adams J, Franks S, Polson DW, Mason HD, Abdulwahid NA, Tucker M, Morris DV, Price J, Jacobs HS. Multifollicular ovaries: clinical and endocrine features and response to pulsatile gonadotrophin-releasing hormone. Lancet 1985; ii:1375–8.
14 Adams J, Polson DW, Franks S. Prevalence of polycystic ovaries in women with anovulation and idiopathic hirsutism. Br Med J 1986; 293:355–9.
15 Franks S. Polycystic ovary syndrome: a changing perspective. Clin Endocrinol 1989; 31:87–120.
16 Mason HD, Sagle M, Polson DW, Kiddy D, Dobriansky D, Adams J, Franks S. Reduced frequency of luteinizing hormone pulses in women with weight loss-related amenorrhoea and multifollicular ovaries. Clin Endocrinol 1988; 28:611–18.
17 Saxton DW, Farquhar CM, Rae T, Beard RW, Anderson MC, Wadsworth J. Accuracy of ultrasound measurements of female pelvic organs. Br J Obstet Gynaecol 1990; 97: 695–9.
18 Polson DW, Adams J, Wadsworth J, Franks S. Polycystic ovaries—a common finding in normal women. Lancet 1988; i:870–2.
19 Wilroy RS, Givens JR, Wiser WL, Coleman SA, Andersen RN, Summitt RL. Hyperthecosis: an inheritable form of polycystic ovarian disease. Birth Defects, original article: (1975) Series XI 81–5.
20 Hague W, Adams J, Reeders S, Peto TEA, Jacobs HB. Familial polycystic ovaries: a genetic disease. Clin Endocrinol 1988; 29:593–606.
21 Kiddy DS, Hamilton-Fairley D, Seppala M, Koistinen R, James VHT, Reed MJ, Franks S. Diet-induced changes in sex hormone-binding globulin and free testosterone in women with normal or polycystic ovaries: correlation with serum insulin and insulin-like growth factor-I. Clin Endocrinol 1989; 31:757–64.

Section 2
Central Nervous System—Pituitary–Ovarian Axis

Chapter 3
Hypothalamic–Pituitary Abnormalities in Polycystic Ovary Syndrome

MARCO FILICORI & CARLO FLAMIGNI

Excessive secretion of luteinizing hormone (LH) is one of the most common features of the polycystic ovary syndrome (PCO). However, the specific role of hypothalamic or pituitary derangements remains to be clarified. Great efforts have been devoted to investigations of the pathogenetic role of this endocrine abnormality in PCO. The fundamental question to be resolved is whether the endocrine and clinical disorder of PCO depends primarily upon abnormal secretion of LH or whether the hypothalamic–pituitary disorder is a consequence of dysfunctional ovarian function or other associated disorders (e.g. adrenal hyperfunction). Putative neurotransmitters and drugs that affect hypothalamic function have been utilized to assess possible hypothalamic derangements associated with this disorder. The use of gonadotropin-releasing hormone (GnRH) analogs and of exogenous pulsatile administration of GnRH also provides interesting information as to the role of hypothalamic–pituitary function in PCO.

Hypothalamic function

Several neurotransmitters are probably involved in the control of GnRH and, thus, the secretion of gonadotropins. Various studies have addressed the issue of neurotransmitter-related abnormalities in PCO. Dopamine (DA) lowers serum concentrations of LH in women and its activity appears to be directly proportional to endogenous estrogen levels [1,2]. Furthermore, the capability of DA to lower serum levels of LH is related to baseline concentrations of LH, so that DA causes a more profound suppression of LH levels when circulating levels of LH are elevated. Quigley *et al.* [3] found that administration of DA resulted in a significant reduction of LH levels in PCO. Moreover, in this study the degree of reduction of LH levels appeared to be proportional to the initial levels of LH present in each patient. Excretion of homovanillic acid (a urinary metabolite of DA) was found to be low in women with PCO [4]. These results suggest that DA activity may be reduced in PCO and that this central derangement may be responsible for the excessive levels of LH typical of patients with PCO. However, Barnes *et al.* [5] found subsequently that, when subjects were matched for weight and estrogen secretion, the degree of LH suppression achieved through infusion of DA was similar in patients with PCO and in normal controls. In the same study, metoclopramide (an antagonist of receptors for DA) did not affect gonadotropin secretion but increased prolactin levels to a greater degree in women with PCO than in controls. Rosen and Lobo [6] studied the effect of disulfiram, a compound that should increase hypothalamic levels of DA via inhibition of the conversion of DA to norepinephrine (NE). Administration of disulfiram did not affect mean LH levels or pulsatile LH secretion in normal women and in three out of five women with PCO. However, in two women with PCO, disulfiram significantly lowered the LH response to exogenous GnRH. Taken together, these data suggest that inadequate hypothalamic secretion of DA is not a fundamental pathogenetic component in most cases of PCO. However, similar to the situation encountered in normal women at the time of the midcycle surge or in postmenopausal subjects, markedly high concentrations of LH may be related to inappropriately low rates of DA secretion. Convincing evidence against a major disturbance related to DA in PCO also comes from studies of the results of treatment with bromocriptine (BCP) of these patients. Steingold *et al.* [7] and Murdoch *et al.* [8] did not find changes in LH secretion after 1, 2 or 12 months of BCP administration; the latter investigation was a double-blind placebo study. Furthermore, Buvat *et al.* [9] did not see any overall hormonal or clinical improvement in 55 women with PCO treated in a double-blind placebo protocol for 6 months. Although about half of their patients with PCO developed reduced levels of LH, this reduction was not accompanied by significant changes in concentrations of testosterone (T). Significant reduction of LH and T levels during treatment with BCP were reported by Falaschi *et al.* [10] and by Murdoch *et al.* [8] in 12 and 11 patients with PCO, respectively. However, improvement of hirsutism and of menstrual disturbances were only reported in two of the cases studied by Murdoch *et al.* [8]. Thus, these data confirm that if any DA-related derangement of LH secretion exists in PCO, this disorder is probably limited to a minority of patients with PCO.

Finally, the possibility that secretion of NE may be abnormal in PCO was suggested by the finding of reduced urinary levels of 3-methoxy-

4-hydroxyphenylglycol (a metabolite of NE) in such subjects [11]. However, infusion of NE did not increase levels of circulating LH in normal women [12] and administration of thymoxamine (an α_1-adrenoceptor antagonist) only modestly increased the amplitude of LH pulses in women with PCO [13]. Thus, it is unlikely that NE is a critical contributor to dysfunctional LH secretion in PCO.

Abnormalities in the secretion of gonadotropins

The sensitivity of pituitary gonadotropins to exogenous GnRH is clearly increased in patients with PCO as compared to that in normal women in the follicular phase of the cycle [14]. This abnormality is probably related to the excessive plasma levels of estrone or unbound estradiol present in this disorder. Episodic secretion of LH is also markedly abnormal in PCO. Although the exact frequency of LH peaks is still the subject of some controversy, there is a general agreement as to an increment in the amplitude of LH pulses in patients with PCO (Table 3.1). Three out of five studies [15,16,19] of pulsatile patterns of LH secretion revealed a significantly higher frequency of pulsatile release of LH in women with PCO than in normal women at various stages of the

Table 3.1 Parameters of the pulsatile secretion of LH (amplitude and frequency) from five studies of normal controls and women with PCO.

	Controls			PCO	
	Cycle stage	Frequency (min)	Amplitude (IU/l)	Frequency (min)	Amplitude (IU/l)
Burger *et al.* [15]	FP	60	3.0	50*	5.8*
Filicori *et al.* [16]	EFP	94 ± 4	6.4 ± 0.4	55 ± 2*	10.9 ± 1.4*
	MFP	67 ± 3	5.1 ± 0.8		
	LFP	71 ± 4	7.2 ± 1.2		
Kazer *et al.* [17]	EFP	60 ± 1	6.2 ± 0.8	60 ± 2	12.1 ± 2.7*
	MFP	60 ± 2	6.4 ± 0.6		
Venturoli *et al.* [18]	MFP	66 ± 19	5.2 ± 1.8	62 ± 11	11.6 ± 3.7*
Waldstreicher *et al.* [19]	EFP	94 ± 4	6.4 ± 0.4	58 ± 2*	13.6 ± 2.7*
	MFP	67 ± 3	5.1 ± 0.8		
	LFP	71 ± 4	7.2 ± 1.2		

* Denotes statistically significant difference between controls and women with PCO ($P < 0.05$).
Stages of the menstrual cycle at which pulse studies were performed in controls: FP, follicular phase; EFP, MFP, and LFP, early, mid, and late follicular phases, respectively.

follicular phase. The issue of disturbed LH pulse frequency is not purely academic. It has been shown that an exact GnRH pulse frequency is essential for appropriate synthesis of the mRNA for LH [20] and that a lower than normal GnRH frequency results in a blunted midcycle LH surge and anovulation [21]. Excessively rapid, pulsatile administration of GnRH (every 30 min) during the follicular phase of the normal menstrual cycle results in an increase in mean levels of circulating LH and of the ratio of LH to follicle-stimulating hormone (FSH) and may cause luteal phase defects [22]; such abnormalities are common findings in patients with PCO.

Circadian rhythmicity in levels of LH may be abnormal in PCO, in particular during adolescence. Zumoff *et al.* [23] reported an increase in levels of LH in five teenage women desynchronized from their normal sleep period. This increase in levels of LH occurred 7–8 hours after awakening from night sleep. Similar findings were reported by Porcu *et al.* [24] who studied 12 adolescent women with high or normal levels of LH; a deranged circadian rhythmicity of LH was found only in the high-LH group (five women). These studies suggest that an abnormal chronobiological secretion of LH may occur in some adolescent women and that this derangement may be somehow related to the development of PCO. However, in several of these subjects a normalization of gonadotropin secretion occurred within 1–2 years. Thus, the exact role of this derangement is still uncertain.

Use of analogs of GnRH and pulsatile GnRH

Analogs of GnRH (GnRH-A) block the pituitary secretion of gonadotropins and thus induce a pharmacologic and reversible hypogonadotropic condition in patients with PCO. Levels of gonadal steroids are low during treatment with GnRH-A and improvement of acne and hirsutism occurs within a few months. Unfortunately, the low estrogen levels that develop during administration of GnRH-A prevent the prolonged use of these compounds because of potential risks of osteoporosis.

Levels of gonadotropins, estrogens, and testosterone promptly return to pretreatment values when GnRH-A is discontinued [25]. However, most subjects with PCO and disorders of their menstrual cycle remain anovulatory after treatment with GnRH-A in spite of the temporary hypogonadotropic condition created by GnRH-A [25]. In PCO, pulsatile administration of GnRH alone (without pretreatment with GnRH-A) causes further abnormalities in levels of gonadotropins and steroids and results in ovulation only in around 40% of cycles [16,26,27]. Conversely, we demonstrated that when suppression by GnRH-A is immediately followed by pulsatile administration of GnRH, ovulation occurs in a high percentage of previously anovulatory patients with PCO [16,26].

The improvement in the response of patients with PCO to this drug regimen is probably related to the profound depletion of pituitary reserves of LH, to increments of the FSH/LH ratio in the follicular phase [16], and to the lowering of intraovarian concentrations of androgens achieved with GnRH-A. Thus, the more physiologic pattern of LH levels achieved with pulsatile GnRH after suppression by GnRH-A permits us to stimulate optimally the secretion of gonadal steroids and folliculogenesis. Nevertheless, our studies also indicate that abnormalities of gonadal function may persist even after profound suppression of gonadotropins for 8 weeks. Ovarian volume decreases during exposure to GnRH-A and usually it does not return to within the limits encountered in normal women. In spite of follicular phase levels of LH that are only slightly greater than those in hypogonadotropic patients (Fig. 3.1), levels of testosterone increase rapidly across the follicular phase of pulsatile-GnRH cycles induced after suppression by GnRH-A and return to presuppression concentrations by the time of ovulation. Consecutive cycles of pulsatile GnRH, induced without repeating the suppression by GnRH-A, are not as effective as the first cycle after treatment with GnRH-A in restoring ovulation [26]. Thus, it seems that dysfunctional ovarian function promptly returns when normal levels of LH are restored.

Summary

PCO is a nonhomogeneous and elusive disorder. It is likely that, at present, various etiopathogenetic entities are grouped together under the PCO label and that no single conclusion can be applied to all of these entities. The issue of whether PCO is primarily a hypothalamic or a gonadal disorder is still unresolved.

Although disturbances of hypothalamic neurotransmitters may exist in PCO (particularly in patients with high circulating levels of LH), a primary role for such disturbances appears to be unlikely in most patients with PCO. Little controversy exists as to the essentially deranged nature of the secretion of LH and this abnormality is undoubtedly a critical component of the endocrine and ovulatory disorders of PCO. Nevertheless, in adult patients with PCO, excessive episodic secretion of LH appears to affect an already dysfunctional ovary.

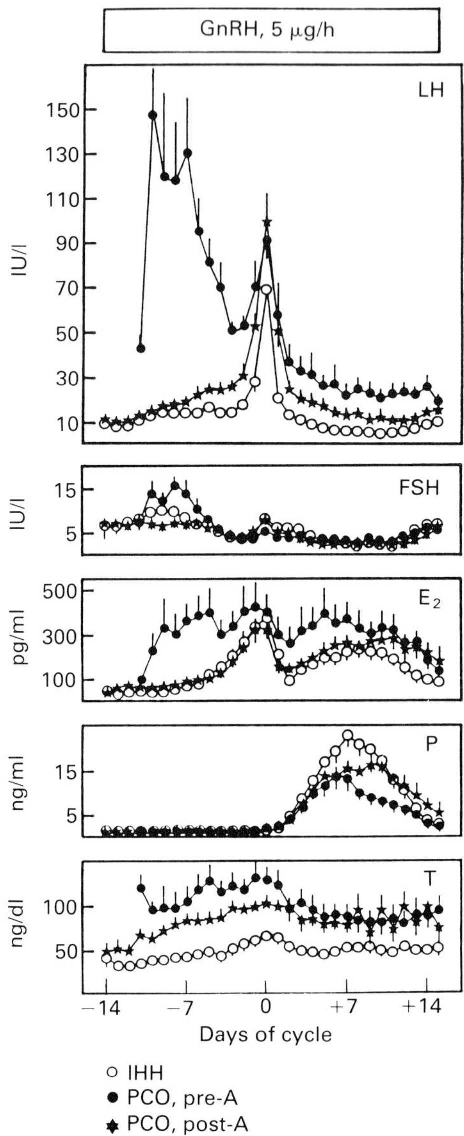

Fig. 3.1 Daily concentrations of gonadotropins and gonadal steroids in different ovulatory disorders treated with pulsatile GnRH (5 μg every 60 min). IHH, primary hypogonadotropic amenorrhea; PCOD pre-A, patients with PCOD without pretreatment with GnRH-A; PCOD post-A, patients with PCOD after suppression with GnRH-A. E2, estradiol; P, progesterone; T, testosterone. (Reprinted, with permission, from Filicori *et al.* [26], © by The Endocrine Society.)

Acknowledgment

We wish to thank Ms Silvia Arsento for excellent secretarial assistance.

References

1 Judd SJ, Rakoff JS, Yen SSC. Inhibition of gonadotropin and prolactin release by dopamine: effect of endogenous estradiol levels. J Clin Endocrinol Metab 1978; 47:494–8.

2 Judd SJ, Rigg LA, Yen SSC. The effects of ovariectomy and estrogen treatment on the dopamine inhibition of gonadotropin and prolactin release. J Clin Endocrinol Metab 1979; 49:182–4.
3 Quigley ME, Rakoff JS, Yen SSC. Increased luteinizing hormone sensitivity to dopamine inhibition in polycystic ovary syndrome. J Clin Endocrinol Metab 1981; 52:231–4.
4 Shoupe D, Lobo RA. Evidence for altered catecholamine metabolism in polycystic ovary syndrome. Am J Obstet Gynecol 1984; 150:566–71.
5 Barnes RB, Mileikowsky GN, Cha KY, Spencer CA, Lobo RA. Effects of dopamine and metoclopramide in polycystic ovary syndrome. J Clin Endocrinol Metab 1986; 63: 506–9.
6 Rosen GF, Lobo RA. Further evidence against dopamine deficiency as the cause of inappropriate gonadotropin secretion in patients with polycystic ovary syndrome. J Clin Endocrinol Metab 1987; 65:891–5.
7 Steingold KA, Lobo RA Judd HL, Lu JKH, Chang J. The effect of bromocriptine on gonadotropin and steroid secretion in polycystic ovarian disease. J Clin Endocrinol Metab 1986; 62:1048–51.
8 Murdoch AP, McClean KG, Watson MJ, Dunlop W, Taylor PK. Treatment of hirsutism in polycystic ovary syndrome with bromocriptine. Br J Obstet Gynaecol 1987; 94:358–65.
9 Buvat J, Buvat-Herbaut M, Marcolin G, Racadot A, Fourlinnie JC, Beuscart R, Fossati P. A double-blind controlled study of the hormonal and clinical effects of bromocriptine in the polycystic ovary syndrome. J Clin Endocrinol Metab 1986; 63:119–24.
10 Falaschi P, Rocco A, Del Pozo E. Inhibitory effect of bromocriptine treatment on luteinizing hormone secretion in polycystic ovary syndrome. J Clin Endocrinol Metab 1986; 62:348–51.
11 Lobo RA, Granger LR, Paul WL, Goebelsmann U, Mishell DR. Psychological stress and increases in urinary norepinephrine metabolites, platelet serotonin, and adrenal androgens in women with polycystic ovary syndrome. Am J Obstet Gynecol 1983; 145:496–503.
12 Barnes RB, Cha KY, Lee DG, Lobo RA. Modulation of luteinizing hormone immunoreactivity and bioactivity by dopamine but not norepinephrine in women. Am J Obstet Gynecol 1986; 154:445–50.
13 Paradisi R, Venturoli S, Capelli M, *et al.* Effects of α_1-adrenergic blockade on pulsatile luteinizing hormone, follicle-stimulating hormone, and prolactin secretion in polycystic ovary syndrome. J Clin Endocrinol Metab 1987; 65:841–6.
14 Rebar R, Judd HL, Yen SSC, Rakoff J, Vandenberg G, Naftolin F. Characterization of the inappropriate gonadotropin secretion in polycystic ovary syndrome. J Clin Invest 1976; 57:1320–9.
15 Burger CW, Korsen T, van Kessel H, van Dop PA, Caron FJM, Schoemaker J. Pulsatile luteinizing hormone patterns in the follicular phase of the menstrual cycle, polycystic ovarian disease (PCOD) and non-PCOD secondary amenorrhea. J Clin Endocrinol Metab 1985; 61:1126–32.
16 Filicori M, Campaniello E, Michelacci L, Pareschi A, Ferrari P, Bolelli GF, Flamigni C. Gonadotropin-releasing hormone (GnRH) analog suppression renders polycystic ovarian disease patients more susceptible to ovulation induction with pulsatile GnRH. J Clin Endocrinol Metab 1988; 66:327–33.
17 Kazer RR, Kessel B, Yen SSC. Circulating luteinizing hormone pulse frequency in women with polycystic ovary syndrome. J Clin Endocrinol Metab 1987; 65:233–6.
18 Venturoli S, Porcu E, Fabbri R, *et al.* Episodic pulsatile secretion of FSH, LH, prolactin, oestradiol, oestrone, and LH circadian variations in polycystic ovary syndrome. Clin Endocrinol 1988; 28:93–107.
19 Waldstreicher J, Santoro NF, Hall JE, Filicori M, Crowley WF, Jr. Hyperfunction of the hypothalamic–pituitary axis in women with polycystic ovarian disease: indirect

evidence for partial gonadotroph desensitization. J Clin Endocrinol Metab 1988; 66:165–72.
20 Haisenleder DJ, Khoury S, Zmeili SM, Papavasiliou S, Ortolano GA, Dee C, Duncan JA, Marshall JC. The frequency of gonadotropin-releasing hormone secretion regulates expression of α and luteinizing hormone β-subunit messenger ribonucleic acids in male rats. Mol Endocrinol 1987; 1:834–8.
21 Filicori M, Flamigni C, Campaniello E, Ferrari P, Meriggiola MC, Michelacci L, Pareschi A, Valdiserri A. Evidence for a specific role of GnRH pulse frequency in the control of the human menstrual cycle. Am J Physiol 1989; 257:E930–E936.
22 Soules MR, Clifton DK, Bremner WJ, Steiner RA. Corpus luteum insufficiency induced by a rapid gonadotropin-releasing hormone-induced gonadotropin secretion pattern in the follicular phase. J Clin Endocrinol Metab 1987; 65:457–64.
23 Zumoff B, Freeman R, Coupey S, Saenger P, Marrowitz M, Kream J. A chronobiologic abnormality in luteinizing hormone secretion in teenage girls with the polycystic-ovary syndrome. N Engl J Med 1983; 309:1206–9.
24 Porcu E, Venturoli S, Magrini O, Bolzani R, Gabbi D, Paradisi R, Fabbri R, Flamigni C. Circadian variations of luteinizing hormone can have two different profiles in adolescent anovulation. J Clin Endocrinol Metab 1987; 65:488–93.
25 de Ziegler D, Steingold K, Cedars M, Lu JKH, Meldrum DR, Judds HL, Chang RJ. Recovery of hormone secretion after chronic gonadotropin-releasing hormone agonist administration in women with polycystic ovarian disease. J Clin Endocrinol Metab 1989; 68:1111–17.
26 Filicori M, Flamigni C, Campaniello E, Valdiserri A, Ferrari P, Meriggiola MC, Michelacci L, Pareschi A. The abnormal response of polycystic ovarian disease patients to exogenous pulsatile gonadotropin-releasing hormone: characterization and management. J Clin Endocrinol Metab 1989; 69:825–31.
27 Eshel A, Abdulwahid NA, Armar NA, Adams JM, Jacobs HS. Pulsatile luteinizing hormone-releasing hormone therapy in women with polycystic ovary syndrome. Fertil Steril 1988; 49:956–60.

Chapter 4
Neuroendocrine Investigation of Polycystic Ovary Syndrome: New Approaches

JANET E. HALL , ANN E. TAYLOR,
KATHRYN A. MARTIN & WILLIAM F. CROWLEY JR

Polycystic ovary syndrome (PCO) is a poorly defined syndrome that involves various combinations of neuroendocrine, steroidogenic, morphologic and metabolic abnormalities. A prominent feature of a clear subset of patients with this disorder is deranged neuroendocrine control of gonadotropin secretion by gonadotropin-releasing hormone (GnRH), characterized by elevated serum [1,2] and urinary [3] levels of luteinizing hormone (LH) in the presence of normal to low serum levels of follicle-stimulating hormone (FSH) and, hence, an elevated ratio of LH to FSH. In this chapter, we outline several new approaches that we have used to investigate abnormalities in the secretion of GnRH in the pathogenesis of this disorder.

The amplitude of pulsatile secretion of LH from the pituitary has been clearly documented to be elevated in PCO [2,4] and the pituitary sensitivity to exogenous GnRH in such patients is also increased [2]. While it has been widely hypothesized that this augmented response of LH is secondary to abnormal pituitary feedback by circulating estrogens and androgens, attempts to reproduce this abnormality by infusion of either class of steroids have been unsuccessful [5,6]. Maintenance of normal to low levels of circulating FSH in the presence of this increased sensitivity of the gonadotrope to GnRH has been hypothesized to result from either a greater sensitivity of FSH than LH to the estrogen-associated negative feedback [6,7] or to increased levels of circulating inhibin produced by polycystic ovaries preferentially inhibiting FSH [2]. Experience with patients with GnRH deficiency, in whom the dose and frequency of GnRH replacement can be experimentally controlled, has led us to propose an alternative and unifying hypothesis for the abnormal gonadotropin dynamics in PCO.

Responses of levels of gonadotropin to increasing GnRH pulse frequency

The effect of increasing the frequency of administration of a fixed and "physiologic" dose of GnRH on secretion of LH and FSH was assessed in five GnRH-deficient men who were given an individualized bolus dose of GnRH that produced LH pulse amplitudes within the middle of the range for normal men when administered intravenously [8]. In the presence of levels of sex steroids that remained unchanged for the duration of these studies, mean levels of LH increased progressively as the interpulse interval for administration of GnRH decreased from 120 to 15 min, while those of FSH remained constant (Fig. 4.1). When the mean levels of LH and FSH were normalized to account for the increment in gonadotropin secretion that would have been predicted from an increase in the frequency of stimulation by GnRH, it became apparent that increasing the frequency of administration of GnRH within the selected time frame resulted in a relative loss of responsiveness of the gonadotrope (desensitization), which was considerably more marked in the case of FSH than in that of LH (Fig. 4.2). Thus, early desensitization

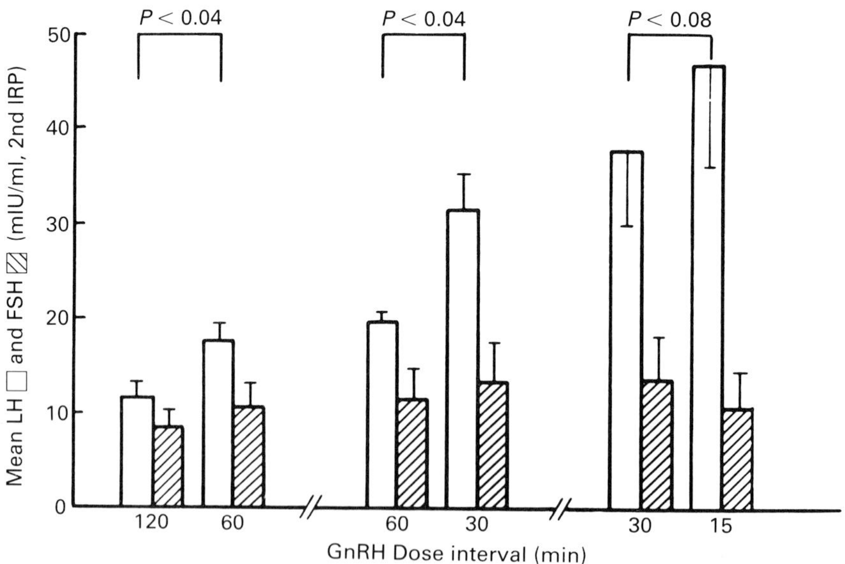

Fig. 4.1 Mean (±SEM) concentrations of LH and FSH during three 12-hour admissions in five GnRH-deficient men who received pulsatile GnRH at the dose intervals indicated. Note the preferential secretion of LH over FSH at higher frequencies of GnRH. Serum levels of LH increased with acute changes in frequency of administration of GnRH, but not with chronic changes. (Reprinted, with permission, from Spratt *et al.* [8], © by The Endocrine Society.)

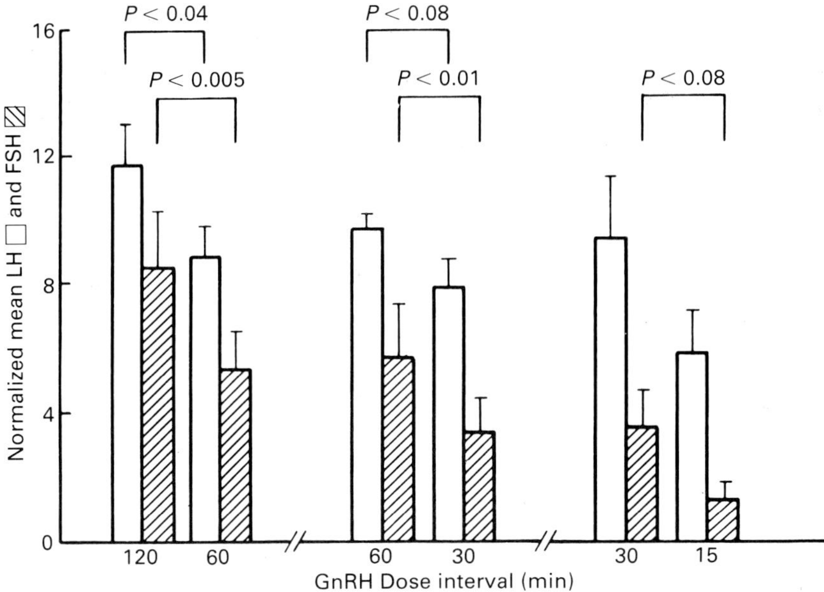

Fig. 4.2 Mean (±SEM) concentrations of LH and FSH normalized to account for the increase in gonadotropin secretion that would be expected with the increased frequency of administration of GnRH. Normalized levels of LH and FSH decreased acutely, but not chronically. This effect was greater for FSH than for LH. (Reprinted, with permission, from Spratt *et al.* [8], © by The Endocrine Society.)

of the gonadotrope, caused by an increased frequency of a fixed and physiologic amount of GnRH, leads to an increase in mean levels of LH, a marked reduction in the response of the gonadotrope to each bolus of GnRH, a relatively fixed level of FSH, and a resultant high ratio of levels of LH to FSH. With maintenance of this increased frequency of administration of GnRH over 7 days, responsiveness did not continue to decrease, but remained constant [8].

The frequency hypothesis

From the foregoing observations in men with GnRH deficiency in whom both gonadal feedback and the bolus dose of GnRH could be kept relatively constant, we hypothesized that an increased frequency of GnRH secretion is sufficient to account for the abnormal gonadotropin dynamics that are characteristic of a subset of patients with PCO. Thus, if it could be demonstrated that (i) the frequency of GnRH secretion is increased in patients with PCO in comparison to that in normal women in whom the sex-steroid environment is closely matched, and (ii) this increased frequency is sustained over time, this finding alone could explain the increased levels of LH and normal levels of FSH seen in this subset of patients with PCO. The hypothesis that a modest increase in GnRH pulse frequency sustained over time produces a state of partial pituitary desensitization with differential effects on levels of LH and FSH would not require that circulating levels of inhibin be elevated in patients with PCO to account for the low levels of FSH. This hypothesis would also imply that decreasing the frequency of pulsatile secretion of GnRH in patients with PCO would restore normal gonadotropin dynamics and facilitate ovulation.

Increased LH pulse frequency in PCO

To examine the frequency of secretion of pulses of GnRH in PCO, 12 women with the disorder were studied for 12–24 hours, with samples taken for analysis at 10-min intervals [4]. All patients included in these studies had (i) enlarged and polycystic ovaries on ultrasound or direct examination, (ii) a history of oligomenorrhea/amenorrhea, (iii) hyper-androgenemia with or without hirsutism, and (iv) an elevated ratio of LH to FSH that was greater than 2.4 (2 SD above that observed in normal women in the early follicular phase (EFP) of ovulatory menstrual cycles) [9]. The women were all euthyroid and normoprolactinemic and had baseline levels of 17-hydroxyprogesterone and dehydro-epiandrosterone sulfate (DHEAS) within the normal range. In these patients with PCO, serum levels of estradiol were similar to those in women in the EFP, but lower than those in women in the midfollicular (MFP) and late follicular (LFP) phases, while serum estrone levels were greater in the PCO patients than in normal women in the EFP and MFP, but lower than those of women in the LFP. Hence, gonadotropin levels were compared to those in normal women at all stages of the follicular phase [9]. Mean serum levels of LH were higher in women with PCO than in normal women at all stages of the follicular phase, while levels of FSH were indistinguishable in women with PCO and normal women in the follicular phase. The amplitude of LH pulses was significantly elevated in women with PCO over that found at each stage of the follicular phase (Fig. 4.3a). The LH pulse frequency in PCO was also increased significantly in comparison to that found during the normal EFP, MFP or LFP (Fig. 4.3b). In addition, a striking similarity of patterns of secretion of LH and FSH with an increased amplitude and frequency of LH pulses was seen in four patients with PCO in whom repeat studies were performed at intervals of 2–4 months.

Our results revealed that a significant increase in LH pulse frequency

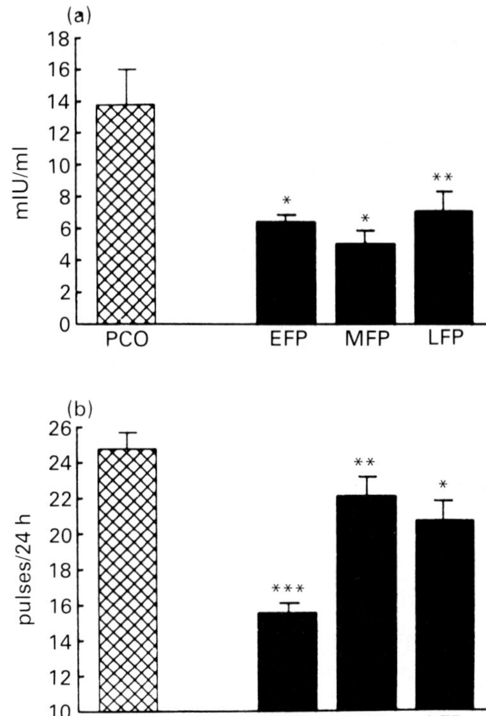

Fig. 4.3 Mean (±SEM) amplitude and frequency of pulses of LH in women with PCO and normal women in the early, mid, and late follicular phase (EFP, MFP and LFP) as indicated. $*P < 0.01$; $**P < 0.005$; $***P < 0.0005$. (Reprinted, with permission, from Waldstreicher *et al.* [4], © by The Endocrine Society.)

exists in PCO in comparison to the frequency in normal women at all stages of the follicular phase, implying an increase in the frequency of pulsatile secretion of GnRH. The increase in pulse frequency is relatively modest, although consistent, and would appear to be sustained over time in individual patients. While our findings are in agreement with some studies by other investigators [2,10], other groups have failed to confirm these observations [11]. Therefore, to corroborate our findings of an increase in GnRH pulse frequency as suggested by an increase in the frequency of pulsatile release of LH in patients with PCO, we have used an additional marker of GnRH secretion.

Free α-subunit as a marker of GnRH secretion

The glycoprotein hormones secreted from the gonadotrope and thyrotrope are comprised of a common α-subunit and a β-subunit that is distinct and confers specificity on intact LH, FSH and thyroid-stimulating hormone (TSH). The α-subunit is also secreted in an uncombined or free form (FAS) and its secretion is known to be controlled by both thyrotropin-releasing hormone (TRH) and GnRH. Exogenous administration of both GnRH and TRH results in increases in serum levels of FAS [12,13]; FAS is also elevated in the serum of castrates and hypothyroid patients and levels can be normalized by the administration of estrogen and thyroid hormone, respectively [14]. While previous studies have been hampered by cross-reactivity of the assay for FAS with intact hormone, recent studies utilizing a monoclonal antibody specific for FAS, with virtually no cross-reactivity with intact LH, FSH or TSH [15], have demonstrated that men with GnRH deficiency lack the pulsatile secretion of FAS and that long-term administration of GnRH to these patients produces pulses of LH and FAS that are 100% concordant [16]. In normal euthyroid women in the early follicular phase, we have shown that endogenous pulses of FAS are greater than 90% concordant with pulses of LH and that pulsatile secretion of FAS is abolished by administration of a potent GnRH antagonist [17].

While tonic secretion of FAS appears to be controlled by TRH, the pulsatile component of the secretion of FAS appears to be regulated primarily by GnRH. Consequently, pulsatile changes in levels of FAS can serve as a robust marker of GnRH secretion that can corroborate the information about GnRH provided by assessment of pulsatile secretion of LH. Additionally, FAS has a shorter half-life than LH [14], which is advantageous in the assessment of GnRH activity in situations in which pulses are likely to be very frequent, as in women with PCO and during the midcycle gonadotropin surge in normal women. Preliminary

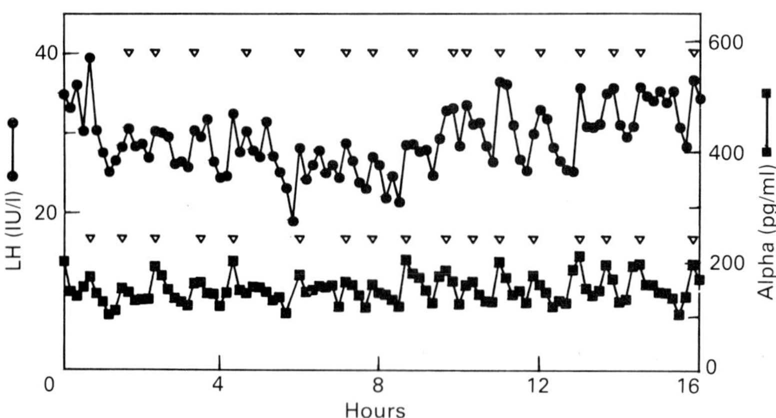

Fig. 4.4 Concordance of pulsatile secretion of FAS (■--■) with that of LH (●--●) in a patient with PCO studied over 16 hours, confirming the hourly frequency of pulsatile secretion demonstrated previously by our group using this second marker of GnRH secretion. Statistically identified pulses are indicated (▽) for both hormones.

studies in women with PCO have demonstrated a remarkable concordance of pulses of FAS and LH (Fig. 4.4), confirming the high frequency of pulsatile secretion of GnRH in a subset of patients with this disorder. We have, therefore, demonstrated an increased frequency of GnRH secretion in patients with PCO using two separate neuroendocrine markers and have demonstrated that this abnormal pattern is sustained over time. It has now been demonstrated that patients with PCO do not have elevated levels of inhibin in comparison with normal women [18]. While evidence indicates that the assay used measures only the α-subunit of inhibin [19], this finding would support the predictions of the frequency hypothesis, as delineated above. This finding is also consistent with data obtained *in vitro* that show that both subunits of inhibin are expressed in the granulosa cells of dominant follicles and corpora lutea, but not the small antral follicles that generally make up most of the population of follicles patients with PCO [20]. Finally, preliminary data indicate that decreasing the frequency of pulses of LH in patients with PCO by administration of exogenous estrogen and progesterone results in normalization of the ratio of LH to FSH [21]. Following discontinuation of the administration of sex steroid in these studies, follicular development occurred in all patients and ovulation in one of them. Taken together, these observations support the hypothesis of a critical role for the increased frequency of pulses of GnRH in the pathogenesis of PCO. They do not, however, address the issue of whether this increase in GnRH pulse frequency is primary or secondary to abnormal steroidogenesis of ovarian or adrenal origin.

Estimation of the quantity of GnRH in PCO

The use of LH pulse frequency as a marker of the frequency of pulsatile secretion of GnRH has been validated in ovine and rat models [22,23] and has been applied extensively to the study of the physiology of GnRH secretion in the human [9,24]. While direct assessment of the amount of GnRH secreted is possible in animal models, such an assessment is not feasible in human studies and additional approaches are required to obtain data about the amount of GnRH secreted in conditions such as PCO, where GnRH secretion is abnormal.

We have proposed that GnRH antagonists can be used to estimate the amount of endogenous GnRH secreted under a variety of physiologic and pathophysiologic circumstances [25]. Use of a GnRH antagonist to assess the total amount of GnRH is derived from pharmacologic considerations similar to those used for the study of endogenous opioids [26]. The same principles can be applied to the assessment of GnRH by assuming that the amount of any unmeasurable ligand present at a given time is directly proportional to the amount of antagonist required to block its effect. Full dose–response curves for the effects of a range of doses of a pure blocker of receptors for GnRH on secretion of LH were constructed for women studied in the EFP. These data then served as a reference for comparisons with data obtained at other stages of the menstrual cycle and in PCO. A dose that results in a 50% effect in the EFP can be used if it is assumed that the dose–response curves generated in different physiologic states are parallel. However, in our studies, full dose–response curves were generated in all situations.

Dose–response curves for LH were established in normal women in the EFP using the NAL-GLU GnRH antagonist (a pure GnRH receptor blocker) [17]. Women studied in the EFP were used as the reference group since the EFP is the stage of the normal cycle during which ovarian influences on the response of levels of LH to GnRH are at their lowest point in the cycle. The NAL-GLU GnRH antagonist was administered as a single subcutaneous injection on days 2 to 5 from the onset of menses. Blood was sampled every 10 min for 4 hours prior to administration of the antagonist, for 8 hours afterwards, and hourly for an additional 16 hours. The nadir for LH was calculated using a six-point moving average (equivalent to 1 hour of sampling, as the nadir for LH occurred within 8 hours of administration of the antagonist during the frequent-sampling portion of the study). The maximum percentage inhibition of LH was then determined by expressing the difference between the mean baseline and the nadir as a percentage of the mean baseline value for each study. A maximal inhibitory effect was achieved for this antagonist at the doses studied, as evidenced by the flattening of the dose–response curves at doses of 50 and 150 μg/kg while a dose of 15 μg/kg produced a submaximal response (Fig. 4.5). These studies have also indicated a remarkable precision in the response of levels of LH to the GnRH antagonist. Similar dose–response relationships were investigated in women at two further stages of the normal menstrual cycle, namely the LFP and the ELP, using the same antagonist [25]. No differences could be detected in percentage inhibition of LH at each of the three above-mentioned doses of antagonist between the EFP and either the LFP or the ELP, despite varying baseline levels of LH and varying degrees of sex-steroid feedback at the pituitary. Studies in the LFP are particularly relevant for comparisons with PCO. Although levels of estradiol in the EFP are generally matched with those in PCO, levels of both estrone and circulating LH are more closely matched with those in PCO in the LFP [4]. Patients with PCO were studied in a similar manner in an attempt to quantitate the overall secretion of GnRH in this

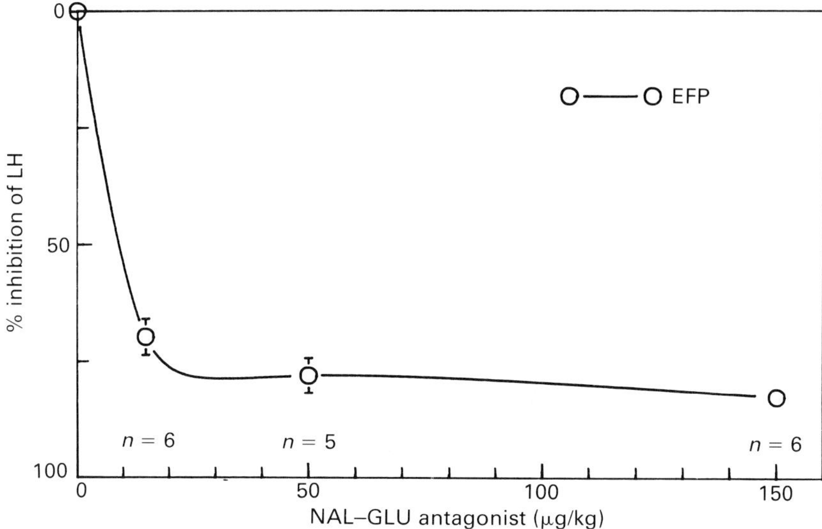

Fig. 4.5 The mean (±SEM) maximum percentage inhibition of LH in response to doses of 15, 50 and 150 μg/kg of the NAL-GLU GnRH antagonist. Where not obvious, "SEM" bars are located within the symbols. (Redrawn, with permission, from Hall *et al.* [17], © by The Endocrine Society.)

disorder [27]. The protocol was identical to that described above for the EFP studies. Administration of the GnRH antagonist was effective in suppressing LH and, to a lesser extent, FSH (Fig. 4.6). Both the amount and duration of suppression of LH were increased with increasing doses of the antagonist. When results were expressed in relation to baseline levels, neither the duration of suppression nor the maximum percentage suppression of LH were different from the reference studies in the EFP at any of the doses of antagonist tested. Therefore, our studies using a GnRH antagonist suggest that the total amount of GnRH secreted in PCO is not increased, despite the increase in frequency of release of GnRH and in the amplitude of pulses of LH that characterize this disorder [27].

Summary

We have hypothesized that the abnormal dynamics of secretion of gonadotropins in PCO, with elevated levels of LH and relatively normal levels of FSH, may result from partial desensitization of the gonadotrope due to a sustained, increased frequency of pulsatile secretion of GnRH. We have now shown, using two separate markers of secretion of GnRH (pulsatile LH and pulsatile FAS), that the frequency of secretion of

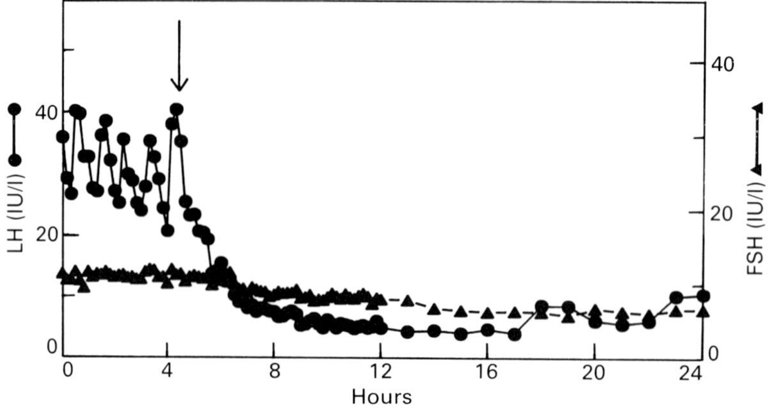

Fig. 4.6 Response of LH (●--●) and FSH (▲--▲) to administration of 50 μg/kg of the NAL-GLU GnRH antagonist at the time indicated by the arrow in a typical patient with PCO. Note the marked suppression of the elevated levels of LH in response to the blockade of GnRH receptors while the response of levels of FSH is relatively modest.

GnRH is, indeed, increased in PCO. In addition, using a GnRH antagonist, we have demonstrated that the total amount of GnRH secreted in PCO is not increased. This latter finding may explain why partial desensitization can be sustained over time, since it is known that the process of desensitization depends on both the frequency and the dose of administered GnRH [28].

Acknowledgments

We would like to acknowledge the extremely valuable clinical contributions of Helen Whitney, RN, and Judy Adams, DMU, in the studies of women with PCO, and the excellent technical support of the technicians in our radioimmunoassay laboratory.

This work was supported by Grants HD-15080, HD-3-2837 and RR-1066 from NIH.

References

1 Yen SSC, Vela P, Rankin J. Inappropriate secretion of follicle-stimulating hormone and luteinizing hormone in polycystic ovarian disease. J Clin Endocrinol 1970; 30:435–42.
2 Rebar R, Judd HL, Yen SSC, Rakoff J, Vandenberg G, Naftolin F. Characterization of the inappropriate gonadotropin secretion in polycystic ovary syndrome. J Clin Invest 1976; 57:1320–29.
3 MacArthur JW, Ingersoll FM, Worcester J. The urinary excretion of interstitial cell hormone and follicle-stimulating activity by women with diseases of the reproductive system. J Clin Endocrinol Metab 1958; 18:1202–15.

4 Waldstreicher J, Santoro NF, Hall JE, Filicori M, Crowley WF Jr. Hyperfunction of the hypothalamic–pituitary axis in women with polycystic ovarian disease: indirect evidence for partial gonadotroph desensitization. J Clin Endocrinol Metab 1988; 66:165–72.
5 Dunaif A. Do androgens directly regulate gonadotropin secretion in the polycystic ovary syndrome? J Clin Endocrinol Metab 1986; 63:215–21.
6 Chang RJ, Mandel FP, Lu JKH, Judd HL. Enhanced disparity of gonadotropin secretion by estrone in women with polycystic ovarian disease. J Clin Endocrinol Metab 1982; 54:490–94.
7 Lobo RA, Granger L, Goebelsmann U, Mishell DB. Elevations in unbound serum estradiol as a possible mechanism for inappropriate gonadotropin secretion in women with PCO. J Clin Endocrinol Metab 1981; 52:156–8.
8 Spratt DI, Finkelstein JS, Butler JP, Badger TM, Crowley WF Jr. Effects of increasing the frequency of low doses of gonadotropin-releasing hormone (GnRH) on gonadotropin secretion in GnRH-deficient men. J Clin Endocrinol Metab 1987; 64:1179–86.
9 Filicori M, Santoro N, Merriam GR, Crowley WF Jr. Characterization of the physiological pattern of episodic gonadotropin secretion throughout the human menstrual cycle. J Clin Endocrinol Metab 1986; 62:1136–44.
10 Buckler HM, Phillips SE, Cameron IT, Healy DL, Burger HG. Vaginal progesterone administration before ovulation induction with exogenous gonadotropins in polycystic ovarian syndrome. J Clin Endocrinol Metab 1988; 67:300–306.
11 Kazer RR, Kessel B, Yen SSC. Circulating luteinizing hormone pulse frequency in women with polycystic ovary syndrome. J Clin Endocrinol Metab 1987; 65:233–6.
12 Spratt DI, Chin WV, Ridgway EC, Crowley WF Jr. Administration of low-dose pulsatile gonadotropin-releasing hormone (GnRH) to GnRH-deficient men regulates free α-subunit secretion. J Clin Endocrinol Metab 1986; 62:102–8.
13 Kourides IA, Weintraub BD, Ridgway EC, Maloof F. Pituitary secretion of free alpha and beta subunits of human thyrotropin in patients with thyroid disorders. J Clin Endocrinol Metab 1975; 40:872–5.
14 Kourides IA, Re RN, Weintraub BD, Ridgway EC, Maloof F. Metabolic clearance and secretion rates of subunits of human thyrotropin. J Clin Invest 1977; 59:508–16.
15 Whitcomb RW, Sangha JS, Schneyer AL, Crowley WF Jr. Improved measurement of free alpha subunit of glycoprotein hormones by assay with use of a monoclonal antibody. Clin Chem 1988; 34:2022–5.
16 Whitcomb RW, O'Dea LStL, Finkelstein JS, Heavern DM, Crowley WF Jr. Utility of free α-subunit as an alternative neuroendocrine marker of gonadotropin-releasing hormone (GnRH) stimulation of the gonadotroph in the human: evidence from normal and GnRH-deficient men. J Clin Endocrinol Metab 1990; 70:1654–61.
17 Hall JE, Whitcomb RW, Rivier JE, Vale WW, Crowley WF Jr. Differential regulation of luteinizing hormone, follicle-stimulating hormone, and free α-subunit secretion from the gonadotrope by gonadotropin-releasing hormone (GnRH): evidence from the use of two GnRH antagonists. J Clin Endocrinol Metab 1990; 70:328–35.
18 Buckler HM, McLachlan RI, MacLachlan VB, Healy DL, Burger HG. Serum inhibin levels in polycystic ovary syndrome: basal levels and response to luteinizing hormone-releasing hormone agonist and exogenous gonadotropin administration. J Clin Endocrinol Metab 1988; 66:798–803.
19 Schneyer AL, Mason AJ, Burton LE, Ziegner JR, Crowley WF Jr. Immunoreactive inhibin α-subunit in human serum: implications for radioimmunoassay. J Clin Endocrinol Metab 1990; 70:1208–12.
20 Schwall RH, Mason AJ, Wilcox JN, Bassett SG, Zeleznik AJ. Localization of inhibin/activin subunit mRNAs within the primate ovary. Mol Endocrinol 1990; 4:75–9.
21 Christman GM, Randolph JF, Kelch RP, Marshall JC. Reduction of Gonadotropin-releasing hormone pulse frequency is associated with subsequent selective follicle-stimulating hormone secretion in women with polycystic ovarian disease. J Clin Endocrinol Metab 1991; 72:1278–85.

22 Clarke IJ, Cummins JT. The temporal relationship between gonadotropin releasing hormone (GnRH) and luteinizing hormone (LH) secretion in ovariectomized ewes. Endocrinology 1982; 111:1737–9.
23 Levine JE, Ramirez VD. Luteinizing hormone-releasing hormone release during the rat estrous cycle and after ovariectomy, as estimated with push-pull cannulae. Endocrinology 1982; 111:1439–48.
24 Reame N, Sauder SE, Kelch RP, Marshall JC. Pulsatile gonadotropin secretion during the human menstrual cycle: evidence for altered frequency of gonadotropin-releasing hormone secretion. J Clin Endocrinol Metab 1984; 59:328–37.
25 Hall JE, Crowley WF Jr. Use of a GnRH antagonist as a physiologic probe of GnRH secretion in women. Program of the 72nd Annual Meeting of the Endocrine Society, Atlanta, Ga, 1990, p. 350 (Abstract).
26 Cicero TJ, Wilcox CE, Bell RD, Meyer ER. Naloxone-induced increases in serum luteinizing hormone in the male: mechanisms of action. J Pharmacol Exp Ther 1980; 212:573–8.
27 Hall JE, Taylor AE, Martin KA, Crowley WF Jr. Response of patients with polycystic ovarian disease to GnRH antagonist administration. Clin Res 1990; 38:342A.
28 Weiss J, Duca KA, Crowley WF Jr. Gonadotropin-releasing hormone-induced stimulation and desensitization of free α-subunit secretion mirrors luteinizing hormone and follicle-stimulating hormone in perfused rat pituitary cells. Endocrinology 1990; 127: 2364–71.

Chapter 5
Neuroendocrine Abnormalities in Polycystic Ovary Syndrome: an Overview

GEORGE R. MERRIAM

Discussion in this section centered on two questions: what neuroendocrine abnormalities can be demonstrated in patients with polycystic ovary syndrome (PCO); and what evidence supports or undercuts the belief that these changes are primary, rather than secondary to the abnormal steroid milieu and lack of ovarian cyclicity.

Gonadotropin abnormalities

Among the many abnormalities that have been described, those which have been found most frequently include elevated levels of luteinizing hormone (LH) or an elevated LH/follicle-stimulating hormone (FSH) ratio, an increased LH pulse frequency, and an altered diurnal rhythm of LH secretion. The incidence of these findings, however, varies widely among different studies. In part this may reflect the different selection criteria for choosing patients from a heterogeneous population for study. At one time, for example, an elevated LH/FSH ratio was proposed as a major criterion for the diagnosis of polycystic ovary syndrome (PCO), and if this is used all patients will naturally have this abnormality.

Lobo and Crowley discussed how selection criteria might account for the differences between the different series: Crowley most often uses patients with clearly elevated LH levels to try to obtain a more homogeneous group, and thus the incidence of other abnormalities in his studies strictly applies only to that group. In Lobo's series, many patients who meet other diagnostic criteria for PCO do not have elevated LH levels or even LH/FSH ratios, although an exaggerated response to gonadotropin-releasing hormone (GnRH) is a more consistent finding. Further, patients with elevated LH on screening evaluation may have normal gonadotropins on repeated evaluation, indicating that a high LH is not a constant even in individual subjects. Because the entry criteria for different studies vary, it is not possible to pool the different series to obtain a good estimate of the prevalence of abnormal LH by meta-analysis.

A second abnormality described by several investigators is an increased LH pulse frequency. In the study of Waldstreicher *et al.* [1] summarized in Chapter 4, an increased LH pulse frequency was a consistent finding and was confirmed by a similarly elevated frequency of α-subunit pulses. The studies surveyed by Filicori and Flamigni (Chapter 3), however, indicate that while LH pulse amplitude is usually elevated, an increased LH pulse frequency is not always found, occurring in about half of the papers summarized.

These differences could also reflect differences in patient selection criteria, if a frequency increase were more common in patients with clearly elevated LH. As Merriam pointed out, the increase could also be artifactual. Most of the statistical criteria used for defining pulses include an amplitude cutoff, and any process that increases pulse amplitude could magnify small subthreshhold peaks to an amplitude at which they are accepted as significant; thus a change in pulse amplitude could cause an apparent change in pulse frequency, without there being any real change in the frequency of episodic GnRH secretion. This could perhaps reconcile the apparent paradox implied in Hall's studies with GnRH antagonists, which suggest an increase in pulse frequency but no increase in the amount of GnRH secreted (Chapter 4).

A third abnormality reported by several groups is an alteration in the circadian rhythm of gonadotropin secretion. Ralph Kazer noted that normal women have reduced levels of LH at night during the early follicular phase of the cycle [2], but that this reduction is absent in PCO patients. These findings have been confirmed by several other investigators, but Rosenfield reported that it was not a consistent abnormality in his series.

Despite the large number of earlier studies suggesting a central abnormality of dopamine regulation in PCO patients, which gave rise to several trials of therapy with bromocriptine and other dopaminergic agonists, no participants advocated the dopamine hypothesis in this session. The generally negative results of controlled therapy trials with dopaminergic agonists have provided little encouragement to believe that this is an important abnormality.

Although most of the discussion centered on possible abnormalities in LH, Merriam and Franks briefly addressed the question of whether alterations in FSH might be equally important. Although earlier studies had suggested that FSH levels might be reduced in PCO, most current reports find immunoassayable levels of FSH to be normal despite the high LH/FSH ratio. However, Franks and others have shown that treatment with small supplemental doses of FSH is frequently successful in inducing ovulation. This apparent paradox might be explained by levels being insufficient for coordinated follicular maturation in individual patients but still within population normal ranges, or by alterations in the biologic activity of FSH not reflected in radioimmunoassay levels. Several groups have reported that alterations in either the pattern of GnRH secretion or in the sex steroid milieu can affect the glycosylation of gonadotropins and thus their biologic activity. This has not yet been extensively studied in PCO.

Neuroendocrine changes: primary or secondary?

The second focus for discussion was the issue of whether these neuroendocrine abnormalities could be primary and drive the ovarian abnormalities in PCO, or whether they are themselves secondary to ovarian or other abnormalities. Clear answers to these questions are made difficult by the heterogeneity of patients with PCO, and by the possible (but unproven) establishment of "vicious circles" in which the central and ovarian abnormalities seem to reinforce each other.

Several kinds of strategies have been used to try to separate these possibilities, particularly gonadotropin suppression with GnRH agonist or antagonist analogs, gonadotropin stimulation with pulsatile GnRH, and administration of steroid agonists or antagonists, either as drugs or by studies of patients with primary abnormalities of steroid production.

Ovarian steroid hormone secretion is not autonomous in idiopathic PCO, and it is not surprising that suppression of gonadotropin secretion reduces androgen levels in these patients. The dose–response studies of gonadotropin suppression with GnRH antagonists reported by Crowley (Chapter 4) suggest that the quantity of GnRH secreted in PCO does not differ from normal. Furthermore, Filicori reported that ovarian volume in patients placed on GnRH agonist analog suppression for 2 months did not return to normal, suggesting that some abnormality persists even without gonadotropin elevation, although several participants argued that this may not have been a long enough time to reverse all secondary ovarian changes. Crowley noted the report by Judith Adams of a patient with a craniopharyngioma who had ultrasonographic findings compatible with PCO despite undetectably low gonadotropins. Merriam reported the findings of Levy-Toledano and himself that acromegalic patients frequently had ultrasonographic findings of PCO despite low gonadotropins, in the setting of elevated levels of growth hormone and insulin-like growth factor 1 (IGF-1). Thus the increased LH seen in some PCO patients is hard to attribute to increased GnRH secretion, and the persistence of morphologic abnormalities in the ovaries in the setting of low gonadotropins does not support the idea of a primary central defect.

Several participants reported experience with administering pulsatile GnRH to PCO patients. In other settings, for example hyperprolactinemic amenorrhea, a normal ovarian response to GnRH treatment has served as evidence that the limiting abnormality is central, not ovarian. The relatively low (approximately 40%) rate of success with GnRH in PCO reported by Filicori, an experience shared by Lobo and other participants, would seem to point away from a central lesion; but the established ovarian abnormalities cloud interpretation of this finding. Filicori reported his experience with resting the ovary with 2 months of GnRH analog suppression of gonadotropins, followed by pulsatile GnRH therapy. When GnRH analog is given and the patient allowed to recover spontaneously, ovarian function drifts back to its abnormal baseline state [3]. However, when patients are given pulsatile GnRH immediately after ending suppression, PCO patients frequently have a normal initial response, and the success rate for ovulation induction is much improved (Chapter 3). This would be compatible with correction of an abnormal central signal, although McKenna wondered how it was possible that a lower exogenous pulse frequency could override a faster endogenous one in PCO.

Unfortunately, this encouraging early response is not sustained after the first cycle; Filicori reported that on continued pulsatile GnRH treatment, androgen levels rose progressively, and the success rate for a second ovulation fell to 50%, a rate not much higher than that in unprimed PCO patients. Chang and other participants commented that this abnormal response to a pulse pattern that is highly successful in hypothalamic amenorrhea does not point to a primary hypothalamic abnormality in PCO.

It still remains possible that a primary or secondary defect is present at the pituitary level. Studies reporting an ovarian response to small increases in FSH, either as given directly by Franks and colleagues or as induced indirectly by Marshall and colleagues [4], are suggestive, but have not yet been conducted for several consecutive cycles to determine if that effect too will wear off.

Crowley and Merriam noted that if an elevated pulse frequency were the cause of the abnormality, it should in principle be possible to induce PCO by applying pulsatile GnRH at an elevated frequency. Early studies of Knobil and colleagues [5] had shown that raising the GnRH pulse frequency could increase the LH/FSH ratio. Crowley related his experience that altering the pulse frequency could alter the ovarian response, but the only report of a specific abnormality induced by a high pulse frequency was Soules' report of inducing luteal phase deficiency (LPD) with high-frequency pulsatile GnRH [6]. Merriam reported his colleagues' experience with administering different GnRH pulse frequencies for three consecutive cycles to patients with hypothalamic amenorrhea: both abnormally high and low pulse frequencies were less successful in inducing ovulation, but the fast frequencies induced neither LPD nor PCO [7].

Thus these studies with pulsatile GnRH also do not support the belief that there is a primary abnormality in GnRH secretion responsible for PCO. Effects at the pituitary level have not been excluded but seem unlikely to be primary. Since PCO is a chronic condition, it was suggested that experiments in which an elevated GnRH pulse frequency was given to monkeys for an extended period of time would provide useful information.

The final group of observations discussed were of studies or experiments in which steroid hormone levels were directly altered. Several observers have noted that patients with 21-hydroxylase deficiency (see Chapter 13) or ovarian tumors [8] can develop many of the features of PCO, including an elevated LH/FSH ratio. If the gonadotropin abnormality can be induced by a primary steroid abnormality, but not vice versa, it suggests that abnormal gonadotropin secretion is not likely to be the primary abnormality in idiopathic PCO either.

The specific class of steroid hormones primarily driving these changes is uncertain; both androgen and estrogen levels are elevated, with the generally high levels of LH stimulating aromatization of precursor androgens. Dunaif reported preliminary studies in which estrogen infusions increased the LH pulse amplitude in human subjects, but noted that Billiar and colleagues had not observed the induction of PCO in macaques given long-term implants of estradiol or estrone. As Crowley noted, he and Dunaif had attempted to treat PCO with the aromatase inhibitor testolactone, but with very variable results: some patients were improved, others not [9]. The review of abnormalities in steroidogenesis continued in a later session (see Chapters 7, 9, and 12).

This discussion ended with the general consensus that while abnormalities in gonadotropin levels and patterns are common in PCO, the weight of evidence does not currently suggest that these are the primary abnormalities responsible for the disease. Some of the experiments proposed may help make it possible to draw a more definitive conclusion.

References

1 Waldstreicher J, Santoro NF, Hall JE, Filicori M, Crowley WF. Hyperfunction of the hypothalamic–pituitary axis in women with PCOD. J Clin Endocrinol Metab 1988; 66:165–72.

2 Kazer RR, Kessel B, Yen SSC. Circulating LH pulse frequency in women with polycystic ovary syndrome. J Clin Endocrinol Metab 1987; 65:233–6.

3 de Ziegler D, Steingold K, Cedars M, Lu JKH, Meldrum DR, Judd HL, Chang RJ. Recovery of hormone secretion after chronic GnRH agonist administration in women with PCOD. J Clin Endocrinol Metab 1989; 68:1111–17.

4 Christman GM, Randolph JF, Kelch RP, Marshall JP. Reduction of GnRH pulse frequency induces preferential FSH stimulation and follicular development in women with PCOD. The Endocrine Society Annual Meeting, 1989, p. 270 (Abstract).

5 Knobil E. The neuroendocrine control of the menstrual cycle. Recent Prog Horm Res 1980; 36:53–88.

6 Soules MR, Clifton DK, Bremner WJ, Steiner RA. Corpus luteum insufficiency induced by a rapid GnRH-induced gonadotropin secretion pattern in the follicular phase. J Clin Endocrinol Metab 1987; 65:457–64.

7 Letterie GS, Coddington CC, Collins RL, Muir-Nash J, Loriaux DL, Merriam GR. Ovulation induction using pulsatile GnRH: effectiveness of different pulse frequencies. American Fertility Society–Canadian Society for Andrology and Fertility, October 1986, Abstract 335.

8 Dunaif A, Scully RE, Andersen RN, Chapin DS, Crowley WF. The effects of continuous androgen secretion on the hypothalamic–pituitary axis in woman: evidence from a luteinized ovarian thecoma. J Clin Endocrinol Metab 1984; 59:389–93.

9 Dunaif A, Longcope C, Canick J, Badger T, Crowley WF. Effects of the aromatase inhibitor testolactone on gonadotropin release and steroid metabolism in PCOD. J Clin Endocrinol Metab 1985; 60:773–80.

Section 3
Genetics of Steroidal Abnormalities

Chapter 6
Elucidating the Genetics of Polycystic Ovary Syndrome

JOE LEIGH SIMPSON

Familial aggregates of women with polycystic ovary syndrome (PCO) are observed not infrequently. Affected sibs, concordantly affected monozygotic twins, and affected mother–daughter pairs have long been recognized [1–6]. However, studies are far from definitive, because none have taken into account the genetic heterogeneity of the disorder clinically labelled as PCO. This chapter addresses the heritability of PCO. The thesis is that success in elucidating the genetics of this disorder will not be achieved until attention is paid to the existence of genetic heterogeneity.

Formal genetic studies

The first formal study of PCO was conducted in 1968 by Cooper and associates [7] at the University of Minnesota. Matched-pair analysis was performed on 18 individuals with the "Stein–Leventhal syndrome." Like most other studies to be cited in the section, adult-onset adrenal hyperplasia was not excluded, or even actually appreciated at the time. Ethnic origin of subjects was not stated, although most if not all were apparently white. Histories of oligomenorrhea were elicited from 4 of 13 mothers of subjects, but from 0 of 13 control mothers. Oligomenorrhea occurred more commonly in sisters of subjects (9/19) than in sisters of controls (1/18). Hirsutism was likewise more common in relatives. When subjected to culdoscopy (this 1968 study was conducted before the availability of laparoscopy), 8 women with Stein–Leventhal syndrome were detected among 12 first-degree relatives studied. Male relatives showed an increased prevalence of "pilosity." The investigators proposed autosomal dominant inheritance with decreased penetrance.

In the 1970s, Givens, Cohen, Wilroy and others at the University of

Tennessee at Memphis concluded in a series of reports that PCO was inherited in X-linked dominant fashion. Diagnostic criteria consisted of hirsutism and polycystic or bilaterally enlarged ovaries. In the first report (1971), two kindreds of multiple generations were reported, with affected females usually showing so-called ovarian hyperthecosis [8]. In one kindred, some affected females experienced myocardial infarction in their fifth decade; in 1988 Givens added the observations that acanthosis nigricans, insulin resistance, and hypertension were present in many family members [9]. In 1975 a third kindred was reported, again showing affected members in more than one generation [10]. In this family, several females had grand mal seizure, whereas a 46,XY male showed maturational arrest of spermatogenesis (Fig. 6.1). Another male had Klinefelter syndrome (47, XXY). In 1975 Wilroy *et al.* [11] provided information on those families characterized by having more than one affected relative. (Information was not sought on families in which only a single family member was known to be affected.) Ethnic origin was not stated formally, but most subjects were apparently black. After excluding the index case, Wilroy *et al.* [11] noted that 47% of female offspring of affected females were considered affected. Of offspring of males having elevated ratios of serum levels of LH to FSH, 89% of daughters were affected (Table 6.1). That almost all daughters of affected males were affected is consistent with X-linked dominant inheritance.

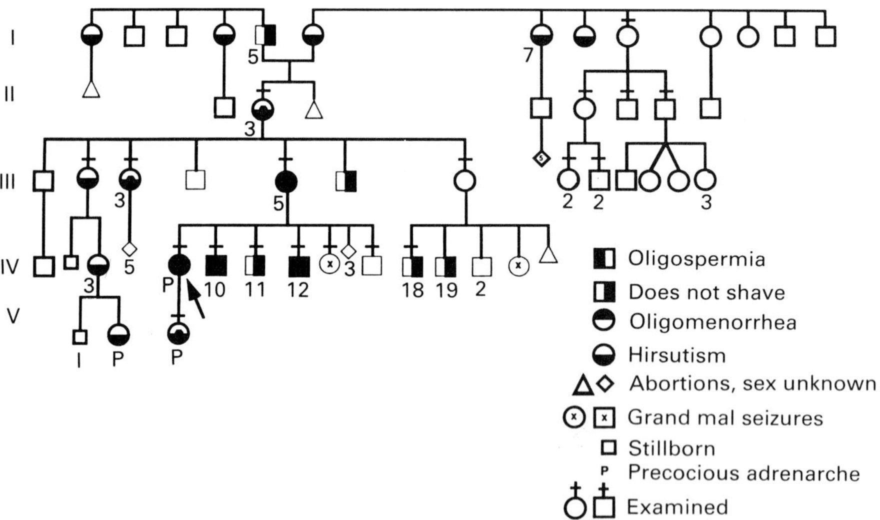

Fig. 6.1 A kindred study from the University of Tennessee showing multiple family members with PCO. Several males showed testicular abnormalities. (Modified from Cohen *et al.* [10].)

Table 6.1 Pattern of affected PCO relatives in families in which more than a single member had PCO. (Modified from Wilroy *et al.* [11].)

	Maternal	Paternal	Maternal and paternal
Sibships	28	15	5
Affected members	39	41	9
Total members	93	47	10
Percentage affected	47%	87%	90%

The Memphis studies of Givens and colleagues [8–11] made it clear that PCO was heritable; however, it was equally clear that their population was very heterogeneous, including cases with and without insulin resistance and lipid abnormalities, as well as cases with and without grand mal seizures. Furthermore, no information concerning the presence or absence of adrenal enzyme deficiency was available. A further problem is the uncertainty with respect to the composition of the original sample. To what extent were the families studied representative of the general population? Were unwitting selection biases operative?

A third major study is that of Ferriman and Purdie [12] from the United Kingdom. Investigators studied 707 patients with "hirsutism and/or oligomenorrhea both with and without infertility." Frequency of various abnormalities in relatives was tabulated and stratified according to the phenotype of the index case. Of the 707 women, information on ovarian size was available in 467, as assessed by gynecography (an air-contrast method now considered of uncertain accuracy). Of these 467, 45 had "identifiable disorders," defined to include ". . . adrenal, pituitary or hypothalamic disorders." Family history was available in 381 of the remaining 422 cases. Of the 381 women, about 60% showed enlarged, "presumed polycystic ovaries." The frequency of oligomenorrhea and infertility was then sought among first-degree relatives (sibs, parents, offspring) and compared to the same parameters in a control group of 179 normal women. Subjects were further stratified into those with or without hirsutism, as well as into those with or without enlarged ovaries. Familial tendencies proved greatest among hirsute women having enlarged ovaries; however, far fewer than 50% of relatives were similarly affected (Table 6.2). In contrast to the Minnesota population of Cooper and associates [7], baldness proved significantly more frequent in relatives of hirsute women than in either relatives of controls or relatives of nonhirsute women with enlarged ovaries. Ferriman and

Table 6.2 Numbers of affected relatives stratified according to clinical characteristics of proband with PCO. (Modified from Ferriman and Purdie [12].)

Group		Total no. of patients	Number with first-degree female relatives suffering from:		
Body hair growth	Ovarian size		Hirsutism	Oligomenorrhea	Infertility
Hirsute	Enlarged	188	38	30	19
	Normal	96	13	15	10
Nonhirsute	Enlarged	45	1	8	5
	Normal	45	1	7	3
Controls		179	7	8	8

Purdie concluded that a "modified dominant" disorder exists in some families. Such a condition was said to be characterized by hirsutism, oligomenorrhea, and infertility; polycystic ovaries in females or premature balding in males may or may not also coexist. By contrast, a second group of women was considered to be characterized by oligomenorrhea, infertility, and sometimes enlarged ovaries; however, neither hirsutism nor premature male baldness was common.

In 1987 Lee *et al.* [13] reported a kindred in which each of four affected individuals showed premature pubarche, hirsutism and amenorrhea (proband; mother and her dizygotic twin sister; proband's mother's father's mother). Levels of 17α-hydroxyprogesterone after stimulation by adrenocorticotropic hormone (ACTH) proved either normal or of the magnitude observed in heterozygotes for congenital adrenal hyperplasia (CAH). "Attenuated" CAH was, therefore, not considered present. The authors concluded that the disorder was not linked to HLA; however, this conclusion was based on a single affected individual, two other affected individuals being HLA-A identical (Fig. 6.2). By contrast, Mandel *et al.* [14] found no evidence for HLA association or linkage to PCO.

The most recent familial studies, from St Mary's Medical School and Middlesex Hospital in London, relied upon ultrasound diagnosis of polycystic ovaries. Adams *et al.* [15] defined PCO on the basis of 10 or more 2–8-mm cysts associated with increased ovarian stroma. In 92% of women fulfilling this ultrasound diagnosis of PCO, at least one endocrine marker of PCO was said to be present—elevated levels of luteinizing hormone (LH), testosterone (T), androstendione (A), or an increased ratio of serum LH to follicle-stimulating hormone (FSH). When these criteria were applied, 87% of oligomenorrheic women were given

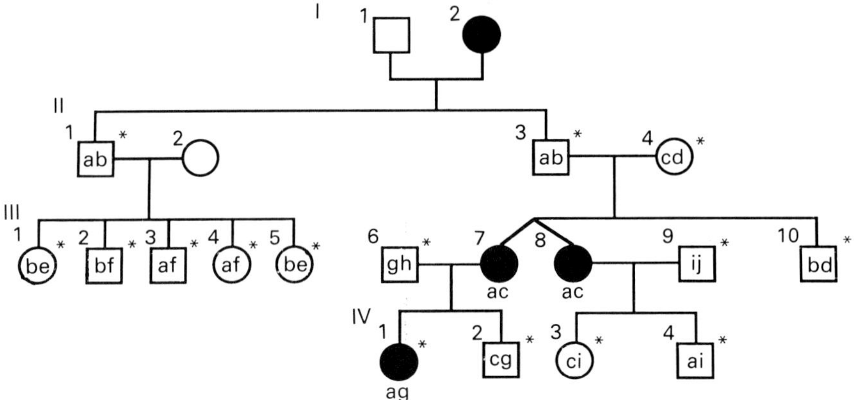

Fig. 6.2 Pedigree showing four females with PCO. Two had the same HLA haplotypes but a third did not. (a) A2, C7, BW6, DR6; (b) A11, C51, CW1, BW4, DR6; (c) A2, C7, BW6, DR2; (d) A30, C13, CW6, BW4, DR7; (e) A3, C40, CW3, BW6, DR6; (f) A23, C44, CW4, BW4, DR6; (g) A3, C14, BW6, DR4; (h) A32, C7, BW6, DR2; (i) A2, C44, CW4, BW4, DR7; (j) A1, C17, BW4, DR3. (Modified from Lee *et al.* [13].)

a diagnosis of PCO, as were 90% of the hirsute yet ovulatory women. Later, familial studies were conducted by Hague *et al.* [16] in 50 women with symptoms of PCO and in 17 women with CAH. One hundred and thirty-seven postmenarcheal, premenopausal female relatives of these probands were examined by ultrasonography. Familial PCO was observed in 56 of the 61 pedigrees (92%) in which sufficient family members were available for study. Surprisingly, the frequency of PCO in the relatives of women with CAH was no different from that found in the nonadrenal PCO group. In the latter, 24 of 36 (67%) mothers of probands and 45 of 52 (87%) sisters of probands were affected. The proportion of females affected in all sibships (segregation ratio) was 107 of 133 (80.5%). This segregation ratio is significantly different from ratios predicted for either autosomal dominant or X-linked dominant modes of inheritance. Mechanisms that might account for such a segregation ratio include meiotic drive due to a gene that causes segregation distortion, vertical transmission of an infectious agent, environmental factors such as the effect of maternal androgens during pregnancy on gonadal development, or genetic imprinting due to mitochondrial factors or vicissitudes of methylation.

The studies of Adams *et al.* [15] and Hague *et al.* [16] might have benefited from assurances about the representative nature of their samples. Another major question concerns the specificity of their diagnostic criteria, perhaps an arguable point given that 22% of their population fulfilled the stated ultrasonographic criteria for PCO [17].

Pitfalls in published studies

The studies cited above make it clear that heritable tendencies exist in essential PCO. The mode or modes of inheritance remain unclear, but some facts are clear. Familial aggregates indicate that dominant tendencies are far more plausible than recessive tendencies. Although studies looking for defects in adrenal enzymes were usually not performed, it can be assumed that homozygosity for such a defect is not responsible for familial aggregates because enzyme deficiencies are usually autosomal recessive. (A formal possibility is pseudoautosomal dominant inheritance, vertical transmission then being due to homozygous individuals mating with heterozygous individuals.) Heterozygosity for an enzyme defect also remains a possibility.

Heritability due to a single dominant gene seems unlikely. Far fewer than 50% of symptomatic, first-degree relatives are usually affected. Most clinicians have the impression that no more than 5–10% of first-degree relatives are symptomatic [18]. In their search [8] for linkage between PCO and HLA, Mandel *et al.* [14] studied 23 subjects with PCO in Los Angeles; only 4 had an affected relative (a sister in each case; one patient with an affected mother as well). Thus, possible explanations for extant genetic data include: (i) a single dominant gene of low penetrance or highly variable expressivity; (ii) polygenic inheritance; or (iii) etiologic heterogeneity, i.e. existence of one or more genetic forms and one or more nongenetic forms.

Potential approaches to the genetic analysis of PCO

Several different approaches can be envisioned for elucidating the genetics of complex traits such as PCO. Different approaches must be contemplated because it remains unclear whether PCO is a single monogenic entity, a polygenic (quantitative) trait or a genetically heterogeneous group of disorders.

Monogenic inheritance of a single entity

If diagnostic criteria were not in doubt, one could very easily study the genetics of PCO. One would only have to identify affected individuals and perform classical segregation analysis; deduce the mode of inheritance on the basis of the ratio of affected to unaffected relatives, merely taking into account ascertainment biases which could be accomplished most simply by excluding the index case.

If the mode of inheritance became clear, the next goal would be to localize the gene to a particular chromosome. In X-linked conditions the chromosomal location is self-evident, but for autosomes it is not. If a discrete gene product existed, one could theoretically utilize *in situ* hybridization to determine the gene's chromosomal location. In the absence of a discrete gene product—the situation for PCO—one must attempt to link the gene to other loci. This approach is well illustrated for 21-hydroxylase deficiency (see Chapter 13), which is linked on chromosome 6 to HLA. However, the polymorphic loci need not be DNA that translates into protein. Rather, one can seek linkage to loci that encode for anonymous DNA, taking advantage of the limitless variations in sequence that humans possess with respect to their repetitive DNA. Although of no phenotypic significance, these differences produce changes with respect to whether a given restriction endonuclease will or will not act at a particular site, namely restriction fragment length polymorphisms (RFLP). So long as the minority locus is relatively frequent (i.e. polymorphic), an RFLP is potentially useful for linkage analysis. Many anonymous DNA probes are known, often having been generated by using flow cytometry to sort metaphases into chromosome-specific components. Search of the available probes has revealed many useful RFLPs and a stated purpose of the Human Genome project is to identify polymorphic genetic markers 0.1 centimorgans apart throughout the genome [19].

How does one determine whether two or more genes are linked or not? Data concerning their segregation are ordinarily pooled from several families, with weight given to the differing amounts of information in the various families. The maximum likelihood for a given recombination is calculated, and a maximum-likelihood ratio, termed theta (θ), is derived. If θ is greater than 3.0, linkage is said to exist. If no recombination occurs between two tested loci, values of θ of 3.0 can be achieved with 10 informative matings. If linkage is not so tight, more matings are required to show linkage. If markers on both sides (5′ and 3′) of the gene exist, fewer matings may be required to prove linkage.

Polygenic inheritance

Different approaches would be necessary if PCO proved to be polygenic. Indeed, PCO is a quantitative trait, i.e. it shows continuous phenotypic variation. This characteristic makes PCO a genuine candidate for polygenic etiology. Moreover, *clinical* recurrence rates in PCO are not those expected for monogenic traits but, rather, are nearer to the 1–5% that is characteristic of polygenic traits.

If PCO were polygenic, segregation analysis based on monogenic models would not prove informative because familial aggregates are too uncommon. Instead, alternative approaches would be necessary. One possibility would be to perform linkage analysis under expectations of several different modes of inheritance, with the hope that a single strong genetic relationship would become evident. Another approach would be to compare the risk in relatives of probands to the risk in relatives in the general population. When a comparison is made of rates of recurrence between first- , second- and third-degree relatives, the slope for decreasing risk of recurrence as the degree of relationship decreases will differ among polygenic, autosomal recessive and autosomal dominant models.

Several investigators have developed linkage-analysis models suitable for quantitative (polygenic) traits [20–24]. As one recent example, Risch [20–22] defined a risk ratio lambda (λ), the risk in relatives of a proband vs. the risk in the population; λ was set as a direct indicator of the mode of inheritance. For monogenic traits, $\lambda - 1$ decreases by a factor of 2 with each degree of relationship. If a trait were 10 times more frequent among offspring of probands (first-degree relatives) than in the general population, $\lambda - 1 = 9$. For half-sibs or uncles and aunts of probands (second-degree relatives) $\lambda - 1 = 4.5$; for third-degree relatives (first cousins) $\lambda - 1 = 2.25$. As defined, λ holds for disorders characterized by reduced penetrance or admixtures with phenocopies; however, use of λ does not distinguish between different modes of inheritance. Nonetheless, this approach could theoretically be applied to PCO if multiple diagnostic criteria were decided upon and if these criteria were segregating independently.

In quantitative linkage analysis one chooses a polymorphic trait for testing and then searches for identity by descent. Does an affected grandparent have the same marker as an affected granddaughter? If so, the marker could be, but is not necessarily, related to the disease in question, through linkage in that particular family. Power to detect such linkage is greatest for grandparent/grandchild pairs. Power decreases progressively for cousin, half-sib, uncle, niece and sib comparisons. Ott [24] showed that if $\lambda = 5$ and $\theta = 0.1$, a power of 98% is achieved with 100 grandparent/grandchild pairs; however, power is only 30% with 100 sib/sib pairs [24]. In PCO, the most logical practical approach from a clinical standpoint would involve analysis of cousin pairs, for their ages would in general be similar and would thus allow verification of similar endocrine status. Is complex genetic linkage analysis feasible for PCO? Naturally, it is tantalizing to think that a mainframe or less powerful computer could produce an answer to a seemingly unfathomable clinical question. Unfortunately, for PCO this approach would probably be doomed without well-defined diagnostic criteria. Current models of quantitative linkage analysis assume a binary distribution, i.e. affected vs. nonaffected individuals. Although, as noted above, quantitative linkage models handle vicissitudes of penetrance and phenocopies well, they cannot handle varied expressivity. However, varied expressivity is characteristic of PCO. Quantitative linkage analysis also cannot take into account different modes of inheritance, but PCO is observed both in families with dominant tendencies as well as in families that show autosomal recessive tendencies (i.e. enzyme deficiencies). Thus, quantitative linkage analysis is unlikely to be useful in PCO.

Genetic heterogeneity

This author suggests that by far the most fruitful investigative approach to elucidating the genetics of PCO is to treat the disorder not as a single entity, but rather as many entities. Polycystic ovary syndrome should be split up as far as phenotype and demography permit. Consider a related endocrine example in which such an approach proved fruitful: etiologies of gonadal dysgenesis include monosomy X, structural abnormalities of the X-chromosome, X-linked recessive form(s) (XY gonadal dysgenesis), autosomal recessive forms (XX gonadal dysgenesis), and phenocopies [25,26]. The several different cytochrome P-450 adrenal enzymes (scc, 3β-ol, 17α, 21-, 11β-) (see Chapter 7) are all genetically distinct, but all may cause genital ambiguity [27]. It is unreasonable to expect PCO to prove less complex.

The consequence of our failing to take into account genetic heterogeneity is our unwitting pooling of individuals who have several different disorders. Even if sophisticated genetic studies are performed, the likelihood of finding an informative result will be greatly diminished if different modes of inheritance exist, to say nothing of the concomitant existence of nongenetic factors (e.g. increased body fat leading to increased serum levels of estrone through increased peripheral conversion of androstenedione to estrone, with anovulation and PCO arising secondarily). However, heterogeneity for PCO is already established, adult-onset deficiency in 21-hydroxylase being an unequivocal cause. Different mutant genes causing phenotypically indistinguishable PCO should be assumed.

For investigative purposes, this author suggests that we first establish discrete diagnostic criteria for PCO, even if they are seemingly arbitrary. For heuristic purposes we might divide PCO into forms associated with insulin resistance and those that are not, forms associated with prepuberal obesity and those that are not, and forms associated with adrenal hyperplasia and those that are not. If unusual phenotypic characteristics exist in a given family (e.g. seizures, lipid abnormalities), we should further stratify those families as discrete entities, and we should consider taking ethnic origin into account as well. For example, PCO associated with insulin resistance and obesity should be studied separately in blacks and whites.

If X-linked tendencies appear evident, we should search for linkage with known X-linked loci (e.g. using existing RFLPs). If autosomal tendencies appear evident, we should be prepared to seek linkage with markers that represent all autosomes. A reasonable start is to begin testing for linkage to genes that might plausibly be related to control of androgens or gonadotropins. Examples include adrenal steroid enzymes, androgen receptors, 5α-reductase, FSH, LH, gonadotropin-releasing hormone (GnRH), insulin and insulin receptors, and epidermal growth factor (EGF). The task will prove laborious, but eventually should prove successful if one or more monogenic forms of PCO exist.

References

1 Goldzeiher JW, Green JA. The polycystic ovary. I. Clinical and histologic features. J Clin Endocrinol 1962; 22:326–8.

2 Jeffcoate TNA. The androgenic ovary, with special reference to the Stein–Leventhal syndrome. Am J Obstet Gynecol 1964; 88:143–56.

3 McDonough PG, Mahesh VB, Ellegood JO. Steroid, follicle-stimulating hormone and luteinizing hormone profiles in identical twins with polycystic ovaries. Am J Obstet Gynecol 1972; 113:1072–6.

4 Judd HL, Scully RE, Herbst AL, Yen SSC, Ingersol FM, Kliman B. Familial hyperthecosis: comparison of endocrinologic and histologic findings with polycystic ovarian disease. Am J Obstet Gynecol 1973; 117:976–82.

5 Case records of the Massachusetts General Hospital (Case 43481). N Engl J Med 1957; 108:257–62.

6 Simpson JL. Genetic aspects of gynecological disorders occurring in 46,XX individuals. Clin Obstet Gynecol 1972; 15:157–82.

7 Cooper HE, Spellacy WN, Prem KA, Cohen WD. Hereditary factors in Stein–Leventhal syndrome. Am J Obstet Gynecol 1968; 100:371–87.

8 Givens JR, Wiser WL, Coleman SA, Wilroy RS, Andersen RN, Fish SA. Familial ovarian hyperthecosis: a study of two families. Am J Obstet Gynecol 1971; 11:959–72.

9 Givens JR. Familial polycystic ovarian disease. Endocrinol Metab Clin North Am 1988; 17:1–17.

10 Cohen PN, Givens JR, Wiser WL, Wilroy RS, Summitt RL, Coleman SA, Andersen RN. Polycystic ovarian disease, maturation arrest of spermatogenesis and Klinefelter's syndrome in siblings of a family with familial hirsutism. Fertil Steril 1975; 26:1228–38.

11 Wilroy RS, Givens JR, Wiser WL, Coleman SA, Andersen RN, Fish SA. Hyperthecosis—an inheritable form of polycystic ovarian disease. In: Bergsma D, ed. Genetic forms of hypogonadism. Birth Defects 1975; 11(5):81–5.

12 Ferriman D, Purdie AW. The inheritance of PCO and possible relationship to premature balding. Clin Endocrinol 1979; 11:291–300.

13 Lee PA, Migeon CJ, Bias WB, Jones GS. Familial hypersecretion of adrenal androgens transmitted as a dominant, non-HLA linked trait. Obstet Gynecol 1987; 69:259–65.

14 Mandel FP, Chang RJ, Dupont B, Pollack MS, Levine LS, New MI, Lu JKH, Judd HL. HLA genotyping of family members and patients with familial polycystic ovarian disease. J Clin Endocrinol Metab 1982; 56:862–4.
15 Adams J, Polson DW, Franks S. Prevalence of polycystic ovaries in women with anovulation and hirsutism. Br Med J 1986; 293:355–9.
16 Hague WH, Adams J, Reeders ST, Peto TEA, Jacobs HS. Familial polycystic ovaries: a genetic disease. Clin Endocrinol 1988; 29:593–605.
17 Polson DW, Wadsworth J, Adams J, Franks S. Polycystic ovaries—a common finding in normal women. Lancet 1988; i:870–2.
18 Simpson JL, Golbus M, Martin A, Sarto G. Genetics in Obstetrics and Gynecology. New York: Grune and Stratton, 1982.
19 Watson JD. The human genome project: past, present and future. Science 1990; 248:44–9.
20 Risch N. Linkage strategies for genetically complex traits. I. Multilocus models. Am J Hum Genet 1990; 46:222–8.
21 Risch N. Linkage strategies for genetically complex traits. II. The power of affected relative pairs. Am J Hum Genet 1990; 46:229–41.
22 Risch N. Linkage strategies for genetically complex traits. III. The effect of markers of polymorphism on analysis of affected relative pairs. Am J Hum Genet 1990; 46:242–53.
23 Bishop DT, Williamson JA. The power of identity-by-state methods for linkage analysis. Am J Hum Genet 1990; 46:254–65.
24 Ott J. Cutting a Gordian knot in linkage analysis of complex human traits. Am J Hum Genet 1990; 46:219–21.
25 Simpson JL, Rebar RW. Normal and abnormal sexual differentiation and development. In: Becker KL, ed. Principles and Practice of Endocrinology and Metabolism. Philadelphia: JB Lippincott Co, 1990, pp. 710–39.
26 Simpson JL. Human disorders of sex differentiation and the genetic control of sex differentiation. In: Pasqualini JR, Scholler R, eds. Hormones and Fetal Pathophysiology. New York: Marcel Dekker (in press).
27 Simpson JL. Disorders of gonads and internal reproductive ducts. In: Emery AEH, Rimoin DL, eds. Principles and Practice of Medical Genetics, 2nd edn. Edinburgh: Churchill Livingstone, 1990, pp. 1593–1616.

Chapter 7
Regulation of Expression of Genes that Encode Steroidogenic Enzymes in the Ovary

EVAN R. SIMPSON, JAN M. McALLISTER, MARKUS LAUBER, MICHELLE DEMETER & MICHAEL R. WATERMAN

The secretion of steroid hormones by the ovary is highly episodic in nature and occurs in a precisely coordinated fashion that is controlled, at least in part, by the gonadotropins. Examination of the steroidogenic pathway (Fig. 7.1) reveals that most of the steps are catalyzed by various members of what is now regarded as a superfamily of genes that are known collectively as cytochrome P-450 [1]. The first step, namely the conversion of cholesterol to pregnenolone, is catalyzed by cholesterol side-chain cleavage cytochrome P-450 ($P\text{-}450_{scc}$). The subsequent conversion of C_{21} steroids, first to the 17α-hydroxylated steroids and then to C_{19} androgens, is catalyzed by 17α-hydroxylase cytochrome P-450 ($P\text{-}450_{17\alpha}$). Subsequently, the conversion of C_{19} steroids to the corresponding C_{18} steroids or estrogens is catalyzed by aromatase cytochrome P-450 ($P\text{-}450_{arom}$), so called because this reaction involves aromatization of the A-ring of the androgens to give the phenolic A-ring characteristic of estrogens. Also participating in the steroidogenic pathway are dehydrogenases, namely the 3β-hydroxysteroid dehydrogenase and 17β-hydroxysteroid dehydrogenase.

Characterization of cytochrome P-450 species involved in ovarian steroidogenesis

The amino acid sequences of all of the steroidogenic cytochrome P-450 species have been deduced, in large part, from nucleotide sequences of the corresponding cDNAs. A number of sequence homologies are apparent, not only within the steroidogenic P-450s but also when the various species are compared to the cytochrome P-450 family in general. Thus, for example, toward the carboxy-terminus there is a heme-binding region that is responsible for association with the

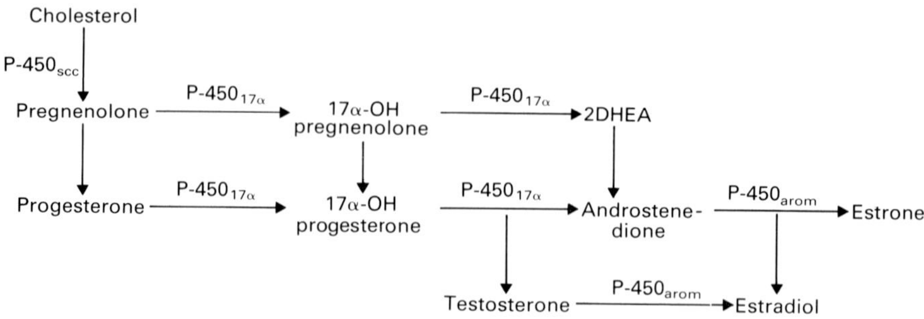

Fig. 7.1 Schematic diagram of the steroidogenic pathways that lead to the biosynthesis of estrogen. The steps catalyzed by various steroidogenic members of the cytochrome P-450 superfamily are indicated.

Human cytochrome P-450$_{arom}$	F G F G P R G C A G K Y I A
Chicken cytochrome P-450$_{arom}$	F G F G P R G C V G K F I A
Human cytochrome P-450$_{C21}$	F G C G A R V C L G E P V A
Bovine cytochrome P-450$_{C21}$	F G C G A R V C L G E C L A
Human cytochrome P-450$_{17\alpha}$	F G A G P R S C I G E I L A
Bovine cytochrome P-450$_{17\alpha}$	F G A G P R S C V G E M L A
Bovine cytochrome P-450$_{scc}$	F G W G V R Q C V G R R I A
Bovine cytochrome P-450$_{11\beta}$	F G F G V R Q C L G R R V A

Fig. 7.2 Amino acid homologies of the heme-binding region of steroidogenic forms of cytochrome P-450. The cysteine that forms the fifth coordinating ligand of the heme iron is underlined.

protoporphyrin IX prosthetic group (Fig. 7.2). Within this region, there is a cysteine common to all cytochrome P-450 species, which is believed to form the fifth coordinating ligand for the heme iron.

Expression of steroidogenic P-450s throughout the ovarian cycle

Characterization of cDNA inserts complementary to mRNA that encodes these steroidogenic enzymes has permitted their use as probes in Northern analysis to determine the expression of these enzymes throughout the ovarian cycle [2]. It has been found that, in the bovine ovary, P-450$_{17\alpha}$ is expressed in follicles but levels of the mRNA decline precipitously to become undetectable after ovulation, consistent with the observation that throughout the luteal phase the bovine ovary does not secrete androgens or estrogens (Fig. 7.3). In contrast, in the human

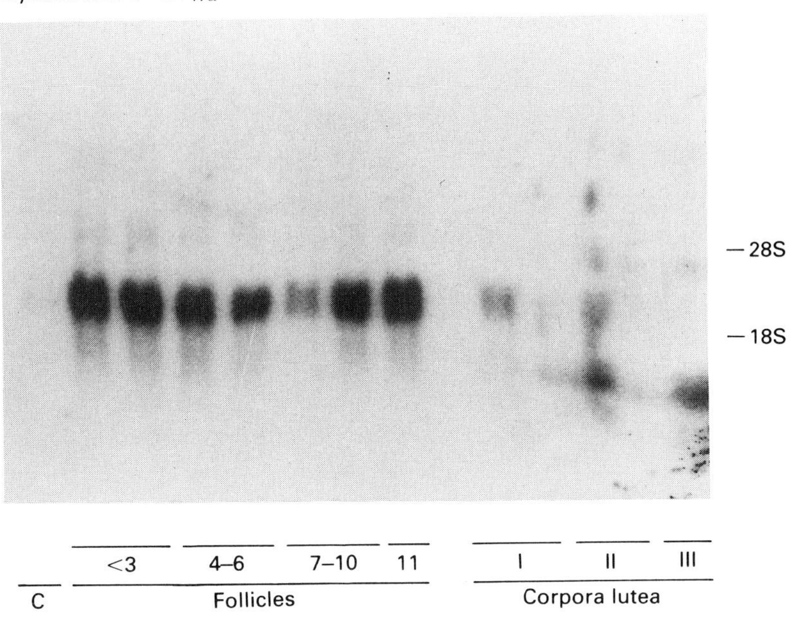

Fig. 7.3 Expression of mRNA that encodes P-450$_{17\alpha}$ throughout the bovine ovarian cycle. RNA was extracted from bovine follicles and corpora lutea as indicated. Poly A^+ RNA was prepared and subjected to Northern analysis as described [2]. The classification of corpora lutea at stages I, II and III follows that of Ireland *et al.* [10].

ovary, P-450$_{17\alpha}$ is expressed both in follicles and in corpora lutea [3]. In a similar fashion, in the human ovary, P-450$_{arom}$ is also expressed both in follicles and in corpora lutea, an observation consistent with the fact that in the human the corpus luteum secretes estrogens to about the same extent as the preovulatory follicle. By contrast, in both species the expression of P-450$_{scc}$ increases enormously following luteinization, consistent with the massive increase in progesterone secretion that occurs with the formation of the corpus luteum. Thus, we may conclude that the pattern of secretion of steroid hormones throughout the ovarian cycle can be explained, in large part, in terms of the differential expression of the enzymes responsible for their biosynthesis.

Regulation of expression of steroidogenic enzymes *in vitro*

In our attempts to understand the mechanisms whereby the expression of steroidogenic enzymes occurs, human granulosa cells [4] and human thecal cells [5] have been maintained in culture in order to determine the effects of various potential regulatory factors on the expression of these steroidogenic enzymes. Utilizing human thecal cells in culture, we found that 17α-hydroxylase activity in these cells was stimulated by human chorionic gonadotropin (hCG) and by forskolin. Moreover, such stimulation was blocked by the presence of a number of growth factors in the culture medium, notably transforming growth factor-β, fibroblast growth factor, and epidermal growth factor, as well as the phorbol ester, TPA. By contrast, insulin-like growth factor 1 (IGF-1) stimulated the activity of 17α-hydroxylase in these cells. When pregnenolone was used as a substrate (Fig. 7.4) the initial product was 17α-hydroxypregnenolone, which then was further converted to dehydroepiandrosterone (DHEA) [5]. However, when progesterone was utilized as substrate, the principal product was 17α-hydroxyprogesterone, and little androstenedione was formed. This result is consistent with the known properties of the human and bovine P-$450_{17\alpha}$ enzymes when their cDNAs are expressed in COS-1 monkey kidney tumor cells, namely that the 17,20-lyase activity of the enzyme is inactive toward Δ^4-3-ketosteroids and is only active towards Δ^5-3β-hydroxysteroids [6].

The conclusion from these observations is that the pathway for the formation of androstenedione and, indeed, testosterone in the human ovary, involves the prior formation of DHEA and that, since granulosa cells appear to contain higher levels of 3β-hydroxysteroid dehydrogenase than do the thecal cells [5], it may well be that the bulk of the androstenedione and testosterone formed is a consequence of DHEA being synthesized in the thecal cells and then passing into the granulosa cells for oxidation to the corresponding Δ^4-3-one compound.

Expression of chimeric constructs that contain regions of the P-450_{scc} and P-$450_{17\alpha}$ genes upstream from the transcriptional start sites

In recent years, the genes for the various steroidogenic forms of cytochrome P-450 have been cloned and characterized (Fig. 7.5). In order to understand at the molecular level the mechanisms whereby regulatory factors control the expression of these steroidogenic P-450 genes, we have prepared chimeric constructs that contain a series of deletions of the 5′-untranslated regions of the bovine genes for P-450_{scc} [7] and P-$450_{17\alpha}$ [8]. These fragments have been fused upstream from the reporter gene, chloramphenicol acetyltransferase (CAT), as well as the β-globin gene. Such chimeric constructs have been used to transfect primary cultures of bovine luteal cells [9], as well as those of bovine

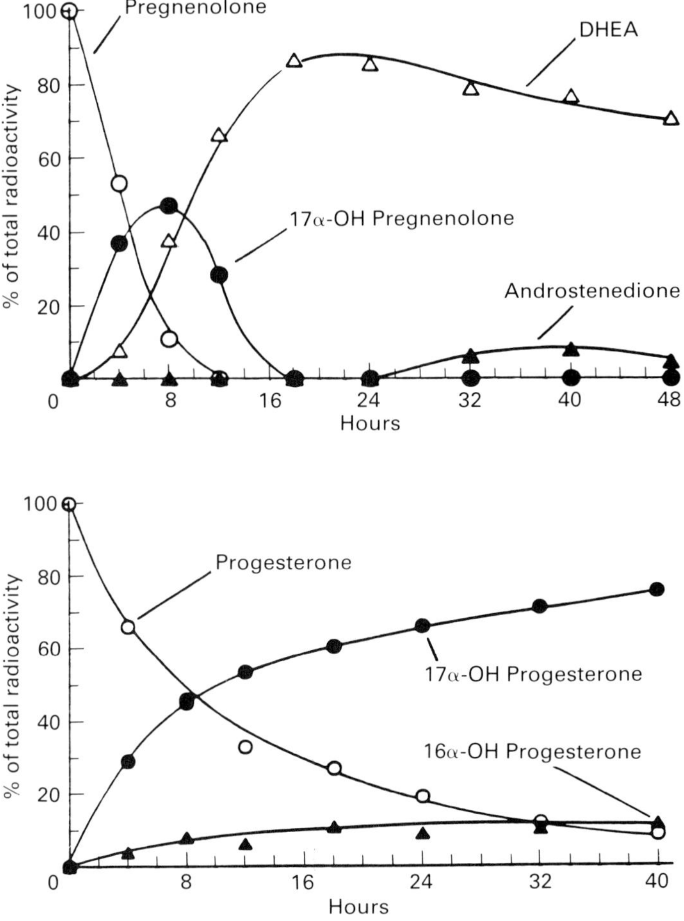

Fig. 7.4 17α-Hydroxylase activity of human thecal cells cultured in the presence of forskolin (25 μM) for 72 hours [5]. The top panel shows an experiment in which pregnenolone (1 μM) was used as substrate; the lower panel shows an experiment in which progesterone (1 μM) was used as substrate.

thecal cells. The results indicate that such constructs, which contain 5′-untranslated regions of the bovine P-450_{scc} gene can confer responsiveness to cyclic adenosine monophosphate (cAMP) on the CAT reporter gene in bovine luteal cells. Moreover, this property appears to be confined to the region between −186 and −100 base pairs upstream from the start of transcription. This region also confers responsiveness to cAMP on the CAT reporter gene when used to transfect bovine adrenocortical cells and mouse adrenal tumor Y1 cells [7]. However, corresponding constructs that contain 5′-upstream regions of the

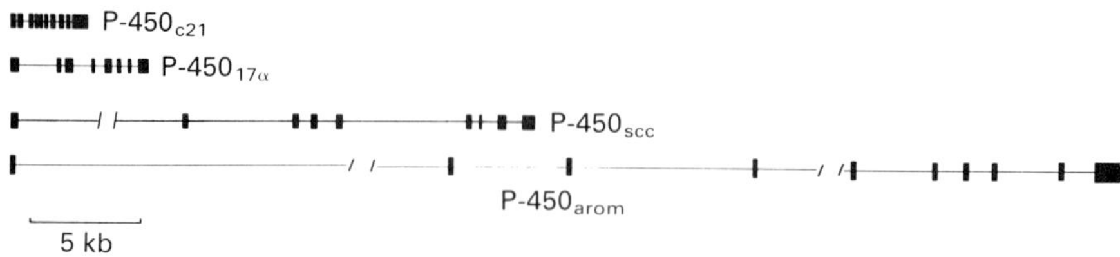

Fig. 7.5 Schematic diagram showing the relative sizes of the genes that encode P-450_{C21}, P-$450_{17\alpha}$, P-450_{scc}, and P-450_{arom}. The number of exons varies between 8 and 10, but the size of the introns varies considerably. In each case the heme-binding region is encoded by the last exon.

P-$450_{17\alpha}$ gene were not expressed in bovine luteal cells, even though they were expressed in bovine thecal cells. These results are consistent with the concept that the differential expression of P-450_{scc} and P-$450_{17\alpha}$ in the bovine ovary after luteinization, whereby a dramatic increase in expression of P-450_{scc} and a decrease in the expression of P-$450_{17\alpha}$ occur, are the result of the differential expression of transcriptional factors in the thecal and luteal cells, which are responsible for interacting with the responsive elements in the 5′-upstream region of these genes.

Summary

In the final analysis, a complete understanding of the molecular basis of polycystic ovarian disease and other ovarian disorders will depend on the elucidation of cellular and molecular mechanisms whereby the expression of the steroidogenic enzymes is regulated. Such studies are in their infancy but, nonetheless, there are already intriguing suggestions that ultimately the differential expression of the transcriptional elements that interact with the steroidogenic P-450 genes will prove of great consequence in determining the switching on and off of these activities throughout the ovarian cycle. The regulation of these transcriptional factors ultimately depends upon the differentiation-associated factors that determine the changes in cell function, size, and morphology that occur during development and throughout the cycle. An understanding of the control mechanisms responsible for regulation of steroidogenesis in the normal ovary will, in turn, lead to an understanding of the pathophysiologic sequelae that underline the etiology of syndromes such as PCO.

Acknowledgments

The authors gratefully acknowledge the skilled editorial assistance of Sandra Finley. This work was supported in part by USPHS grants nos. HD13235 and DK28350. J.M.M. was supported, in part, by USPHS Training grant no. T32-HD07190.

References

1 Nebert DW, Nelson DR, Adesnik M, *et al.* The P-450 superfamily: updated listing of all genes and recommended nomenclature for the chromosomal loci. DNA 1989; 8:1–13.

2 Rodgers RJ, Waterman MR, Simpson ER. Levels of messenger ribonucleic acid encoding cholesterol side-chain cleavage cytochrome P450, 17α-hydroxylase P450, adrenodoxin and low-density lipoprotein receptor in bovine follicles and corpora lutea throughout the ovarian cycle. Mol Endocrinol 1987; 1:274–9.

3 Doody KJ, Lorence MC, Mason JI, Simpson ER. Expression of mRNA species encoding steroidogenic enzymes in human follicles and corpora lutea throughout the menstrual cycle. J Clin Endocrinol Metab 1990; 70:1041–5.

4 McAllister JM, Mason JI, Byrd W, Trant JM, Waterman MR, Simpson ER. Proliferating human granulosa-lutein cells in long-term monolayer culture: expression of aromatase, cholesterol side-chain cleavage and 3β-hydroxysteroid dehydrogenase. J Clin Endocrinol Metab (in press).

5 McAllister JM, Kerin JFP, Trant JM, *et al.* Regulation of cholesterol side-chain cleavage and 17α-hydroxylase/lyase activities in proliferating human theca interna cells in long-term monolayer culture. Endocrinology 1989; 125:1959–66.

6 Zuber MX, Simpson ER, Waterman MR. Expression of bovine 17α-hydroxylase cytochrome P450 cDNA in nonsteroidogenic (COS1) cells. Science 1986; 234:1258–61.

7 Ahlgren R, Simpson ER, Waterman MR, Lund J. Characterization of the promoter/regulatory region of the bovine CYP11A ($P450_{scc}$) gene: basal and cAMP-dependent expression. J Biol Chem 1990; 265:3313–19.

8 Lund J, Ahlgren R, Wu D-H, Kagimoto M, Simpson ER, Waterman MR. Transcriptional regulation of the bovine CYP17 ($P450_{17\alpha}$) gene. J Biol Chem 1990; 265:3304–12.

9 Lauber M, Ahlgren R, Waterman MR, Simpson ER. Characterization of the 5′-regulatory region of cytochrome $P450_{scc}$ expressed in bovine luteal cells in primary culture. 72nd Annual Meeting of the Endocrine Society, Atlanta, Ga, 1990, p. 291 (Abstract).

10 Ireland JJ, Murphee RL, Cowlson PB. Accuracy of predicting stages of bovine estrous cycle by gross appearance of the corpus luteum. J Dairy Sci 1980; 63:155–63.

Chapter 8
Genetics of Steroidal Abnormalities: an Overview

FLORENCE P. HASELTINE

The physiologic effects of excessive androgens clearly differ among individuals and depend on many factors. What participants have attempted is to discuss the basic principles that need to be considered whenever PCO and related disease syndromes are discussed. When the syndrome was first noted, a large range of symptoms was attributed to androgen excess, for example the presence of acne or evidence of irregular menstrual periods. The superimposed genetic variability among individuals' tendencies towards development of acne, and the sensitivity of individual women to androgens in the regulation of their menstrual cycles, would render this syndrome difficult enough to study even if there were only a single genetic defect. It became clear during the discussion that the only way for an individual group of researchers to study PCO was to look at a defined population. Meaningful studies can be done on defined groups of patients. However, each study population differs, so that information from one group of researchers does not always help when another study group is examined.

Joe Leigh Simpson explains the ways in which geneticists approach a set of syndromes that have both genetic variability and phenotypic variability, namely genetic heterogeneity. The realization that the androgen-related syndromes can derive from specific mutations that can be localized on the genome and that the effects of these different mutations must be considered on a background of other genetic traits gives the clinician hope that each affected woman can be eventually accurately assessed and individually treated.

Evan Simpson's discussion centers on the some of the known pathways for production of androgens and their effects. One of the truly exciting areas that will surely be developed further in the future involves the details of the production of androgens and the associated physiology. The male often has such high levels of androgens available that the subtle effects of androgens are not appreciated. However, in the female the effects of androgens are more diverse. The cytochrome P-450 system in the ovary, which converts progesterone to estrogen and androgen, is highly regulated. The production of the mRNAs that control the protein synthesis necessary to produce the cytochrome P-450 enzymes is tightly regulated and is tied to ovulation. When we are able to elucidate the basic regulation of these steroid-conversion enzymes, their expression, and the effects of various mutations, we will have a better understanding of the abnormalities that plague women with excessively high levels of androgens. Furthermore, it is important that we examine the many mutations that can affect the actual proteins, as well as the mutations that affect the regulation of their expression, and the differences between the regulation of expression in the ovary and in the adrenal glands.

The time will come when the physiology of androgen metabolism is fully understood. The corresponding nucleotide sequence will be known for every enzyme, receptor, and regulator of androgen metabolism. Then it will be possible to define the disorder in each woman by reference to a specific genetic category. However, we may still find that women with identical genetic makeups experience varying degrees of severity of the syndrome, with these differences being the result of environmental factors and life style. Researchers must also not ignore differences that arise from inheriting the syndrome from the mother or the father, and the effects of early prenatal priming exposure to steroid hormones, early pregnancies, choice of birth control, stress and other unmeasurable factors. The variability in symptomatology, heritability, and effects of extraneous factors may confound researchers, but continuation of the steady progress made to date should eventually result in effective therapy for all affected individuals.

Section 4
Ovarian Function in Polycystic Ovary Syndrome

Chapter 9
Ovarian Steroidogenic Abnormalities in Polycystic Ovary Syndrome: Evidence for Abnormal Coordinate Regulation of Androgen and Estrogen Secretion

ROBERT L. ROSENFIELD, DAVID A. EHRMANN, RANDALL B. BARNES, DEBORAH F. BRIGELL & DONALD W. CHANDLER

Ovarian function in polycystic ovary syndrome

Background

Polycystic ovary syndrome (PCO) is a common and heterogeneous disorder which, in its full-blown state, is characterized by menstrual abnormalities, hirsutism, and obesity. We have proposed a new model for the pathogenesis of the syndrome in which functional, gonadotropin-dependent ovarian hyperandrogenism is central [1]. We recently developed a practical method for evaluating ovarian function that permitted us to test this model. The results of this clinical research suggest that excessive formation of androstenedione (AD) via 17-hydroxyprogesterone (17-PROG) in response to luteinizing hormone (LH) is typical of most cases of PCO [2]. Abnormal regulation of steroidogenesis seems to be the basis of the problem [3].

We found that ovarian secretory capacity could be tested rapidly after inducing a rise in levels of endogenous gonadotropins by the administration of a test dose of the potent agonist of gonadotropin-releasing hormone (GnRH), nafarelin (Syntex Laboratories, Inc., Palo Alto, CA) [2]. We then examined the response to nafarelin in PCO (which we have equated with functional ovarian hyperandrogenism, as defined primarily by results of a dexamethasone (dex) test, namely plasma levels of testosterone (T) of 7.6 pg/ml or more with normal adrenocortical suppression after 4 days administration of low-dose dex). Our results demonstrated that patients with PCO (n = 8) typically had masculinized pituitary–gonadal responses to nafarelin [2]. That is, their responses resembled those of males in several ways. Both groups had greater early responses in terms of serum LH and lesser responses in terms of follicle-stimulating hormone (FSH) ($P < 0.05$), and these responses were followed by significantly greater responses in terms of plasma levels of 17-PROG and androgen than those of normal women in the early follicular phase of the menstrual cycle (Fig. 9.1). Performance of the nafarelin test coincident with the dex suppression test demonstrated that the steroid-related responses to nafarelin were not due to concomitant adrenal secretion. Furthermore, the responses to nafarelin were similar in all respects to those obtained when dex was not administered. Although a small increase in ovarian secretion of 17-hydroxypregnenolone by PCO ovaries could be discerned during coincidental dex suppression, measurement of responses of levels of dehydroepiandrosterone (DHEA) or androstenediol revealed no other abnormalities on the Δ^5-pathway (Fig. 9.2).

There was no evidence of a block in the steroidogenic pathway. Rather, the responses of all steroids on the pathway between progesterone (PROG) and estradiol (E_2) tended to be exaggerated in PCO.

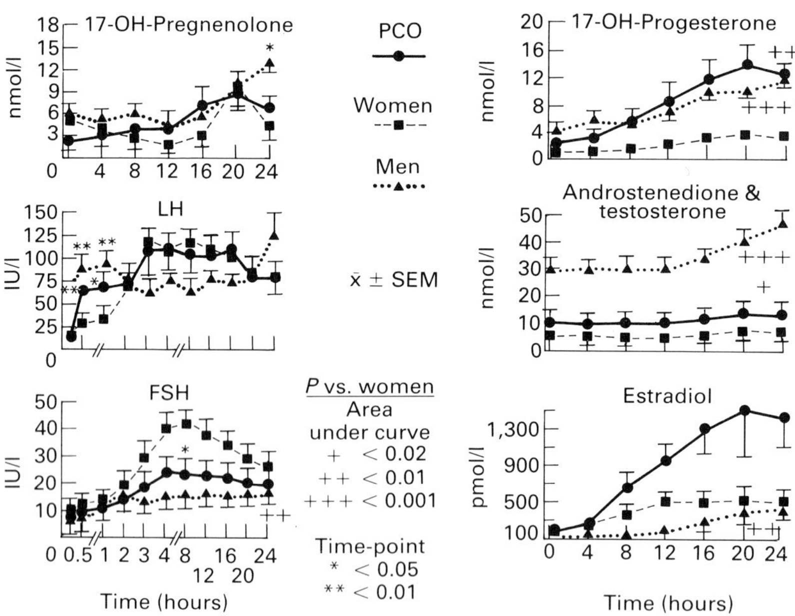

Fig. 9.1 Responses to nafarelin of normal men ($n = 5$) and patients with PCO ($n = 5$) compared with those of normal females in the follicular phase ($n = 9$). Nafarelin (100 µg, injected subcutaneously) was administered immediately after the 0-min sample was taken. Plasma concentrations of LH, FSH, 17-hydroxypregnenolone, 17-PROG, androgen (androstenedione plus testosterone), and estradiol are shown over the subsequent 24-hour period. The statistical comparisons of the responses at the various time points are shown only when the areas under the response curve are not significantly different among groups. All P-values are two-tailed. (Modified, with permission, from Barnes *et al.* [2].)

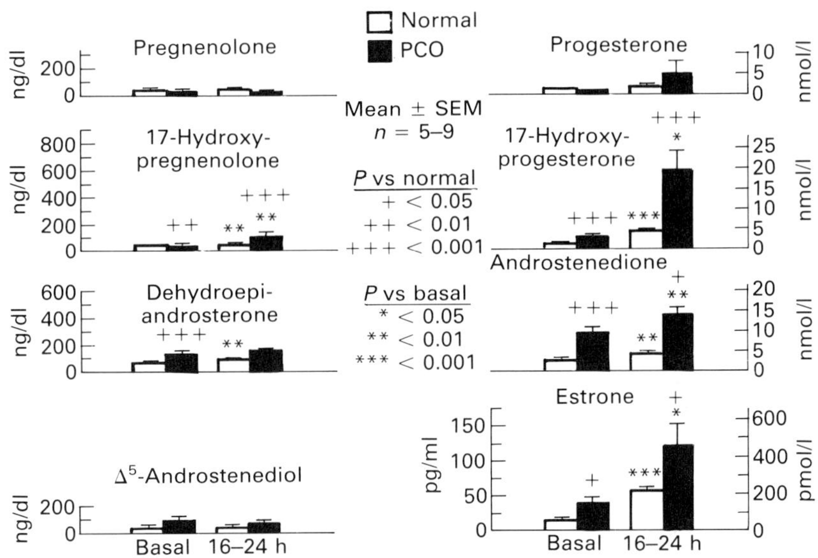

Fig. 9.2 Steroid levels before and after (maximal response at 16–24 hours) administration of 100 μg of nafarelin. Nine normal women in the follicular phase and five patients with PCO (nine for pregnenolone) were studied. Treatment with dexamethasone was begun at a dosage of 2 mg daily, in divided doses, 4 days prior and continued for 24 hours after administration of nafarelin. The layout is in accordance with the steroidogenic pathway, with biosynthesis of steroids proceeding from pregnenolone in the upper left through two alternate pathways (Δ^5-path on the left, Δ^4-path on the right) toward estrone in the lower right. Levels of pregnenolone were measured at Endocrine Sciences, after extraction and high-pressure liquid chromatography, by a radioimmunoassay using an antiserum against pregnenolone-20-oxime. The method was sensitive to 0.69 nmol/l. The coefficient of variation of the assay at these plasma levels averaged 12%. Other data for steroids are from Barnes *et al.* [2]. All *P*-values are two-tailed.

The levels of 17-PROG in response to nafarelin in women with PCO were consistently greater than normal: peak concentrations ranged from 8.2 to 36 nmol/l in PCO and were 6.4 nmol/l (224 ng/dl) or lower in normal women. Plasma levels of AD postnafarelin were elevated in most cases ($P < 0.05$). Furthermore, levels of estrone seemed to rise more rapidly than, and out of proportion to, AD in response to nafarelin: levels of estrone rose threefold, whereas levels of AD rose by only 50%; during treatment with dex, the increase in levels of estrone was significantly greater than that in normal women ($P < 0.05$). These results are not those that would be expected if peripheral conversion of AD to estrone were central to the pathogenesis of PCO [3].

In most cases of PCO (6/8), the oversecretion of 17-PROG and AD was associated with an elevated response of levels of LH to nafarelin. Patients with PCO resembled men in that they had higher blood levels of 17-PROG and AD, as well as greater early responses in terms of levels of LH, 17-PROG, and AD to nafarelin, than did normal women. These data were compatible with gonadal secretion of 17-PROG and AD being regulated similarly in women with PCO and in men.

The responses to nafarelin testing in typical women with PCO contrasted with those in a woman with PCO known to be secondary to Δ^5-3β-hydroxysteroid dehydrogenase (3β-ol) deficiency, in whom a block in ovarian steroidogenesis was demonstrable. Plasma levels of Δ^5-3β-hydroxysteroids before the enzymatic block increased markedly, whereas plasma levels of the Δ^4-3-ketosteroids 17-PROG and AD—the steroids immediately beyond the block—were low, as were estrone responses (Fig. 9.3).

These results of nafarelin tests appeared to provide an important clue to the etiology of PCO. The hyperresponsiveness of levels of 17-PROG, without evidence of a distal block in steroidogenesis, suggested increased activity in the Δ^4-pathway, commencing at the level of 17α-hydroxylase (17-hydroxylase), and involving 17,20-lyase (17-lyase). Increased activities of earlier enzymes in the biosynthetic path seemed unlikely since levels of 17-hydroxypregnenolone and PROG were not consistently different in women with PCO and normal women.

Recent studies

In order to define how the regulation of enzymatic activity in women with PCO compares with that in normal men and women, we have now analyzed the apparent efficiency of the enzymatically catalyzed reactions from precursor:product relationships of plasma steroids in response to nafarelin. In the above nafarelin tests without pretreatment with dex, concomitant adrenal secretion appeared to cause substantial fluctuations in plasma levels of steroids, which resulted in some seemingly negative responses to nafarelin, making computation of apparent 17-hydroxylase efficiency meaningless. Nevertheless, apparent 17-lyase efficiency could be computed. It can be seen in Fig. 9.4 that responses of levels of 17-PROG to nafarelin increase in the order: normal women < men < PCO. In contrast, responses in terms of plasma levels of androgens (AD + T) are greater in the order: normal women < PCO < men. Furthermore, the ratio of responses of androgens to responses of 17-PROG (whether analyzed in terms of absolute increases or relative increases above baseline) was lower in women with PCO than in men ($P < 0.01$) and in normal women ($P < 0.01$). Thus, the increased formation of androgens in PCO does not seem to be due to increased 17-lyase activity. Instead, gonads in PCO, while overproducing androgen, produce it less efficiently

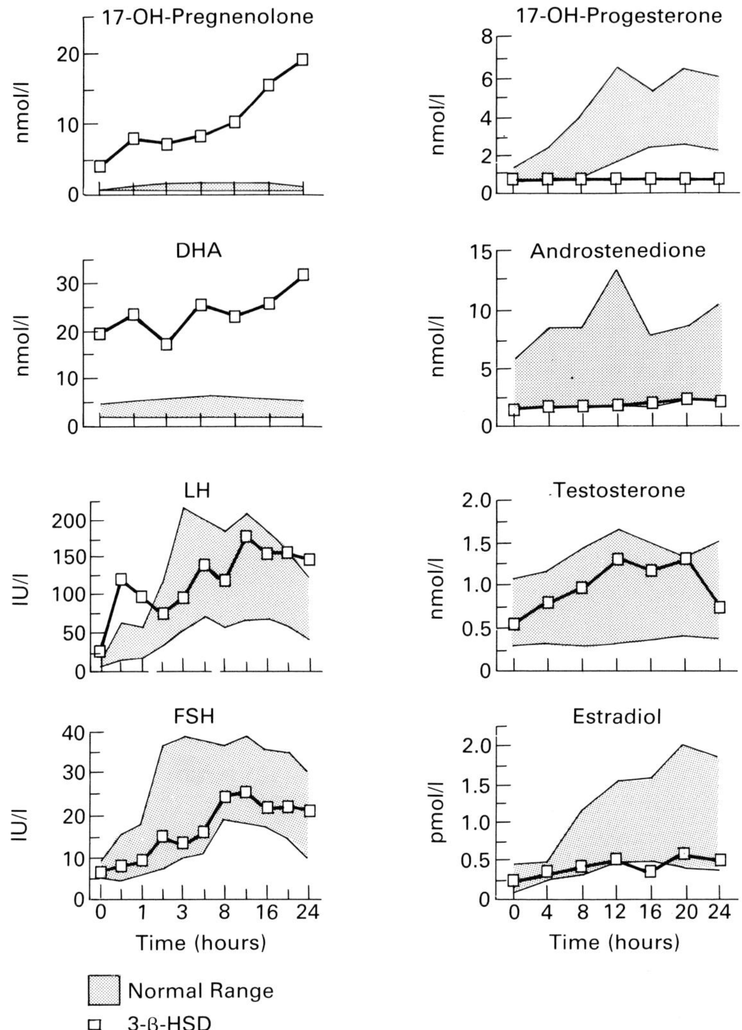

Fig. 9.3 Responses to nafarelin of a woman deficient in 3β-hydroxysteroid dehydrogenase (3-β-HSD) compared with normal women ($n = 9$) during treatment with glucocorticoid. The patient has elevated levels of Δ^5-steroids (17-hydroxypregnenolone and dehydroepiandrosterone) prior to the enzyme block, but low levels of Δ^4-steroids (17-PROG and AD) beyond the block, with a subnormal response in terms of levels of estrone. All of these features are the opposite of the abnormalities in PCO. (Reproduced, with permission of The New England Journal of Medicine, from Barnes *et al.* [2].)

from 17-PROG than do men's gonads. In other words, polycystic ovaries are not functioning like testes.

In order better to assess the first steps in the ovarian steroidogenic pathway, we have now assayed pregnenolone during nafarelin tests of

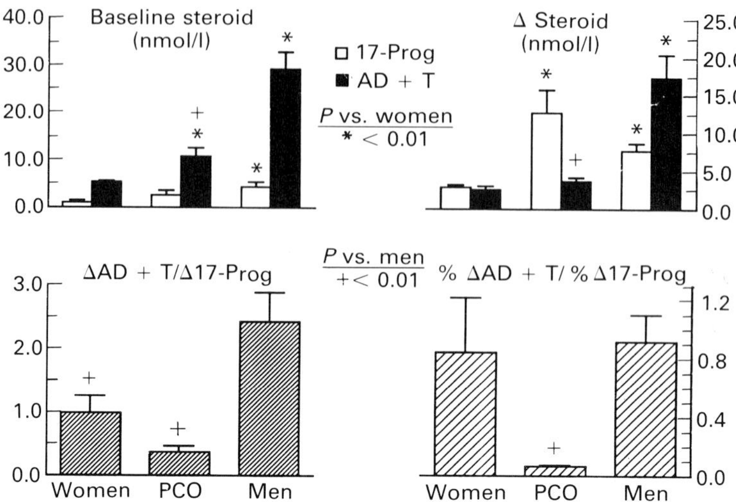

Fig. 9.4 Apparent efficiency of gonadal 17-lyase as judged from plasma levels of 17-PROG and AD in response to nafarelin. In order to compare production of androgen in females and males, who differ in the degree to which AD is converted to T, levels of AD and T have been summed. ΔSteroid, peak level minus baseline concentration; %Δ, level of steroid as a percentage increase. From data in Fig. 9.1 [2]. All *P*-values are two-tailed.

dex-pretreated women. As can be seen in Fig. 9.2 and Table 9.1, plasma levels of pregnenolone were not significantly different in the two groups at baseline and they did not rise in response to nafarelin. This result suggests that there is neither increased enzymatic activity at the level of 20,22-side-chain cleavage nor decreased activity of the enzymatic steps immediately beyond pregnenolone (17-hydroxylase and 3β-ol).

In order to more definitively assess the apparent efficiency of ovarian biosynthesis of androgen in PCO, we have expanded our series of nafarelin tests of subjects pretreated with dex in order to suppress adrenal contributions to plasma levels of steroids. The results are shown in Tables 9.1 and 9.2. As discussed above, there is no abnormality at the level of pregnenolone. Baseline levels and responses in terms of levels of 17-hydroxypregnenolone show modest increases ($P < 0.01$). Although the percentage responsiveness of this steroid is increased ($P < 0.01$), the undetectable baseline levels in normal subjects make this particular parameter suspect and the peak levels achieved are unimpressive (<100 ng/dl). Baseline levels of DHEA are modestly increased ($P < 0.01$). However, in response to nafarelin, plasma levels of DHEA do not rise excessively. Although not statistically significant, the index of 17-lyase activity in the Δ^5-pathway (ΔDHEA/Δ17-hydroxypregnenolone) tends to be low.

Table 9.1 Responses of levels of Δ^5-steroids to nafarelin (dexamethasone-pretreated*). Values are the mean ± SEM.

Group	Pregnenolone† (Preg)		17-Hydroxy-pregnenolone (17-Preg)		DHEA		Percentage increase		Ratio of increases		
	Basal (nmol/l)	Rise‡ (nmol/l)	Basal (nmol/l)	Rise (nmol/l)	Basal (nmol/l)	Rise (nmol/l)	17-Preg	DHEA	ΔDHEA/ Δ17-Preg	ΔAD/ ΔDHEA	Δ17-PROG/ Δ17-Preg
Normal ($n = 11$)	1.26 ±0.16	−0.2 ±0.3	0.69§ ±0.00	0.60 ±0.12	2.24 ±0.22	1.00 ±0.28	90 ±18	50 ±16	5.61 ±4.9	14.9 ±6.9	22.2 ±14.0
PCO ($n = 23$)	1.39 ±0.06	−0.3 ±0.3	0.86 ±0.05	1.49 ±0.20	4.03 ±0.38	1.34 ±0.27	169 ±21	39 ±8	1.16 ±0.29	13.8 ±5.8	21.9 ±10.0
P_2 (t-test)			<0.01	<0.01	<0.01		<0.02				

* dex 0.5 mg q.i.d. × 4 days.
† Subgroups of $n = 9$.
‡ Rise = peak minus basal level.
§ All values below limit of sensitivity of assay, 0.69 nmol/l (23 ng/dl).

Table 9.2 Responses of levels of Δ^4-steroid to nafarelin (dexamethasone-pretreated*). Values are the mean ± SEM.

Group	Progesterone (PROG)		17-Hydroxyprogesterone (17-PROG)		Androstenedione (AD)		Testosterone		Percentage increase			Ratio of increases	
	Basal (nmol/l)	Rise† (nmol/l)	Basal (nmol/l)	Rise (nmol/l)	Basal (nmol/l)	Rise (nmol/l)	Basal (nmol/l)	Rise (nmol/l)	PROG	17-PROG	AD	Δ17-PROG/ΔPROG	ΔAD/Δ17-PROG
Normal ($n = 11$)	0.79‡ ±0.00	1.20 ±0.65	0.85 ±0.06	4.10 ±0.41	2.74 ±0.34	2.20 ±0.39	0.59 ±0.08	0.20 ±0.04	150 ±80	490 ±50	80 ±13	18.1 ±7.3	0.50 ±0.07
PCO ($n = 23$)	0.82 ±0.03	2.40 ±0.52	2.47 ±0.24	13.00 ±1.43	8.34 ±0.65	3.98 ±0.62	2.20 ±0.25	1.04 ±0.18	290 ±60	540 ±50	47 ±6	15.0 ±3.8	0.31 ±0.04
P_2 (t-test)		<0.03§	<0.001	<0.001	<0.04		<0.001	<0.02	<0.04		<0.02		<0.02

* 0.5 mg q.i.d. × 4 days.

† Rise = peak minus basal level.

‡ All values below sensitivity of method, 0.79 nmol/l (25 ng/dl).

§ Mann–Whitney U test.

Abnormalities are more striking in the Δ^4-steroidogenic pathway in women with PCO. Responses in terms of levels of progesterone are modestly increased ($P < 0.03$). The greater relative increase in PCO may be an artifact resulting from overestimation of the basal level in normal subjects. Basal levels of 17-PROG are increased threefold, and responses to nafarelin are increased ($P < 0.001$) proportionally. Baseline levels of AD ($P < 0.04$) and T ($P < 0.001$) are also threefold greater than normal. In response to nafarelin, levels of T rise excessively in women with PCO ($P < 0.02$). However, levels of AD rise only about 50% in these women, whereas they rise about 80% in normal subjects ($P < 0.02$). Indexes of 17-lyase activity in the Δ^4-pathway (such as ΔAD/Δ17-PROG, Table 9.2; or E_2/17-PROG, not shown) are significantly lower than normal ($P < 0.02$).

These analyses, taken together, are compatible with increased efficiency of 17-hydroxylase and high, yet relatively inefficient, 17-lyase activity. Increased efficiency of 17-hydroxylase is suggested by the finding of increased elevation of levels of 17-hydroxypregnenolone and 17-PROG. High 17-lyase activity is suggested by the elevated baseline levels of AD and T, as well as the increased responses of levels of T to nafarelin. 17-Lyase activity seems relatively inefficient since the increase in levels of AD is low relative to baseline or to the increase in levels of the precursor 17-PROG. There is no evidence of a steroidogenic block beyond this step since responses of levels of estradiol and estrone are not hindered; for example ΔE_2 is similar in both the normal women and women with PCO, averaging 1116 and 1372 pmol/l, respectively. The slight elevation of the responsiveness of levels of progesterone seems unlikely to be due to overactivity at earlier steps since no increase in levels of pregnenolone is discernible and ratios indicative of 3β-ol activity are normal. Thus, these studies suggest that polycystic ovaries are functioning in a stimulated but mildly down-regulated state.

Normal regulation of gonadal steroidogenesis

Formation of sex hormones from cholesterol in both sexes requires formation of 17-ketosteroids as intermediates (Fig. 9.5). The requisite 17-hydroxylase and 17-lyase activities appear to be associated with a single enzyme, cytochrome $P\text{-}450_{C17}$ [4] (see Chapter 7). This enzyme is localized to testicular Leydig and ovarian theca-interstitial-stromal ("thecal") cells [5]. This enzyme sequentially converts pregnenolone to 17-hydroxypregnenolone and DHEA. It similarly converts PROG to 17-PROG and, in many species, 17-PROG to AD. In both rodents and humans, there is evidence that 17-ketosteroids are formed by $P\text{-}450_{C17}$

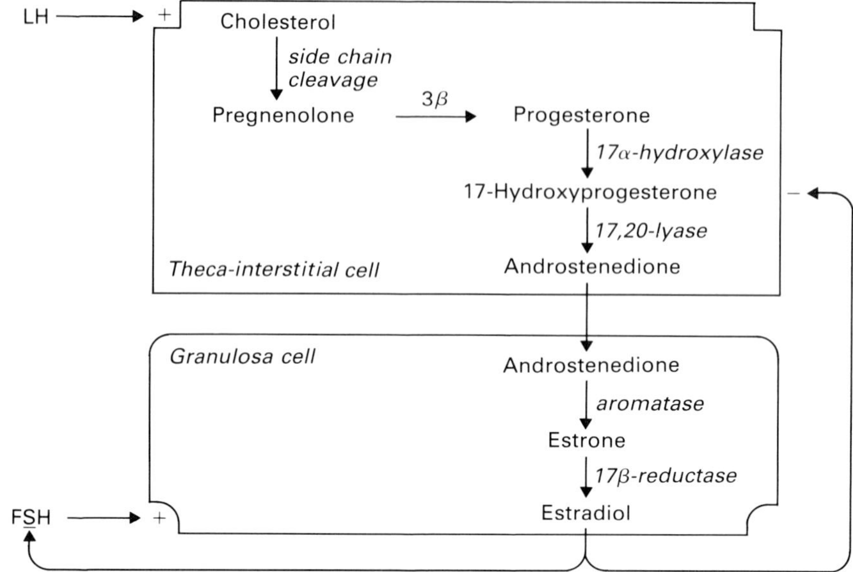

Fig. 9.5 Major factors regulating ovarian biosynthesis of androgen and estrogen. LH stimulates steroidogenesis in thecal cells and FSH stimulates that in granulosa cells. Estradiol is known to exert a sluggish, long-loop, negative feedback effect on release of FSH. The postulated short-loop (paracrine), negative feedback effect of estrogen on thecal 17-lyase activity is emphasized. However, other products of granulosa or thecal cells (such as IGF-1 or T) may be important paracrine regulators. The names of steroidogenic enzymes are italicized: 3β, 3β-hydroxysteroid dehydrogenase/Δ^5-isomerase.

activities in response to LH, that desensitization of the steroidogenic response commences as stimulation by LH increases, and that regulation of this enzyme is crucial to normal ovarian function.

Rodents

In rats, P-450_{C17} binds PROG and converts it sequentially to 17-PROG (by 17-hydroxylation) and AD (by 17-lyase activity). Similarly, this enzyme sequentially converts pregnenolone in the Δ^5-path to 17-hydroxypregnenolone and DHEA.

Small amounts of LH/human chorionic gonadotropin (hCG) up-regulate numbers of receptors for LH [6] and induce P-450_{C17} activities in the testes *in vivo* and in cultured Leydig cells [6–8]. Unlike other steroidogenic enzymes, which are constitutively expressed once they have been induced, expression of P-450_{C17} is critically dependent on the presence of ongoing stimulation by LH. Thus, at low levels of LH, P-450_{C17} is rate-limiting in the synthesis of androgens.

Prolonged or greater stimulation by LH of testes inhibits responsiveness of androgens *in vivo* and *in vitro* [6,9]. Desensitization to LH involves a decrease by LH of the number of LH receptors, an attendant desensitization of adenylate cyclase activity, and postreceptor modulation of steroidogenic enzyme activities, in particular that of P-450_{C17}. Two aspects of postreceptor down-regulation of steroidogenesis have been identified: an "early" inhibition of the formation of pregnenolone and a "late" down-regulation of P-450_{C17} activities. Partial desensitization is characterized by a small decrease in numbers of receptors for LH while secretion of androgens is sustained [6,10]; at this stage, modest inhibition of 17-lyase activity occurs. With greater desensitization, 17-hydroxylase activity decreases [6].

The decrease in 17-hydroxylase/lyase activities in response to hCG appears to be steroid-mediated [11,12]. Both E_2 [6,13] and androgen [11,14] have been incriminated in the inhibition of P-450_{C17}, as will be discussed further in the following section.

Data about the regulation of the production of androgens by ovarian thecal cells are limited, but they are compatible with that defined in testicular Leydig cells. The slight increase in levels of LH prior to the ovulatory surge increases the number of receptors for LH in thecal cells of preovulatory follicles [15]. In small doses LH also induces P-450_{C17} activity and secretion of AD in thecal cells [15–17]. In contrast, a preovulatory surge of LH or hCG inhibits follicular adenylate cyclase [18] and P-450_{C17} activities, in particular that of 17-lyase [19]. Prolonged or excessive exposure to LH also reduces the number of receptor sites for LH in cultured thecal cells from rats [20]. Estradiol rapidly inhibits P-450_{C17} activities both *in vivo* and *in vitro* [17].

Although these studies in the female rat are limited, the results are compatible with the concept that LH in small amounts stimulates rat thecal and Leydig cells, whereas in larger amounts LH desensitizes both cell types to LH itself. Furthermore, this latter effect seems due, in part, to down-regulation of the activities of P-450_{C17}, in particular the 17-lyase component.

Humans

In men, the regulation of secretion of androgens has been extensively characterized *in vivo*. Administration of hCG or LH stimulates secretion of 17-PROG as well as of androgen [21–23]. After injection of a large dose of HCG, plasma levels of 17-PROG initially (for 4 hours) rise in proportion to levels of T. However, levels of 17-PROG and T then diverge: the level of 17-PROG rises to a maximum at 24 hours as that of

T reaches a plateau, then the level of 17-PROG falls as that of T rises to peak at 72–90 hours [21,23]. These data are compatible with the theory that high levels of LH induce a partial block of 17-lyase activity. Estrogen may mediate this apparent partial block: (i) the time-course changes in levels of 17-PROG and E_2 are similar from 4 to 96 hours after administration of hCG [22]; (ii) E_2 rapidly inhibits the response of levels of T to hCG [24]; and (iii) administration of tamoxifen, which competitively inhibits the binding of E_2 to its receptor, inhibits the 17-PROG response to HCG [25]. Nonaromatizable androgen also appears to inhibit the secretion of T directly [26], an effect that has been less well characterized.

In women, data regarding the regulation of secretion of androgens are scanty. It is well known that women do not form as much androgen in response to LH/hCG as do men. Analysis of responses to nafarelin tests shows this expected difference between the sexes (Fig. 9.4) [2]. Normal men also appear to form more androgen from 17-PROG in absolute terms, as indicated by their significantly higher ratios of ΔAD + T/Δ17-PROG. However, men appear to be no more *efficient* than normal women in terms of the formation of androgen from precursor, as indicated by the finding that the sexes are similar in terms of the relative responsiveness of the secretion of androgen and 17-PROG to nafarelin (i.e. the percentage increase above baseline is similar for the androgens and for 17-PROG, resulting in a ratio that approximates 1.0 in both sexes) (Fig. 9.4). These data suggest that men have more androgen-forming enzyme (P-450_{C17}) than women, but that both Leydig and thecal cells operate at about the same level of efficiency. However, no matter how our recent data are analyzed, PCO ovaries operate at subnormal 17-lyase efficiency though androgen formation is high (Fig. 9.4, Table 9.2).

In normal women, the preovulatory rise in serum levels of LH induces a rise in plasma levels of 17-PROG and AD [27]. Administration of hCG to women stimulates plasma levels of AD and T. In PCO, hCG has been found to double the excretion of the 17-PROG-specific metabolite pregnanetriol [28]. Receptor sites for LH in the ovary are reduced in numbers in PCO [29]. All of these responses resemble the situation in males after stimulation by hCG.

From the results described above, it appears that regulation of androgen secretion by human Leydig and thecal cells resembles that in the rat, although the data for women are meager. We believe that the most parsimonious explanation for the observed hyperresponsiveness in PCO to gonadotropins of levels of 17-PROG, AD, and estrone is the hyperfunction of gonadal cytochrome P-450_{C17}, due to abnormal regulation ("dysregulation") of its activities. The molecular mechanisms of regulation of P-450$_{C17}$ have not been definitively elucidated and may differ substantially among species, as discussed below.

Molecular mechanisms of regulation of P-450$_{C17}$ (see Chapter 7)

Induction of P-450$_{C17}$ activities in Leydig cells and levels of the enzyme are critically dependent on LH (acting via cyclic adenosine monophosphate, cAMP) in the mouse [7,8,12]. The situation is similar in cultured rat and human thecal cells [16,30]. The down-regulation of P-450$_{C17}$ induced in Leydig cells by LH is also mimicked by cAMP [9]. However, once established, this metabolic lesion in testes does not correlate with intracellular levels of cAMP or cAMP-dependent protein kinase. Thus, its persistence appears to be independent of and distal to desensitization of adenylate cyclase [6,30,31].

Steroids formed in response to LH/hCG/cAMP appear to mediate the decline in P-450$_{C17}$ activities during desensitization to LH/cAMP [12]. Estradiol seems important in this respect in rat; however, the relevant mechanism is unclear. Dufau *et al.* have reported prevention of the effect of HCG by treatment with an antiestrogen [6]. However, desensitization commences before numbers of receptors for estrogen in Leydig cells decrease significantly [13]. Inhibition by E_2 of thecal secretion of androgen has been shown to be very rapid ($t_{1/2}$ = 10 min), an observation that is compatible with a direct inhibitory effect of E_2 on P-450$_{C17}$ [17]. Estradiol competitively and/or noncompetitively inhibits P-450$_{C17}$ with a K_i of approximately 5 μM (17-lyase) to 20 μM (17-hydroxylase) [32]. The mechanism by which estrogen might act in the human ovary is open to question since hybridization studies *in situ* have failed to detect receptors for E_2 in primate (monkey) follicles or parenchyma [33]. However, as in the case of rat thecal cells [17], secretion from human Leydig cell seems exquisitely sensitive to E_2 [24]. In cultures of rat or mouse Leydig cells, T has an autocrine feedback effect on its own secretion, mediated by the receptor for androgen [11,14]. Steroids seem to modulate P-450$_{C17}$ activities in complex ways. For example, although 17-PROG competitively inhibits 17-hydroxylase activity, 17-hydroxypregnenolone seems to inhibit 17-lyase activity [34].

Recombinant human and bovine P-450$_{C17}$ differ from the enzyme from rat structurally and functionally [35]. Unlike rat P-450$_{C17}$, human and bovine P-450$_{C17}$ convert only relatively small amounts of 17-PROG to AD when they are expressed in nonsteroidogenic cells. In the case of the bovine enzyme, AD is formed from DHEA 7–25% as efficiently as DHEA is formed from 17-hydroxypregnenolone [34], even when cytochrome b_5 is coexpressed as a source of electrons [36] to promote the lyase reaction, which has a lower K_m [4]. This pattern of metabolism is consistent with the pattern of production of steroids by cultured human thecal cells from infertile women [30]. This relatively low 17-lyase activity for Δ^4-steroids has been postulated to be due to a difference in one of the 75 positions at which the amino acids in the polypeptide differ from the rat sequence [35]. Alternatively, it may be due to the absence of a tissue factor that is critical for promoting formation of complexes of P-450_{C17} with enzymes that mediate the transfer of electrons [4].

Paradoxically, the absence of metabolism of PROG or 17-PROG to AD in cultured human thecal or nonsteroidogenic cells contrasts with the situation in fresh ovarian tissue: minced human ovarian tissue from normal women and women with PCO has definitively been shown to convert PROG to 17-PROG to AD efficiently [37,38]. For example, Axelrod and Goldzieher [37] reported that ^{14}C-PROG underwent 30–100% 17-hydroxylation and 3–99% 17,20 cleavage in polycystic ovaries. This result raises the possibility that humans have a Δ^4-17-lyase distinct from P-450_{C17}. If this is so, such an activity does not appear to effect steroidogenesis in either the gonads or adrenal glands in the absence of P-450_{C17} [39].

We favor the concept that a regulatory factor is important for facilitation of the expression of P-450_{C17} lyase activity. The meager data available indicate that LH regulates thecal and Leydig cells of both rodents and humans in a similar manner. This conclusion in turn suggests that P-450_{C17} is involved in the formation of AD from 17-PROG in both species. Thus, the paradoxical difference between metabolism of PROG and 17-PROG by fresh ovarian tissue vs. that by cultured thecal cells is compatible with the requirement for a regulatory factor in tissue that facilitates the expression of this activity. Such a factor might require interaction of thecal cells with other types of cells and might not be expressed in monolayer cultures.

What factors might be involved in modulating the regulation by LH of P-450_{C17} activity? We found that insulin-like growth factor 1 (IGF-1) and insulin augment the stimulation by LH of androgen production by thecal cells [40]. We have shown that this augmentation is associated with induction of receptors for LH and prevention of the reduction in numbers of receptors for LH by LH [20]. Magoffin *et al.* have recently reported that IGF-1 increases levels of P-450_{C17} mRNA and that it reverses the LH-induced down-regulation of levels of P-450_{C17} mRNA [41]. Furthermore, IGF-1 also appears to augment the ability of LH to increase the content but not the activity of this enzyme. Their data suggest that a major mode of action of IGF-1 in counteracting desensitization to LH is by enhancing levels of P-450_{scc} mRNA, enzyme, and activity. Other factors also seem to be involved in modulating the regulation by LH of P-450_{C17} activities. Chasalow *et al.* identified an hCG-induced cytosolic factor in rat Leydig cells that augmented the synthesis of AD from PROG after injection of hCG [31]. It did not, however, overcome the desensitized state. Phospholipids [4] and high-density lipoproteins rich in apoprotein E [3] may play a role in regulating P-450_{C17} activities.

Appropriate regulation of the activities of P-450_{C17} seems to be critical for normal ovarian function. 17-Hydroxylase and 17-lyase activities determine the amount of androgen formed within the ovary. Androgen is a necessary evil insofar as the ovary is concerned. Androgens are, on the one hand, obligate intermediates in the biosynthesis of estrogen. On the other hand, androgens are deleterious to the ovary, being atretogenic [42]. Therefore, it would seem crucial for the function of the ovary that the intraovarian concentration of androgens be kept to the minimum necessary to support biosynthesis of necessary levels of estrogen. Since there is no long-loop, negative feedback system in the female for regulating the secretion of androgens, desensitization to LH would seem to be the primary means of adjusting the ovarian secretion of androgen to that of estrogen. Paracrine (short-loop) feedback regulation of P-450_{C17} activities seems to be the most likely mechanism for this coordination (Fig. 9.5). Thus, PCO seems likely to result from defects in the system of coordinate regulation of the systems for synthesis of androgens and estrogens, such that 17-hydroxylase activity is not appropriately inhibited and excessive ovarian formation of 17-ketosteroids results.

Evidence for abnormal regulation of both ovarian and adrenal steroidogenesis in PCO

A number of pieces of evidence reviewed above suggests that the typical ovarian steroidogenic abnormality in PCO is the result of abnormal regulation (''dysregulation'') of P-450_{C17}. Foremost among the evidence are the data reviewed in the opening section, namely that the increased responsiveness to nafarelin in terms of levels of 17-PROG and AD is compatible with the polycystic ovary functioning in a stimulated but mildly down-regulated state. These steroidogenic abnormalities usually are associated with early hyperresponsiveness of LH.

What might be the nature of the proposed regulatory defect in PCO? Excessive secretion of LH is the major candidate. The elevation of serum concentrations of LH, the low number of ovarian receptor sites for LH, and the steroid-secretory pattern are all compatible with the polycystic ovary being overstimulated and functioning in a state of partial down-regulation. It is possible that, in such cases, the degree of stimulation by LH exceeds the capacity of the ovary to down-regulate.

How might an ovarian regulatory abnormality occur in those cases of PCO in which elevated serum levels of LH are absent, yet similar thecal responses are present? There are several potential mechanisms. First, it is possible that elevated secretion of LH is not reflected in serum concentrations of immunoreactive LH. Second, it is possible that the action of LH on thecal cells is enhanced or amplified without serum concentrations of LH being high. Insulin and IGF-1 are hormones that act synergistically with LH in stimulating the secretion of androgens by thecal cells [40]. These effects are associated with induction of LH receptors, prevention of reduction of receptors for LH by LH, and potentiation of induction by LH of P-450_{C17} [20,41]. Thus, excessive insulin or IGF-1 could interfere with the normal process of desensitization. The recent finding that a 53-kDa IGF-1-binding protein, found in follicular fluid, is an inhibitor of the action of FSH [43] adds support to the concept that IGF-1 is involved in the regulation of ovarian function.

Another possibility is that P-450_{C17} is abnormally up-regulated, as could occur if the enzyme itself were intrinsically abnormal (perhaps with a mutation like that in the rat which would be associated with excessive 17-lyase activity) or if 17-lyase activity were up-regulated, perhaps because of "adrenal rest" tissue in the ovary, perhaps as in the adrenarchal adrenal cortex, by "adrenarche factor".

An increase in adrenal 17-lyase activity occurs during adrenarche (see Chapter 14), according to studies both *in vivo* and *in vitro* [44,45]. Adrenarche, the onset of secretion of 17-ketosteroids in response to adrenocorticotropic hormone (ACTH) which gradually develops peripubertally, is characterized in particular by an increase in formation of DHEA. Adrenarche requires a selective change in the expression of the 17-lyase activity of P-450_{C17}, 17-hydroxylase activity being required throughout life for the biosynthesis of cortisol. P-450_{C17} is encoded by the same gene in both the adrenal gland and the gonads, and it seems to be responsible for secretion of corticoid and sex hormones in humans [4,39]. In addition, the efficiency of 17-hydroxylase and 11β-hydroxylation seems to rise and that of 3β-hydroxysteroid dehydrogenase efficiency seems to fall during adrenarche [44–49]. Sulfokinase activity also increases [50]. The nature of the adrenarche factor(s) that regulate(s) these profound changes in activities of the adrenal steroidogenic enzymes, including P-450_{C17}, is unknown.

Increased responsiveness of adrenal 17-ketosteroids to ACTH is common in PCO. Since the steroidogenic abnormality in many hirsute women also includes evidence of increased 17-lyase activity, we previously termed this abnormality "exaggerated adrenarche" [51]. We subsequently hypothesized that the hyperandrogenic response to ACTH might be due to abnormal regulation of adrenocortical P-450_{C17}, analogous to the dysregulation of ovarian P-450_{C17}. In other words, abnormal regulation of P-450_{C17} function in both the adrenal cortex and the ovary might explain the hyperandrogenic function of both glands. We reviewed our data from patients with PCO retrospectively (patients being identified by dex-suppression test criteria), to test this hypothesis [3]. Patients with PCO were found to have significantly elevated responses to ACTH of levels of 17-PROG, AD, 17-hydroxypregnenolone, and DHEA. These responses to ACTH differed from those of women heterozygous for congenital adrenal hyperplasia due to 21-hydroxylase deficiency. These results are compatible with the hypothesis that coexistent ovarian and adrenal hyperresponsiveness to the respective tropic hormones is due to a similar type of hyperactive dysregulation of P-450_{C17} in the two glands, which leads both to secrete excessive levels of 17-ketosteroids. The exact site of the putative regulatory defect is by no means certain, nor is it clear whether such a defect would be at the level of gene expression of a steroid-binding site on the enzyme, a binding site for some regulatory substance, or a defect(s) in the production of factors that regulate enzymatic function at the transcriptional or translational levels or via allosteric effects.

If the hypothesis is correct that a similar type of dysregulation may coexist in the adrenals and ovaries of patients with PCO, some patients with abnormal responses in terms of levels of 17-PROG to nafarelin will have responses to ACTH compatible with dysregulation rather than enzyme deficiency. We have begun testing this hypothesis prospectively.

Among 20 successive women presenting to our clinics for evaluation of hyperandrogenism who have undergone both dex-prepared nafarelin and ACTH tests, 12 had an abnormal response in terms of levels of 17-PROG to nafarelin, which is typical of PCO (Fig. 9.6). In seven of these patients the response to ACTH was also abnormal (group I). The pattern of responses to ACTH of this group was then compared to that in normal women. These patients had significantly greater responses to ACTH in terms of levels of 17-hydroxypregnenolone, DHEA, and AD than did normal women (Fig. 9.7). Levels of 17-PROG were elevated to a lesser degree ($P < 0.1$), although elevated levels were prominent in our retrospective analysis of data from ACTH tests of women with PCO [3]. Cortisol responses were normal. Thus, the adrenal responds to

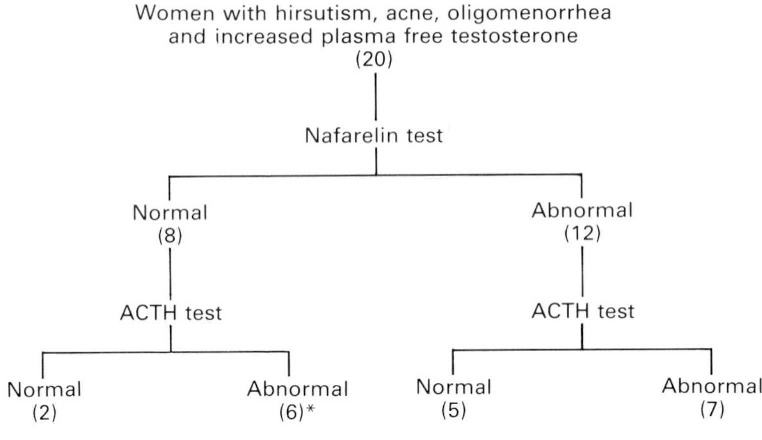

Fig. 9.6 Flow sheet showing the relationships among normal or abnormal responses to nafarelin and ACTH tests in 20 successive hyperandrogenic women. These women were 17–39 years of age, presented at our clinics for hirsutism, acne, or amenorrhea, and were found to have an elevated plasma concentration of free T (>10 pg/ml). Responsiveness to nafarelin was considered abnormal if peak levels of 17-PROG rose beyond 2 SD of normal values (>259 ng/dl) for volunteers 18–35 years of age in the follicular phase similarly pretreated with 2 mg of dexamethasone daily for 4 days (n = 11) without evidence of a steroidogenic block. Responsiveness to ACTH was considered abnormal if levels of two steroid intermediates rose beyond 2 SD of normal (n = 17). The asterisk indicates the one woman whose abnormal response to ACTH was typical of late-onset 21-hydroxylase deficiency.

ACTH with excessive secretion of 17-ketosteroids in a similar way to that in which the ovary responds to LH by excessive secretion of 17-ketosteroids. The pattern is compatible with overactivity of 17-lyase in both the Δ^5- and Δ^4-pathways, and 17-hydroxylase in the Δ^5-path, but not with a blockage of some enzymatic activity. This pattern of response to ACTH is compatible with abnormal regulation of 17-hydroxylase/lyase activities in the adrenal cortex, but it is not compatible with a block in steroidogenesis.

Six women with normal responses to nafarelin had abnormal responses to ACTH. All of these patients were normally dex-suppressible. One of these patients had late-onset congenital adrenal hyperplasia (level of 17-PROG 1 hour post-ACTH of 4756 ng/dl) and was excluded from further analysis. The ACTH test responses were otherwise abnormal in the other five patients with normal responses to nafarelin (group II). The pattern of steroidogenic responses to ACTH was similar in groups I and II (Fig. 9.7). These results are compatible with a regulatory

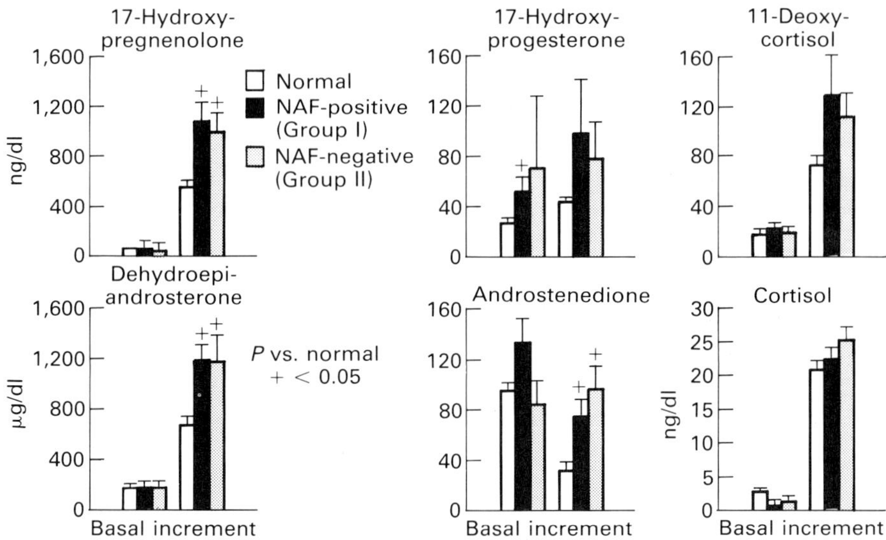

Fig. 9.7 Patterns of steroid levels before and after testing with ACTH in hyperandrogenic women with abnormal responses to ACTH. ACTH (10 μg/m^2) was administered i.v. at 0800, 8 hours after the administration of 1.5 mg of dexamethasone. The figure shows basal steroid levels (post-dex) and the mean of the incremental response (Δ) at 30 and 60 min after administration of ACTH. The group of normal women consisted of 17 volunteers at the early follicular phase, 19–40 years of age. The hyperandrogenic groups consist of women who had abnormal responses in terms of levels of two or more steroid intermediates 30–60 min after administration of ACTH, excluding the one patient found to have late-onset congenital adrenal hyperplasia. The hyperandrogenic patients are grouped according to whether they had a normal response to nafarelin testing (defined in the legend to Fig. 9.6), group I having an abnormal and group II having a normal response. It can be seen that the two hyperandrogenic groups had similar abnormal patterns of responses to ACTH. The most common patterns of abnormal responses to ACTH in these 12 cases were (i) both levels of Δ^5-steroids (17-hydroxypregnenolone and DHEA) and AD elevated ($n = 3$), (ii) levels of both Δ^5-steroids elevated alone ($n = 3$), and (iii) levels of AD plus 11-deoxycortisol elevated ($n = 2$). Levels of 17-PROG were elevated in two other patients, with elevations in levels of both DHEA and AD in one and with an elevation in the level of 11-deoxycortisol in the other. All *P*-values are two-tailed.

defect, not an enzyme deficiency, being the cause of most adrenal hyperandrogenism. The increased responsiveness of levels of 17-hydroxypregnenolone, DHEA, and AD resembles an exaggeration of adrenarche. This apparent dysregulation of adrenocortical steroidogenesis, causing hyperresponsiveness of levels of 17-ketosteroids to ACTH and affecting predominantly the Δ^5-pathway may thus occur alone or in conjunction with a similar regulatory abnormality in the ovary that affects predominantly the Δ^4-pathway.

Diagnostic implications of nafarelin testing

Twenty successive women presenting prospectively to our clinics for evaluation of hyperandrogenism have undergone both a dex-prepared nafarelin test and an ACTH test (Fig. 9.6). The relationship between the plasma level of free T after the dex-suppression test and the responses of levels of 17-PROG to nafarelin in these hyperandrogenic women are shown in Fig. 9.8. The high correlation ($r = 0.748$; $P < 0.001$) supports the concept that poor suppression of plasma levels of free T by dex and hyperresponsiveness of levels of 17-PROG to nafarelin are related manifestations of the same ovarian disorder. The relationship also indicates that there is a spectrum of severity of the disorder and that, in the mildest cases, results of one of the two tests may be slightly

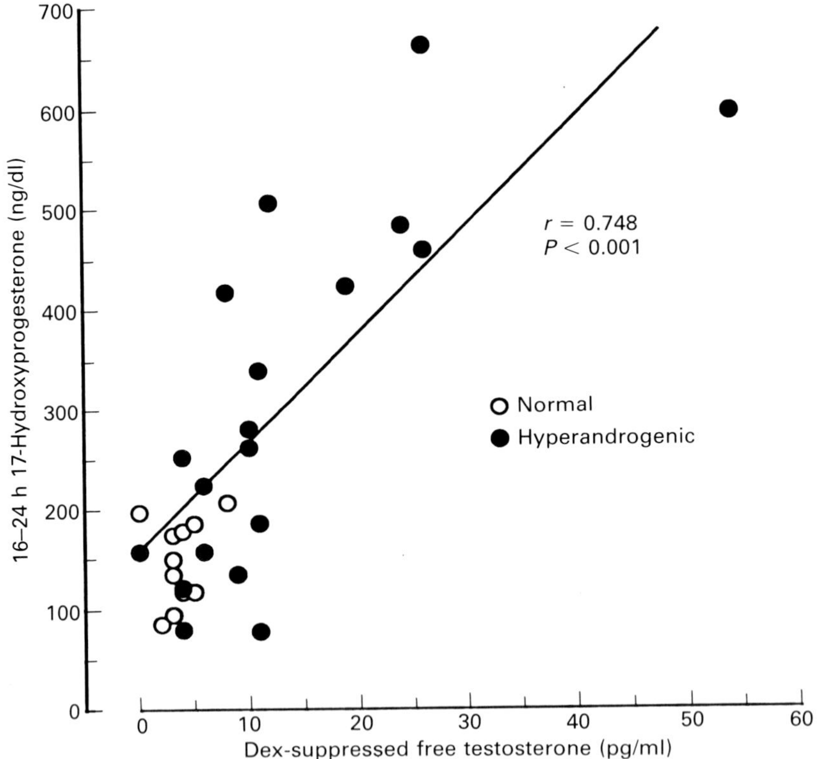

Fig. 9.8 Relationship in hyperandrogenic women between plasma levels of free testosterone after 4 days of dexamethasone (0.5 mg q.i.d.) and the response of levels of 17-PROG (16–24 hour mean) to nafarelin while dex was continued. The coefficient of correlation in hyperandrogenic women is 0.748, $P < 0.001$. Hyperandrogenic women (n = 19) and normal women in the follicular phase (n = 11) (identified in legend to Fig. 9.6).

abnormal while the other is normal. If values more than 2 SD away from values for the normal group are considered abnormal, 12 women had subnormal dex suppressibility (>7.6 pg/ml) and 12 had elevated levels of 17-PROG 16–24 hours postnafarelin (>233 ng/dl). Among the 12 women who met nafarelin test criteria for PCO, 11 also had ovarian hyperandrogenism as judged by criteria of the dex-suppression test. However, the two women with normal responses to both nafarelin and ACTH met dex-suppression test criteria for PCO. In other words, if one considers either nafarelin-test criteria or dex-suppression criteria to define ovarian hyperandrogenism, 14 of the 20 patients had this disorder; of these, 12 were detected by the nafarelin test and 13 were detected by the dex-suppression test, with each test failing to identify 1–2 cases. One of the six hyperandrogenic women with a normal response during dex-suppression testing had an abnormal response during nafarelin testing. These overall results suggest that the sensitivity and specificity of the dex-suppression test and the nafarelin test for ovarian hyperandrogenism are similar, approximating 85% in each case.

The relationship between the response of levels of 17-PROG to nafarelin and LH is less strong. Figure 9.9 shows that there is a weaker correlation between the baseline level of LH and responsiveness of levels of 17-PROG to nafarelin in the hyperandrogenic women ($r = 0.459$; $P < 0.05$). The correlation with the ratio of LH/FSH was similar ($r = 0.505$; $P < 0.05$). Although there is a strong correlation between baseline levels of LH and the mean level of LH 30–60 min after administration of nafarelin ($r = 0.729$; $P < 0.001$), the latter did not correlate with the response of levels of 17-PROG. The finding of normal levels of LH in some of the women with PCO suggests that their ovarian abnormality is intrinsic, i.e. independent of an excess of LH.

We have now extended our comparisons of ovarian responses to nafarelin in patients with PCO and normal female volunteers at the early follicular phase to a total of 18 normal women and 26 patients defined as having ovarian hyperandrogenism by dex-test criteria. A scattergram of peak response is shown in Fig. 9.10. It can be seen that 24 of 26 of these patients had responses in levels of 17-PROG to nafarelin greater than those found in normal women. This analysis suggests a vary small (<10%) overlap between this form of PCO and normality.

There is considerable disparity among endocrinologists when it comes to defining PCO. Many simply define their patients with PCO as hirsute and oligomenorrheic women [52,53]. Others add the criterion of hyperandrogenemia [54], elevation of the LH/FSH ratio [55], or polycystic ovaries [56]. Others require the full-blown syndrome [57,58].

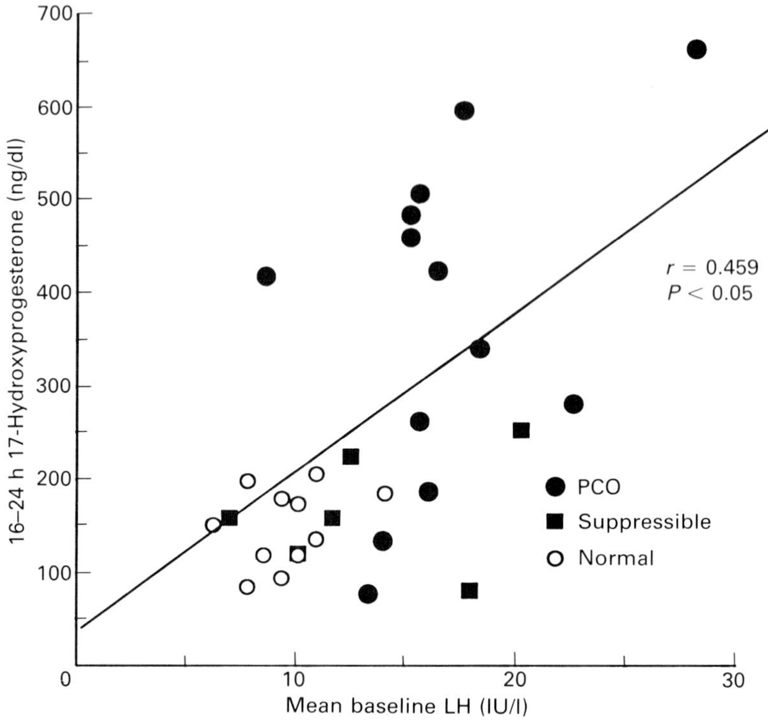

Fig. 9.9 Relationship in hyperandrogenic women between the mean baseline serum concentration of LH during the 1-hour period before the nafarelin test and the mean plasma concentration of 17-PROG 16–24 hours after administration of nafarelin. The same 19 hyperandrogenic and 11 normal women as described in Figs 9.6 and 9.8 were analyzed. Coefficient of correlation = 0.459, $P < 0.05$. However, there is no correlation between these variables within either subgroup of hyperandrogenic women classified by dex-suppression criteria (PCO, abnormal dex-suppression test; suppressible, normal dex-suppression test).

We have previously introduced dex-suppression criteria [59] and we now introduce nafarelin-test criteria.

The discussions during this workshop suggested that the vast majority of investigators in this field agree only upon three empirical criteria for the diagnosis of PCO. These are (i) a complex of symptoms and signs (hirsutism, acne, or anovulatory symptoms), (ii) laboratory documentation of hyperandrogenemia, and (iii) sufficient studies to exclude late-onset congenital adrenal hyperplasia, Cushing's syndrome, prolactinomas, and virilizing tumors (and other rare disorders that may resemble PCO but which have distinct pathogenetic, therapeutic, and prognostic implications). We suspect that different forms of the syndrome will be delineated in women with pure ovarian hyperandro-

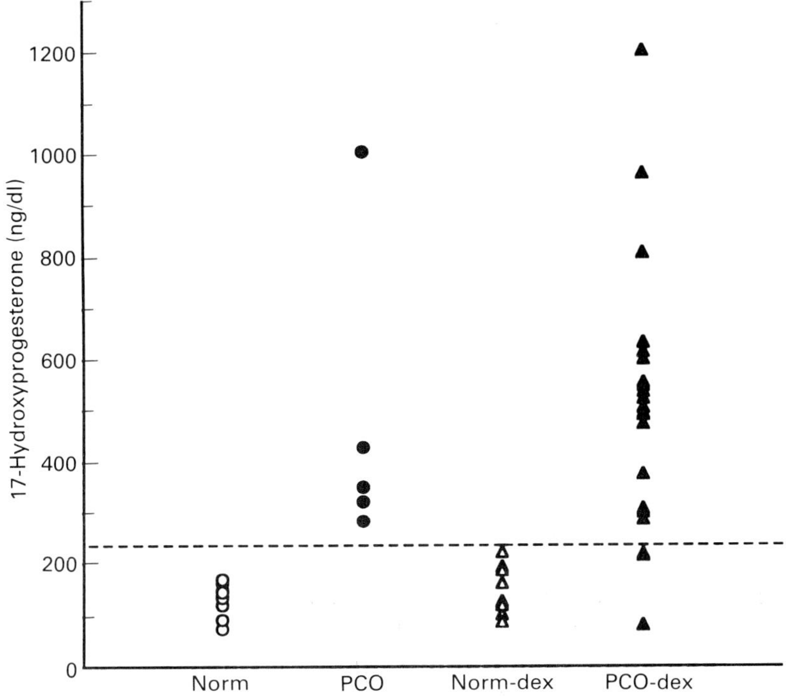

Fig. 9.10 Scattergram showing peak plasma levels of 17-PROG after administration of nafarelin to normal woman in the follicular phase and to subjects with PCO. Nafarelin tests were performed (a) without dex-pretreatment in 7 normal women (Norm) and in 5 women with PCO and (b) after dex-pretreatment in another 11 normal women (NORM-dex) and 21 women with PCO (PCO-dex). The dotted line shows the upper observed limit of the range of peak levels of 17-PROG (224 ng/dl). It can be seen that, among the total of 26 patients with PCO, responses in 24 are above the observed range of responses in the 18 normal volunteers.

Fig. 9.11 Relative roles of the ovary and adrenal in the etiology of hyperandrogenism in women. Our data (Fig. 9.6) suggest that overproduction of androgen in hyperandrogenic women is of ovarian origin in about two-thirds of cases and adrenal origin in about two-thirds (with an overlap that results in mixed ovarian–adrenal origin in about one-third).

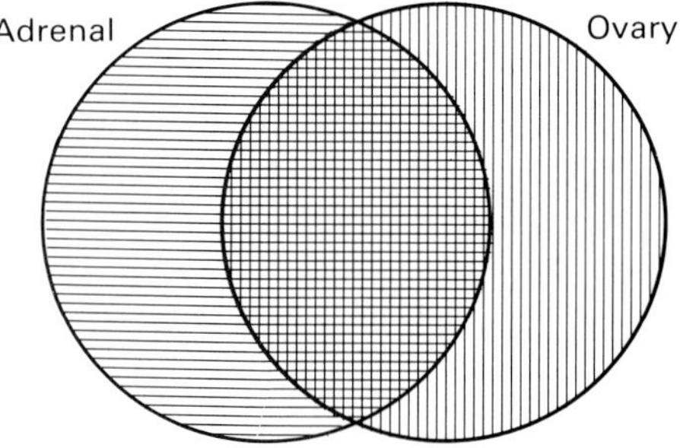

genism (as defined by the nafarelin test), those with pure adrenal hyperandrogenism (as defined by the ACTH test), and in those with mixed ovarian–adrenal hyperandrogenism (Fig. 9.11).

Summary

Polycystic ovary syndrome is here equated with functional ovarian hyperandrogenism, characterized by 17-PROG and AD hyperresponsiveness to a GnRH agonist (nafarelin) test. The proximate cause typically seems to be hyperresponsiveness to LH stimulation of thecal cell 17-hydroxylase activity, with stimulated but relatively inefficient 17-lyase activity, rather than enzyme deficiency. Both of these activities appear to reside on the single androgen-forming enzyme cytochrome P-450_{C17}. The pattern of regulation of these two enzyme activities suggests that the P-450_{C17} of PCO ovaries functions in an excessively stimulated, yet partially down-regulated, state. We postulate that abnormal regulation (dysregulation) of P-450_{C17} activities is the proximate cause of most PCO and may arise either via excessive stimulation by LH or via escape from desensitization to LH. The latter situation may result from an intrinsic intraovarian flaw in the paracrine feedback mechanism by which ovarian androgen and estrogen biosynthesis are coordinated.

Coexistent adrenal 17-ketosteroid hyperresponsiveness to ACTH may be due to a similar type of dysregulation of adrenocortical P-450_{C17}. This theory of abnormal regulation of P-450_{C17} provides a unifying concept that may explain the occurrence of PCO in association with states of elevated or normal LH, adrenal androgenic hyperfunction, and hyperinsulinemia.

To explore the possible utility of nafarelin as a diagnostic test, we prospectively studied 20 successive women who presented to our clinics with hyperandrogenism. Nafarelin and dex-suppression test results correlated strongly ($r = 0.748$; $P < 0.001$). This indicates that both tests reflect related manifestations of ovarian dysfunction. Fourteen women met criteria for ovarian hyperandrogenism by dex or nafarelin test criteria, with each test being abnormal in 12–13 of the 14. Thus, there was approximately 85% correspondence between the tests. These results indicate that ovarian hyperandrogenism is present in about two-thirds of hyperandrogenic women.

Acknowledgments

The authors research was supported in part by USPHS grants HD-06308, RR-00055 and Syntex Research.

References

1 Barnes RB, Rosenfield RL. Polycystic ovary syndrome: pathogenesis and treatment. Ann Intern Med 1989; 110:386–9.
2 Barnes RB, Rosenfield RL, Burstein S, Ehrmann DA. Pituitary–ovarian responses to nafarelin testing in the polycystic ovary syndrome. N Engl J Med 1989; 320:559–65.
3 Rosenfield RL, Barnes RB, Cara JF, Lucky AW. Dysregulation of cytochrome $P450_{C17\alpha}$ as the cause of polycystic ovary syndrome. Fertil Steril 1990; 53:785–91.
4 Miller WL. Molecular biology of steroid hormone synthesis. Endocr Rev 1988; 9:295–318.
5 Voutilainen R, Tapanainen J, Chung B-C, Matteson KJ, Miller WL. Hormonal regulation of $P450_{scc}$ (20,22-desmolase) and $P450_{C17\alpha}$ (17α-hydroxylase/17,20-lyase) in cultured human granulosa cells. J Clin Endocrinol Metab 1986; 63:202–7.
6 Dufau MO, Winters CA, Hattori M, *et al.* Hormonal regulation of androgen production by the Leydig cell. J Steroid Biochem 1984; 20:161–73.
7 Anakwe OO, Payne AH. Noncoordinate regulation of *de novo* synthesis of cytochrome P-450 cholesterol side-chain cleavage and cytochrome P-450 17α-hydroxylase/C17–20 lyase in mouse Leydig cell cultures: relation to steroid production. Mol Endocrinol 1987; 1:595–603.
8 Malaska T, Payne AH. Luteinizing hormone and cyclic AMP-mediated induction of microsomal cytochrome P-450 enzymes in cultured mouse Leydig cells. J Biol Chem 1984; 259:11654–7.
9 Quinn PG, Payne AH. Steroid product-induced, oxygen-mediated damage of microsomal cytochrome P-450 enzymes in Leydig cell cultures. J Biol Chem 1985; 260: 2092–9.
10 Zipf W, Payne AH, Kelch RP. Dissociation of lutropin-induced loss of testicular lutropin receptors and lutropin-induced desensitization of testosterone synthesis. Biochim Biophys Acta 1978; 540:330–6.
11 Hales DB, Sha L, Payne AH. Testosterone inhibits cAMP-induced *de novo* synthesis of Leydig cell cytochrome $P\text{-}450_{17\alpha}$ by an androgen receptor-mediated mechanism. J Biol Chem 1987; 262:11200–6.
12 Rani CSS, Payne AH. Adenosine 3′,5′-monophosphate-mediated induction of 17α-hydroxylase and C_{17-20} lyase activities in cultured mouse Leydig cells is enhanced by inhibition of steroid biosynthesis. Endocrinology 1986; 118:1222–8.
13 Brinkmann A, Leemborg I, Rommarts F, van der Molen H. Translocation of the testicular estradiol receptor is not an obligatory step in the gonadotropin-induced inhibition of C-17,20-lyase. Endocrinology 1982; 110:1834–6.
14 Adashi EY, Hsueh AHW. Autoregulation of androgen production in a primary culture of rat testicular cells. Nature 1981; 293:737–8.
15 Richards JS, Hedin L. Molecular aspects of hormone action in ovarian follicular development, ovulation, and luteinization. Ann Rev Physiol 1988; 50:441–63.
16 Magoffin DA. Evidence that luteinizing hormone-stimulated differentiation of purified ovarian thecal-interstitial cells is mediated by both type I and type II adenosine 3′, 5′-monophosphate-dependent protein kinases. Endocrinology 1989; 125:1464–73.
17 Erickson GF, Magoffin DA, Dyer CA, Hofeditz C. The ovarian androgen-producing cells: a review of structure/function relationships. Endocr Rev 1985; 6:371–99.
18 Lamprecht SA, Zor U, Salomon Y, Koch Y, Ahern K, Lindner H. Mechanism of hormonally induced refractoriness of ovarian adenylate cyclase to luteinizing hormone and prostaglandin E. J Cyclic Nucl Res 1977; 3:69–76.
19 Eckstein B, Greenbaum O, Cohen S. Kinetic studies on ovarian C-17,20-lyase activity: effect of luteinizing hormone surge. Endocrinology 1985; 117:2376–82.
20 Cara JF, Fan J, Azzarello J, Rosenfield RL. Insulin-like growth factor-I enhances LH binding to rat ovarian theca-interstitial cells. J Clin Invest 1990; 86:560–5.
21 Smals AGH, Pieters GFFM, Lozekoot DC, Benraad TJ, Kloppenborg PWC. Dissociated

responses of plasma testosterone and 17-hydroxypregnenolone to single or repeated human chorionic gonadotropin administration in normal men. J Clin Endocrinol Metab 1980; 50:190–3.

22 Smals AGH, Kloppenborg PWC, Pieters GFFM, Losekoot DC, Benraad TJ. Basal and human chorionic gonadotropin-stimulated 17α-hydroxyprogesterone and testosterone levels in Klinefelter's syndrome. J Clin Endocrinol Metab 1978; 47:1144–7.

23 Forest MG, Lecoq A, Saez JM. Kinetics of human chorionic gonadotropin-induced steroidogenic response of the human testis. II. Plasma 17α-hydroxyprogesterone, Δ4-androstenedione, estrone and 17β-estradiol: evidence for the action of human chorionic gonadotropin on intermediate enzymes implicated in steroid biosynthesis. J Clin Endocrinol Metab 1979; 49:284–91.

24 Jones TM, Fang VS, Landau RL, Rosenfield RL. Direct inhibition of Leydig cell function by estradiol. J Clin Endocrinol Metab 1978; 47:1368–73.

25 Smals AGH, Pieters GFFM, Drayer JIM, Boers GHJ, Benraad THJ, Kloppenborg PWC. Tamoxifen suppresses gonadotropin-induced 17α-hydroxyprogesterone accumulation in normal men. J Clin Endocrinol Metab 1980; 51:1026–9.

26 Jones TM, Fang VS, Landau RL, Rosenfield RL. The effects of fluoxymesterone administration on testicular function. J Clin Endocrinol Metab 1977; 44:121–9.

27 Abraham GE. Ovarian and adrenal contributions to peripheral androgens during the menstrual cycle. J Clin Endocrinol Metab 1974; 39:340–6.

28 Rosenfield RL, Ehrlich EN, Cleary RE. Adrenal and ovarian contributions to the elevated free plasma androgen levels in hirsute women. J Clin Endocrinol 1972; 34:92–8.

29 Rajaniemi HJ, Ronnberg L, Kauppila A, Yostalo P, Vihko R. Luteinizing hormone receptors in ovarian follicles of patients with polycystic ovarian disease. J Clin Endocrinol Metab 1980; 51:1054–7.

30 McAllister JM, Kerin JFP, Trant JM, *et al.* Regulation of cholesterol side-chain cleavage and 17α-hydroxylase/lyase activities in proliferating human theca interna cells in long-term monolayer culture. Endocrinology 1989; 125:1959–66.

31 Chasalow F, Marr H, Haour F, Saez JM. Testicular steroidogenesis after human chorionic gonadotropin desensitization in rats. J Biol Chem 1979; 254:5613–17.

32 Onoda M, Hall PF. Inhibition of testicular microsomal cytochrome P-450 (17α-hydroxylase/C-17,20-lyase) by estrogens. Endocrinology 1981; 109:763–7.

33 Hild-Petito S, Stouffer RL, Brenner RM. Immunocytochemical localization of estradiol and progesterone receptors in the monkey ovary throughout the menstrual cycle. Endocrinology 1988; 123:2896–905.

34 Zuber MX, Simpson ER, Waterman MR. Expression of bovine 17α-hydroxylase cytochrome P-450 cDNA in nonsteroidogenic (COS 1) cells. Science 1986; 234:1258–61.

35 Fevold HR, Lorence MC, McCarthy JL, *et al.* Rat $P450_{17\alpha}$ from testis: characterization of a full-length cDNA encoding a unique steroid hydroxylase capable of catalyzing both Δ^4- and Δ^5-steroid-17,20-lyase reactions. Mol Endocrinol 1989; 3:968–75.

36 Estabrook RW, Mason JI, Martin-Wixtrom C, Zuber M, Waterman MR. Some enzymatic vagaries of a bovine adrenal microsomal cytochrome P-450 introduced and expressed in transformed monkey kidney cells. Prog Clin Biol Res 1988; 274:525–40.

37 Axelrod LR, Goldzieher JW. The polycystic ovary. III. Steroid biosynthesis in normal and polycystic ovarian tissue. J Clin Endocrinol 1962; 22:431–40.

38 Dorfman RI, Forchielli E, Gut M. Androgen biosynthesis and related studies. Recent Prog Horm Res 1963; 19:251–73.

39 Yanase T, Sanders D, Shibata A, Matsui N, Simpson ER, Waterman MR. Combined 17α-hydroxylase/17,20-lyase deficiency due to a 7-basepair duplication in the N-terminal region of the cyctochrome $P450c_{17\alpha}$ (CYP17) gene. J Clin Endocrinol Metab 1990; 70:1325–9.

40 Cara JF, Rosenfield RL. Insulin-like growth factor I and insulin potentiate luteinizing hormone-induced androgen synthesis by rat ovarian thecal-interstitial cells. Endocrinology 1988; 123:733–9.
41 Magoffin DA, Kurtz KM, Erickson GF. Insulin-like growth factor I selectively stimulates cholesterol side-chain cleavage expression in ovarian theca-interstitial cells. Mol Endocrinol 1990; 4:489–96.
42 Hillier S, Ross GT. Effects of exogenous testosterone on ovarian weight, follicular morphology and intraovarian progesterone concentration in estrogen-primed hypophysectomized immature female rats. Biol Reprod 1979; 20:261–8.
43 Shimasaki S, Shimonaka M, Ui M, Inouye S, Shibata F, Ling N. Structural characterization of a follicle-stimulating hormone action inhibitor in porcine ovarian follicular fluid. J Biol Chem 1990; 265:2198–202.
44 Rich BH, Rosenfield RL, Lucky AW, *et al.* Adrenarche: changing adrenal response to ACTH. J Clin Endocrinol Metab 1981; 52:1129–36.
45 Schiebinger RJ, Albertson BD, Cassorla FG, *et al.* The developmental changes in plasma adrenal androgens during infancy and adrenarche are associated with changing activities of adrenal microsomal 17-hydroxylase and 17,20-desmolase. J Clin Invest 1981; 67:1177–82.
46 Byrne GC, Perry YS, Winter JSD. Kinetic analysis of adrenal 3β-hydroxysteroid dehydrogenase activity during human development. J Clin Endocrinol Metab 1985; 60:934–9.
47 Dickerman Z, Grant DR, Faiman C, Winter JSD. Intraadrenal steroid concentrations in man: zonal differences and developmental changes. J Clin Endocrinol Metab 1984; 59:1031–6.
48 Cavallero C, Chiappino G. Histochemistry of steroid-3β-ol dehydrogenase in the human adrenal cortex. Experientia 1972; 15:119–20.
49 Dawson IMP, Pryse-Davies J, Snape IM. The distribution of six enzyme systems and of lipid in the human and rat adrenal cortex before and after administration of steroid and ACTH, with comments on the distribution in human foetuses and in some natural disease conditions. J Path Bact 1961; 81:181–95.
50 Kennerson AR, McDonald DA, Adams JB. Dehydroepiandrosterone sulfotransferase localization in human adrenal glands: a light and electron microscopic study. J Clin Endocrinol Metab 1983; 56:786–90.
51 Lucky AW, Rosenfield RL, McGuire J, Rudy S, Helke J. Adrenal androgen hyperresponsiveness to adrenocorticortropin in women with acne and/or hirsutism: adrenal enzyme defects and exaggerated adrenarche. J Clin Endocrinol Metab 1986; 62:840–8.
52 Chang RJ, Nakamura RM, Judd HL, Kaplan SA. Insulin resistance in nonobese patients with polycystic ovary syndrome. J Clin Endocrinol Metab 1983; 57:356–9.
53 Stewart PM, Beastall GM, Shackleton CHI, Edwards CRE. 5α-Reductase activity in polycystic ovary syndrome. Lancet 1990; i:431–3.
54 Dunaif A, Segal KR, Futterweit W, Dobrjansky A. Profound peripheral insulin resistance, independent of obesity, in polycystic ovary syndrome. Diabetes 1989; 38:1165–74.
55 Jialal I, Naiker P, Reddi K, Moodley J, Joubert SM. Evidence for insulin resistance in nonobese patients with polycystic ovarian disease. J Clin Endocrinol Metab 1987; 64:1066–9.
56 Conway GS, Honour JW, Jacobs HS. Heterogeneity of the polycystic ovary syndrome. Clin Endocrinol 1989; 30:459–70.
57 Lobo RA. The role of the adrenal in polycystic ovary syndrome. Semin Reprod Endocrinol 1984; 2:251–62.
58 Waldstreicher J, Santoro NF, Hall JE, Filicori M, Crowley WF Jr. Hyperfunction of the hypothalamic–pituitary axis in women with polycystic ovarian disease: indirect

evidence for partial gonadotroph desensitization. J Clin Endocrinol Metab 1988; 66:165–72.

59 Hatch, R, Rosenfield RL, Kim MH, Tredway D. Hirsutism: implications, etiology, and management. Am J Obstet Gynecol 1981; 140:815–30.

Chapter 10
Folliculogenesis in Polycystic Ovary Syndrome

GREGORY F. ERICKSON

Statement of the problem

Under normal conditions, women produce a single dominant follicle that participates in a single ovulation in each menstrual cycle [1]. This event occurs primarily as a result of two interrelated processes: recruitment (the initiation of primordial follicle growth for the purpose of replenishing the ovaries with a new cohort of developing follicles), and selection (the singling out of one follicle in a cohort to become dominant). In women with polycystic ovary syndrome (PCO), this process does not proceed normally [2,3]. The initial steps in folliculogenesis, namely recruitment and growth to the small antral stages, seem intact in PCO, but the next step, selection of dominant preovulatory follicles, is lacking [4]. This phenomenon leads to an accumulation of large numbers of small Graafian follicles (commonly referred to as cysts) in the ovaries of women with PCO [4–6]. It is easy to see what happens in PCO because the changes are macroscopic; it is less clear how the changes occur. In this chapter, we will examine the course of follicular development in PCO and consider some questions that pertain to the mechanism whereby the development of follicles is arrested.

Normal folliculogenesis

Follicular growth and development in normal women is a very long process [7]. In each cycle, the preovulatory follicle originates from a primordial follicle that was recruited to grow approximately one year earlier (Fig. 10.1). It seems that selection is the last step in this long sequence of events. The actual decision to select the dominant follicle is made at the end of the luteal phase of the preceding menstrual cycle. At this time, each ovary contains a group of small, rapidly growing follicles,

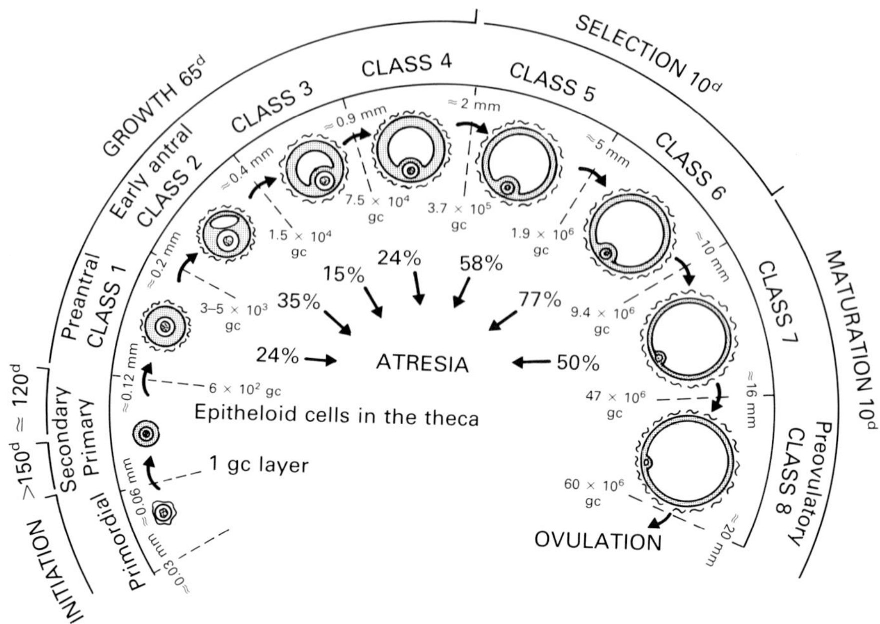

Fig. 10.1 The temporal pattern of folliculogenesis in normal human ovaries. The rates (days = d) and stages (classes 1 to 8) of folliculogenesis and the level of atresia (%) in the eight follicle classes are shown. The number of granulosa cells (gc) and the diameters of corresponding follicle are indicated. (Reprinted with permission of Oxford University Press from Gougeon [7].)

2–5 mm in diameter: it is from this pool that the follicle destined to ovulate in the next cycle is selected (Fig. 10.2). Initially, the chosen follicle is visibly defined only by its size. However, after it reaches 6–8 mm in diameter in the early follicular phase, the mitotic activities in the granulosa and theca cells increase considerably. This sustained capacity for rapid growth and cell division is the difference between the dominant and nondominant follicles: the consequence of the loss of growth potential in nondominant follicles is death by atresia.

At the time of selection, the dominant follicle is a beautifully constructed mass of precisely shaped, precisely located smooth muscle (theca externa), steroidogenic and connective tissue (theca interna) and granulosa cells, all of which form an assemblage around the egg (Fig. 10.3). At this time, the chosen follicle has about one million granulosa and about one million theca interstitial cells [8,9]. These tissues consist of four to six layers of cells, which appear to be dividing rapidly with virtually no evidence of pycnosis. A thin basal lamina, composed of type IV collagen, laminin, and fibronectin, lies between the theca and granulosa cells.

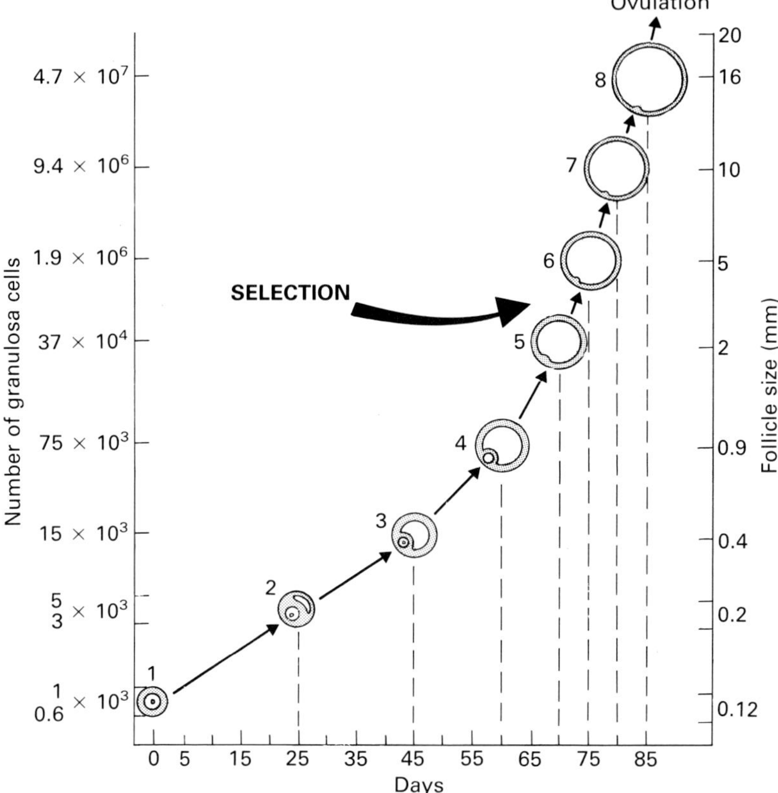

Fig. 10.2 The dominant follicle is selected from a cohort of follicles at stage 5–6 on day 1 of the menstrual cycle. (Modified with permission from Gougeon [7].)

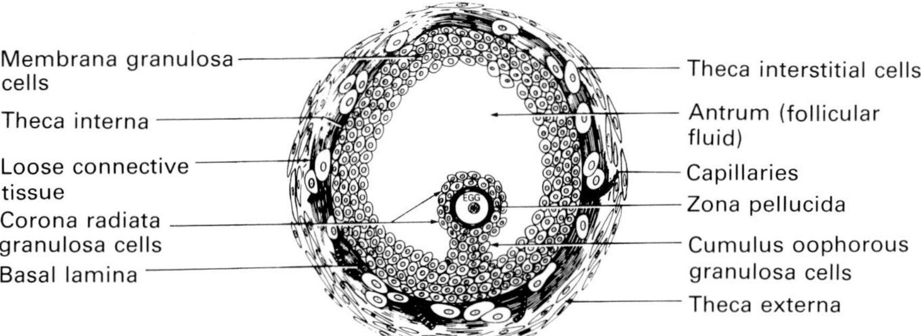

Fig. 10.3 Diagrammatic representation of the histology of a normal healthy human Graafian follicle (4–8 mm in diameter) at the time of selection.

Folliculogenesis in PCO

If one considers that it takes about one year for a human preovulatory follicle to complete its differentiation, it becomes apparent that the errors in folliculogenesis in PCO may reflect a progressive deterioration over a long period of time. What do we know about the pattern of folliculogenesis in PCO?

Evidence suggests the existence of increased numbers of developing follicles in PCO ovaries. In a classical study, Hughesdon [10] found that the number of primordial follicles in polycystic ovaries was within the normal range; however, the number of growing follicles at each stage of development (primary, secondary, tertiary and early Graafian) was about double the normal number in the polycystic ovaries. This hints that the process of folliculogenesis may be aberrant in PCO. How might the number of growing follicles increase in PCO? There are basically two ways in which a build-up of the pool of growing follicles can be achieved: (i) increased recruitment and (ii) decreased atresia. Since the total number of primordial follicles is normal in PCO, we can presume that the increase is not caused by a greater rate of recruitment. Therefore, it is likely that some type of regulatory process acts directly or indirectly on the pool of growing follicles in PCO ovaries to decrease the rate of atresia. This hypothesis provides a reasonable explanation for the phenomenon of follicle build-up in PCO, an event that is clearly abnormal. As seen in Fig. 10.4, the most dramatic consequence of this aberrant process is the accumulation of 20–100 small Graafian follicles in each polycystic ovary [5]. One major question to arise out of this characterization is whether the cohorts of follicles, 4–7 mm in diameter, in polycystic ovaries are normal. The answer to this question requires a comparison between the cell populations in the PCO follicle with the normal population (Fig. 10.3). In the following paragraphs, we will briefly consider the evidence that is available to answer this question. We shall begin with a discussion of the granulosa cells.

Granulosa cells

Mitosis

With regard to structure, one particularly striking difference between the normal and PCO small Graafian follicle is that there is a paucity of follicular granulosa cells in PCO (Fig. 10.5). This difference suggests that PCO granulosa cells have a markedly reduced capacity to proliferate. This raises the question of whether atresia is related to the reduced proliferation of PCO granulosa cells.

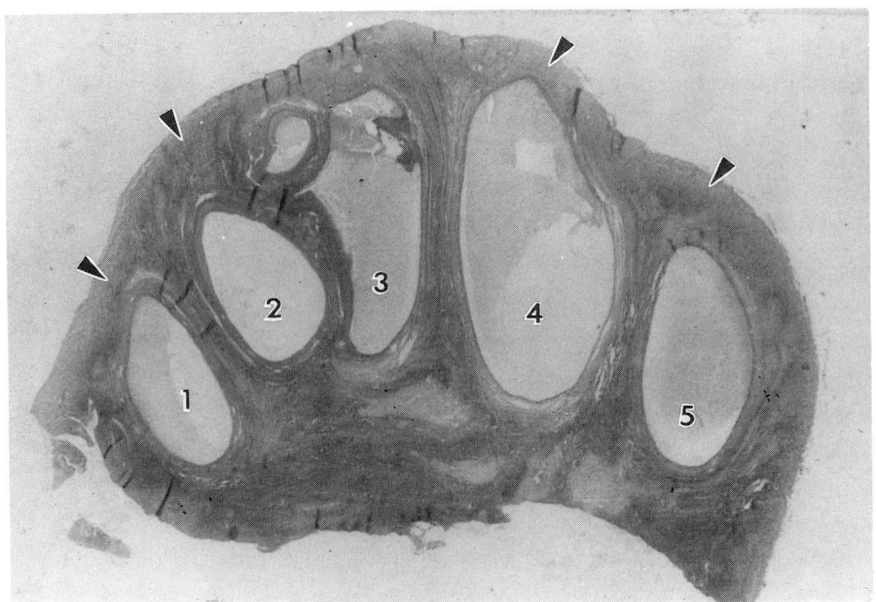

Fig. 10.4 Cross-section of a Stein–Leventhal type of polycystic ovary showing five Graafian follicles, the development of which have been arrested at the small-antral stage (4–7 mm in diameter). Arrowheads show capsular fibrosis.

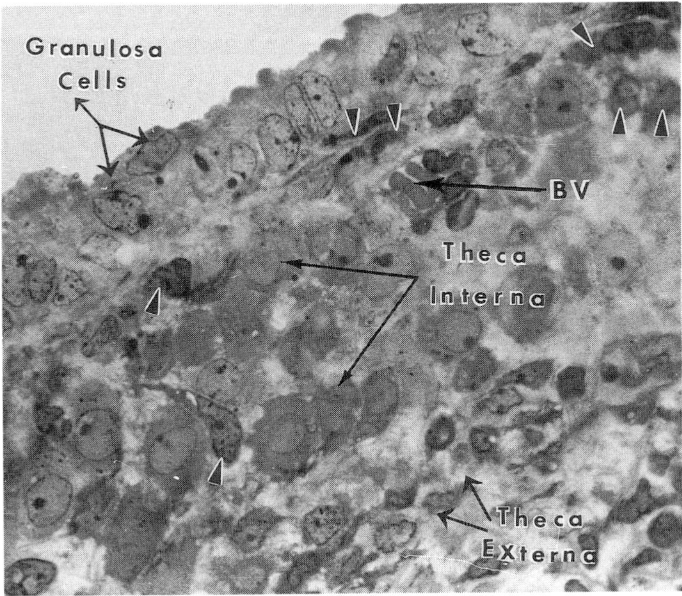

Fig. 10.5 Photograph of section through the wall of a typical PCO follicle arrested at the small-antral stage. There is a single layer of granulosa cells, none of which is dividing. Cell death in the granulosa is not obvious. The theca interna contains numerous fibroblasts (arrowheads), blood vessels (BV), and four to five layers of hypertrophied theca interstitial cells. The theca externa appears poorly developed.

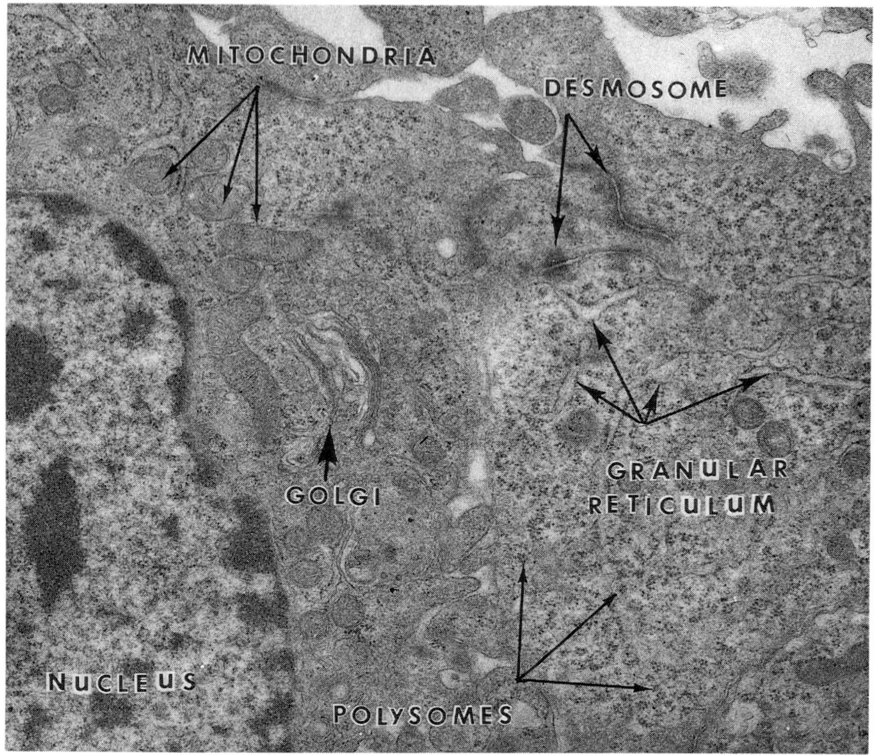

Fig. 10.6 Electron micrograph of granulosa cells of a small PCO follicle (4–7 mm in diameter). Note the well-developed Golgi complex and numerous polysomes. The mitochondria have tubular cristae. The endoplasmic reticulum is the granular type but no agranular reticulum is evident. Desmosomes but no gap junctions are seen.

If one looks closely (Fig. 10.5), there is no evidence of pycnosis (one marker of atresia) or mitosis in the PCO granulosa cells. Indeed, if one examines the ultrastructure of PCO granulosa cells, they appear quite healthy (Fig. 10.6); however, there are some structural features that differ from normal. First, the PCO granulosa cells show an unusual abundance of polysomes. What could this imply? One possibility is that there is aberrant expression of protein production in PCO granulosa cells. Further investigation of this could reveal the absence and/or presence of regulatory proteins that could contribute to the cessation of mitosis. Such aberrant protein expression could also lead to disturbed hormonal production, variation in receptor expression, or receptor function. This is an important area for future investigation. Second, no gap junctions appear between the PCO granulosa cells (Fig. 10.6).

The failure to develop these important intercellular junctions is clearly abnormal and could lead to altered responses of PCO granulosa cells to hormones and growth factors. As such, this could contribute to the paucity of granulosa cells in PCO.

The absence of granulosa cell death supports the theory developed earlier that the PCO follicles may not be atretic in the true sense of the word. This observation suggests that the paucity of PCO granulosa cells occurs primarily as a result of decreased rates of proliferaton as opposed to increased cell death. This leads to the theory that the cessation of mitosis contributes to the lack of follicle selection in PCO. The key question concerns the way in which mitosis is normally controlled in human granulosa cells. Two mitogens, fibroblast growth factor (FGF) and epidermal growth factor (EGF), have been observed to stimulate mitosis in human granulosa cells *in vitro* [11]. Based on this evidence, one explanation for the postmitotic state of PCO granulosa cells is that they are not being stimulated by mitogens, possibly as a result of the failure to synthesize and/or respond to particular growth factors. Remarkably, this situation can be corrected by the administration of a single hormone, follicle-stimulating hormone (FSH), to PCO patients [12]. This result tells us that, under physiologic conditions, FSH may be totally responsible for the stimulation of mitosis in human granulosa cells. Whether this effect of FSH is direct or whether it is controlled indirectly by the production of regulatory molecules, such as growth factors, is unknown. Regardless of the mechanisms, the evidence strongly suggests there is insufficient FSH stimulation in the PCO follicle to support the proliferation of granulosa cells.

It should be mentioned that several lines of evidence indicate that premature entry of luteinizing hormone (LH) into the microenvironment perturbs the selection process in women. Typically, when a dominant follicle is growing, LH is normally excluded from entry into the antral fluid until late in the follicular phase [8]. The significance of keeping LH out of the microenvironment is emphasized by the facts that (i) when LH enters the follicular fluid, granulosa cell mitosis is arrested [13], and (ii) if levels of circulating LH/human chorionic gonadotropin (HCG) are prematurely elevated in the midfollicular phase, development of the dominant follicle is arrested [13–15]. Whether or not the high levels of LH in the blood of women with PCO actually make their way into the follicular fluid is unknown. But, if they do, it seems logical that the PCO granulosa cells could respond to the high level of LH in the follicular fluid by becoming postmitotic. This theory of the contribution of LH to disturbed mitosis in PCO cells needs to be explored.

Control by gonadotropins of P-450$_{aromatase}$ activity

The single most important step in selection of a follicle occurs when one follicle in the cohort acquires the unique capacity to synthesize very large quantities of estradiol (E_2). This process occurs according to the "Two-cell Two-Gonadotropin Principle" (Fig. 10.7). The basis of this

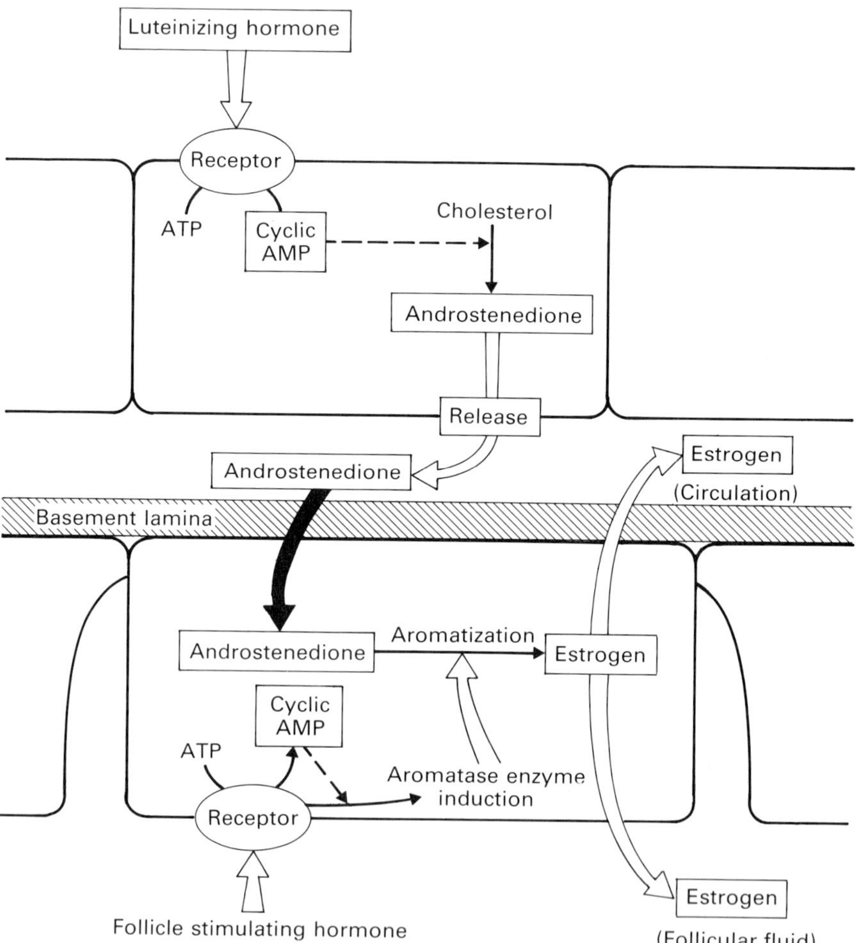

Fig. 10.7 The "Two-cell Two-Gonadotropin Principle" of follicular estrogen biosynthesis. (Reprinted with permission from Erickson GF. Normal ovarian function. Clin Obstet Gynecol 1978; 21:31–52.)

principle is as follows: in response to LH, the theca interstitial cells synthesize and secrete androstenedione (Δ^4A), which diffuses across the basal lamina into the granulosa cells where it is aromatized to E_2 in response to stimulation by FSH. The newly synthesized E_2 is released into both the follicular fluid and the peripheral circulation where it creates a permissive estrogenic microenvironment. As E_2 blood levels rise, the activities of the gonadotropins (FSH and LH) follow a predictable pattern that ultimately causes ovulation at mid cycle [1].

Questions related to this principle are of particular interest to those of us who study PCO because the selection process does not occur and hence the PCO follicle produces very little E_2. To what extent are the theca interstitial cells responsible for the absence of E_2 production by the PCO follicle? If we examine the microenvironment of PCO follicles (Table 10.1), we find very high levels of Δ^4A that are in the normal range. We can conclude, therefore, that there is no deficiency in the ability of LH to stimulate the synthesis of Δ^4A by the PCO theca cells. Thus, we are led to the conclusion that P-$450_{aromatase}$ (P-450_{arom}) is dysfunctional in the PCO follicle. With regard to this issue, there are several possible explanations to account for the limited ability of PCO granulosa cells to aromatize Δ^4A to E_2: (i) an insufficient level of FSH in the microenvironment; (ii) absence of an active signaling system for FSH receptors; (iii) the presence of an FSH inhibitor; and (iv) the presence of a P-450_{arom} inhibitor.

The first of these explanations seems to be unlikely. As recently measured by bioassay [16], PCO follicular fluid seems to contain as much FSH as that found in the normal dominant follicle (Table 10.1). With respect to the second explanation, we know from experiments *in vitro* that FSH produces striking increases in P-450_{arom} activity in PCO granulosa cells, increases that are equal to or greater than those obtained with normal granulosa cells from a size-matched dominant follicle [16,17]. Furthermore, PCO granulosa cells are exquisitely sensitive to FSH; their sensitivity has been found to be five times greater than that of normal cells [16,17]. These results indicate that PCO granulosa cells contain a highly active FSH signaling system, which is able to bring about significant increases in P-450_{arom} activity.

The high level of FSH in the PCO follicle, together with the evidence that FSH can induce maximal P-450_{arom} in PCO granulosa cells *in vitro*, suggests some type of inhibitor must be involved, one that might block FSH signal transmission and/or block the activity of the P-450_{arom} enzyme itself. The theory that there is an FSH inhibitor may have significant validity because it would effectively explain how the differentiation of PCO granulosa cells is blocked in the presence of high levels of FSH activity in the follicular fluid and a highly active FSH receptor and signal transmission system. The classic concept of FSH inhibitors in follicular fluid [18] has recently received new support from the results of studies *in vitro*. It has been reported [19] that the FSH induction of P-450_{arom} in rat granulosa cells can be blocked by a protein that is present in porcine follicular fluid. The FSH inhibitor proved to be the porcine congener of the human growth hormone-dependent insulin-like growth factor-binding protein (IGFBP-3) [20]. The questions that now require an answer are: Does this IGFBP-3 have the same inhibitory effect in human granulosa cells, and what is the relationship between IGFBP-3 and PCO? With regard to a putative aromatase inhibitor, a potentially important molecule to consider is dihydrotestosterone (DHT). In normal healthy and atretic human follicles [21], it has been shown that DHT is present, but the concentrations tend to be low (Table 10.1). If we consider that DHT is capable of blocking P-450_{arom} activity, it becomes apparent that, if high levels of DHT were present in PCO follicles, they would inhibit the synthesis of E_2. This issue needs to be resolved.

Control by growth factors of P-450_{arom} activity

In the past few years, evidence has been obtained that supports the concept that growth factors, most notably IGF-1 and EGF, may be important determinants of the state of P-450_{arom} activity in human granulosa cells. For example, physiologic (nanomolar) amounts of IGF-1 stimulate P-450_{arom} activity in normal human granulosa *in vitro*, and the extent of the stimulation is equal to or greater than that evoked by FSH [17]. Furthermore, IGF-1 and FSH act synergistically to control the level of P-450_{arom} activity in these cells [17]. At the molecular level, IGF-1, like FSH, increases P-450_{arom} activity by stimulating the transcription and translation of the P-450_{arom} gene [22]. Thus, the theory is emerging that there exist at least two hormones that control the expression of P-450_{arom} in human granulosa cells. Although there is no decisive evidence, it has been suggested that IGF-1 plays a role in selection of the dominant follicle in the human ovary by enhancing the ability of FSH to induce granulosa differentiation [17].

A question of obvious importance is the possible role of IGF-1 in the etiology of PCO. In a recent study [16,17], we characterized the response of P-450_{arom} activity to IGF-1 in PCO granulosa cells and found the response to be dramatic and generally normal. From this evidence, it appears that PCO granulosa cells contain a fully functional signal-transduction system, associated with the IGF-1 receptor, which is coupled to the stimulation of P-450_{arom} activity. This evidence, coupled

Table 10.1 The endocrine microenvironment of small human Graafian follicles (based on data in Refs 8, 16, 21, 23).

	Hormone concentration*					
Follicle (4–7 mm)	FSH	LH	IGF-1	Δ^4	E_2	DHT
Normal dominant	2.5	ND	100	800	100–500	2
Normal atretic	ND	ND	100	800	10–50	2
PCO	3.5	?	100	800	10–50	ND

* FSH (mIU/ml); IGH-1 (ng/ml); Δ^4 (androstenedione, ng/ml); E_2 (estradiol, ng/ml); DHT (dihydrotestosterone, ng/ml).
ND, not determined.

with the observation (Table 10.1) that PCO follicles contain large (and near normal) quantities of IGF-1 [23], leads us to conclude that a defect in the IGF-1 signal transduction system may not be a primary cause of PCO.

In this discussion it should be mentioned that, in normal human follicles, virtually all of the IGF-1 in the microenvironment appears to be bound to the IGFBPs, most notably, the small 34-kDa IGFBP-2 [24]. Accordingly, the ability of human granulosa cells to produce the 34-kDa IGF-BP suggests a role of the granulosa in determining the amount of free IGF in the microenvironment [25,26]. Evidence from studies of patients with PCO has pointed to a marked (80%) decrease in the circulating levels of this protein [27]. Recently, Holly *et al.* [28] reported that the concentration of the 34-kDa IGFBP is markedly reduced in the follicular fluid of PCO follicles. Logically, we can propose that there may be abnormally high amounts of free (biologically active?) IGF-1 in the microenvironment of the PCO follicle. Our *in vitro* studies [17] indicate that PCO granulosa cells *in situ* are exquisitely sensitive to FSH, a response that is dependent upon IGF-1 stimulation. Therefore, our results lead to the prediction that there is a high level of IGF-1 bioactivity in the microenvironment of the PCO follicles, which could lead to FSH supersensitivity in PCO granulosa cells. In a broad sense, this theory of "increased free IGF-1" could have important implications for other clinical aspects of PCO, such as hyperandrogenism. Thus, an important future area of investigation is the role of the 34-kDa IGFBP in the etiology of PCO.

Before leaving the subject of growth factors, we should note that EGF is a potent inhibitor of the FSH induction of P-450_{arom} in normal human granulosa cells [22]. Since we propose that FSH action is blocked in PCO, the theory that EGF is the putative inhibitor of FSH needs to be examined.

The basal lamina and connective tissue elements

Several theories that attempt to explain the PCO process as a result of the hyperactivity of connective tissue in PCO ovaries have been proposed [4]. For example, in one theory, ovarian dysfunction in PCO is believed to result from fibrosis of the tunica albuginea caused by a hyperactivity of the capsular fibroblasts [4]. It is clear that the thickness of the ovarian capsule can be strikingly increased in PCO and that this increase could occur as a result of the androgen-stimulated fibroblast activity. However, it seems unlikely that this event *per se* (thickened capsule) contributes to PCO because follicle selection and ovulation can occur despite the presence of the thickened tunica albuginea.

Another theory that has received attention in this area concerns the hyperactivity of the fibroblasts in the theca interna [4]. This theory proposes that androgens stimulate theca fibroblasts to secrete increased amounts of collagen, laminin, and fibronectin. Such hyperactivity would cause an increase in the thickness of the basal lamina, a change that has been found in patients with PCO [4]. In this regard, it has been shown that long-term treatment with testosterone enanthate induces not only a thickened tunica albuginea, but also a marked thickening of the basal lamina, similar to that found in PCO [29]. This observation provides a clear demonstration that elevated levels of androgens can cause hyperactivity of human thecal fibroblasts. How might this theory relate to aberrant folliculogenesis in PCO?

It is generally believed that the basal lamina functions as a highly selective filter, which controls the nature and concentration of the molecules that accumulate in follicular fluid [30]. Vigersky and Loriaux [31] reported that in PCO, unlike the case in normal healthy follicles, there is no difference in the protein composition between the follicular fluid and peripheral plasma. Accordingly, they postulated a disruption of the normal follicular barrier to plasma proteins in PCO. The possible importance of the basal lamina in controlling the accumulation of molecules in the microenvironment is indicated by the results of McNatty [8] who showed the apparent differential entry of various key protein hormones (FSH, LH, prolactin) into the antral fluid during normal follicular growth and development in women. Thus, the obvious question: Could the thickened basal lamina in PCO follicles change the rate of entry of key hormones (like FSH and LH) into the microenvironment, such that their chances of becoming a dominant follicle are destroyed? With regard to PCO follicular fluid, there has never been a thorough characterization of the protein hormones that mediate folliculogenesis. Certainly, this important analysis of PCO follicular fluid needs to be done.

Theca interstitial cells

One of the most important concepts generated by the early studies of PCO was that the arrested Graafian follicles secrete excessive amounts of androgens, most notably Δ^4 [2–6]. Our understanding of the structure/function relationships between hormones and androgen activity have been discussed recently and readers are referred to this review for in-depth discussions of underlying controlling mechanisms [30].

How can small Graafian follicles in PCO ovaries produce such high levels of Δ^4? One possibility is that PCO follicles, 4–7 mm in diameter, contain abnormally large numbers of theca interstitial cells (TIC) relative to normal follicles. If so, it might suggest that hyperplasia of the TIC might cause the hyperandrogenism. It must be emphasized that there is no compelling evidence in the literature that proves this concept, e.g. either morphometric studies of numbers of TIC or their mitotic rates in PCO. The resolution of this question is important because the concept implies that aberrant mitosis of TIC may ultimately be part of the etiology of PCO. Assuming that the PCO TIC indeed exhibit increased mitosis, there must be some growth factor responsible for this function. At this point, virtually nothing is known about the underlying mechanism that controls mitosis and cell division in any population of TIC, human or animal. Clearly, it is important to determine whether hyperplasia of TIC is involved in PCO and what hormones or growth factors might elicit the putative hyperplasia.

Second, it is possible that PCO TIC exhibit hyperandrogenism because they respond differently to hormones. At the biochemical level, we know that both the basal and the response to LH is greater in each TIC when compared to normals [4]. On the basis of this knowledge, it seems that each individual TIC in the PCO follicles is hyperactive, at least in regard to Δ^4 production. Since LH levels are high in PCO patients, it seems logical to predict that PCO TIC might be resistant to LH-induced desensitization and down-regulation of receptors for LH. Clearly, LH and its receptor are profoundly important for correct androgen production by human TIC during folliculogenesis. To what degree aberrant regulation of these functions is causal to PCO should continue to be a major focus of biologic and clinical investigations.

Both insulin and IGF-1 might be important in the hypertrophy and hyperactivity of TIC in PCO. A particularly important advance in our field occurred with the discovery that the action of LH in human TIC can be significantly amplified by insulin and IGF-1 [30,32,33]. In animal models, there is evidence that the amplification is associated with an up-regulation of the number of receptors for LH in TIC. Clinical results indicate that insulin levels can be elevated in patients with PCO [32,33]. In such PCO patients, the high levels of circulating insulin would be expected to enhance the capacity of TIC to respond to LH and thereby engender a constitutively hyperandrogenic TIC. What about the role of IGF-1? Although excellent evidence exists in animals [34], there is no decisive proof that IGF-1 promotes excessive androgen production by human TIC. Certainly, it will be important to determine whether IGF-1 is a physiologic regulator of androgen production by human TIC and whether aberrant IGF-1 functions are involved in TIC hyperactivity in PCO. In this regard, it is interesting to consider, once again, the fact that circulating and peripheral levels of the 34-kDa IGF-BP are significantly reduced in women with PCO. As discussed in the section on granulosa cells, apparently all the IGF-1 in the interstitial fluid is normally bound to the 34-kDa protein [24]. Accordingly, the evidence might suggest that the interstitial fluid in the theca interna contains more free IGF-1 molecules than can act on the TIC to stimulate Δ^4 production. Ultimately, the role of IGF-1 and its binding proteins in normal and PCO TIC must be established by both *in vitro* and *in vivo* studies.

Theca externa

As stated earlier, the developing human follicle is normally surrounded by an outer layer of smooth muscle cells designated the theca externa (Fig. 10.3). Evidence indicates that the human theca externa is innervated by autonomic nerves [30]. Can an alteration in this tissue account for PCO? At the present time, this question cannot be answered because nothing is known about theca externa function in any species. It was pointed out earlier (Fig. 10.5) that the PCO follicles appear to contain a poorly developed theca externa. This feature could suggest aberrant development of theca externa in PCO and that nerves could possibly be involved. Does this aberration alter the normal pattern of follicle growth and development? Perhaps it would be prudent to explore this subject in a comprehensive manner in both the normal and PCO state. There could perhaps be some surprises.

The oocyte

One final question to be answered involves the extent to which PCO eggs are normal. During the first stages of folliculogenesis, up to approximately the cavitation stage (0.4 mm), the oocytes in PCO follicles appear histologically to be perfectly normal (Fig. 10.8). This is suggested by the fact that PCO eggs have completed their growth and measure about 120 μm in diameter; they are arrested at the germinal vesicle (dictyate) stage of meiosis; they have synthesized a noncellular zona pellucida; and they are in contact with the prospective cumulus and corona radiata granulosa cells (Fig. 10.8). Thus, no obvious defect can be identified in PCO eggs during preantral follicle growth [35]. However, work done by several investigators indicates that PCO eggs in the small Graafian follicles manifest degenerative properties. Sanyal *et al.* [36] have shown that a high percentage (77%) of oocytes within the 4–7-mm PCO follicles are degenerating. As expected, their potential for normal meiotic maturation *in vitro* was severely reduced [8,37]. These findings raise the question of whether there are functional defects in PCO eggs and whether they mediate at least in part the aberrant folliculogenesis seen in PCO. It is noteworthy that recent evidence in the rat suggests that the oocyte is able to regulate important functions of the follicle [38]. Hence, the question: How much of the program of follicle selection and atresia is contained within the human egg itself? The resolution of this fundamental question should be a future goal of human ovary research, both in normal ovaries and PCO.

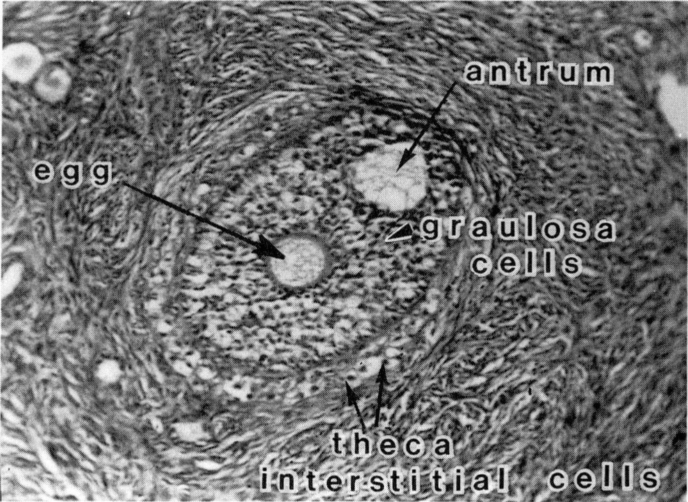

Fig. 10.8 Light micrograph of a developing PCO follicle at the early-antrum stage (0.4 mm in diameter). The relative amounts and general organization of the granulosa cells appear normal. A fully grown oocyte with zona pellucida is visible. The theca is unusually well developed and the theca interstitial cells appear hypertrophied and hyperplastic. With the exception of the changes in the theca, the PCO preantral follicle seems normal.

Summary

In this chapter, structural comparisons in combination with related functional studies have given rise to the novel concept that an inhibitor molecule in the PCO microenvironment may prevent the selection of a dominant follicle by blocking the physiologic responses of the PCO granulosa cells to FSH. Apparently, the action of the inhibitor is reflected in the failure of PCO granulosa cells to express active P-450_{arom} enzyme molecules. If this concept is true, what might the inhibitor be? Analogy with animal data hints that the inhibitor may be an IGFBP. Further investigation of this theory could reveal the nature of new regulators that may have important physiologic and clinical implications.

References

1 Erickson GF. The ovary: basic principles and concepts. In: Felig P, Baxter JD, Broadus AE, Frohman LA, eds. Endocrinology and Metabolism. New York: McGraw-Hill Book Co., 1987, pp. 905–51.
2 Goldzieher JW. Polycystic ovarian disease. Fertil Steril 1981; 35:371–94.
3 Yen SSC. The polycystic ovary syndrome. Clin Endocrinol 1980; 12:177–208.
4 Erickson GF, Yen SSC. New data on follicle cells in polycystic ovaries: a proposed mechanism for the genesis of cystic follicles. Semin Reprod Endocrinol 1984; 2:231–43.
5 Goldzieher JW, Green JA. The polycystic ovary. I. Clinical and histological features. J Clin Endocrinol 1962; 22:325–38.
6 Franks S. Polycystic ovary syndrome: a changing perspective. Clin Endocrinol 1989; 31:87–120.
7 Gougeon A. Dynamics of follicular growth in the human: a model from preliminary results. Hum Reprod 1986; 2:81–7.
8 McNatty KP, Moore-Smith D, Osathanondh R, Ryan KJ. The human antral follicle: functional correlates of growth and atresia. Ann Biol Anim Biochem Biophys 1979; 19:1547–58.
9 Gougeon A. Qualitative changes in medium and large antral follicles in the human ovary during the menstrual cycle. Ann Biol Anim Biochem Biophys 1979; 19:1461–8.
10 Hughesdon PE. Morphology and morphogenesis of the Stein–Leventhal ovary and of so-called "hyperthecosis." Obstet Gynecol Surv 1982; 37:59–77.
11 Gospodarowicz D, Bialecki H. Fibroblast and epidermal growth factors are mitogenic agents for cultured granulosa cells of rodent, porcine, and human origin. Endocrinology 1979; 104:757–64.
12 Mahesh VB, Greenblatt RB. Physiology and pathogenesis of the Stein–Leventhal syndrome. Nature 1961; 191:888–90.
13 Delforge JP, Thomas K, Roux F, Carneiro J, Ferin J. Time relationships between granulosa cell growth and luteinization, and plasma luteinizing hormone discharge in human. I. A morphometric analysis. Fertil Steril 1972; 23:1–11.
14 Tamada T, Matsumoto S. Suppression of ovulation with hCG. Fertil Steril 1969; 20:840–8.
15 Friedrich F, Kemeter P, Salzer H, Breitenecker G. Ovulation inhibition with human chorionic gonadotropin. Acta Endocrinol 1975; 78:332–42.
16 Erickson GF, Magoffin DA, Cragun JR, Chang RJ. The effects of insulin, and insulin-like growth factors I and II on estradiol production by granulosa cells of polycystic ovaries. J Clin Endocrinol Metab 1990; 70:894–902.

17 Erickson GF, Garzo VG, Magoffin DA. Insulin-like growth factor I regulates aromatase activity in human granulosa and granulosa luteal cells. J Clin Endocrinol Metab 1989; 69:716–24.
18 Lee DW, Sheldon RM, Reichert LE. Identification of low and high molecular weight follicle stimulating hormone receptor binding inhibitors in human follicular fluid. Fertil Steril 1990; 53:830–5.
19 Ui M, Shimonaka M, Shimasaki S, Ling N. An insulin-like growth factor-binding protein in ovarian follicular fluid blocks follicle stimulating hormone stimulated steroid production by ovarian granulosa cells. Endocrinology 1989; 125:912–16.
20 Shimasaki S, Shimonaka M, Ui M, Inouy S, Shibata F, Ling N. Structural characterization of a follicle-stimulating hormone action inhibitor in porcine ovarian follicular fluid. J Biol Chem 1990; 265:2198–202.
21 Brailly S, Gougeon A, Milgrom E, Bomsel-Helmreich O, Papiernik E. Androgens and progestins in the human ovarian follicle: differences in the evolution of preovulatory, healthy nonovulatory and atretic follicles. J Clin Endocrinol Metab 1981; 53:128–34.
22 Steinkampf MP, Mendelson CR, Simpson ER. Effects of epidermal growth factor and insulin-like growth factor I on the levels of mRNA encoding aromtase cytochrome P450 of human ovarian granulosa cells. Mol Cell Endocrinol 1988; 59:93–9.
23 Eden JA, Jones J, Carter GD, Alaghband-Zadeh J. A comparison of follicular fluid levels of insulin-like growth factor-I in normal dominant and cohort follicles, polycystic and multicystic ovaries. Clin Endocrinol 1988; 29:327–36.
24 Seppala M, Wahlstrom T, Koskimies AI, Tenhunen A, Turanen EM, Koistinen R, Huhtaniemi I, Bohn H, Stenman UH. Human preovulatory follicular fluid luteinized cells of hyperstimulated preovulatory follicles and corpus luteum contain placental protein 12. J Clin Endocrinol Metab 1984; 5B:509–10.
25 Suikkari AM, Jalkanen J, Koistinen R, Butzow R, Ritves O, Ranta T, Seppala AM. Human granulosa cells synthesize low molecular weight insulin-like growth factor-binding protein. Endocrinology 1989; 124:1088–90.
26 Koistinen R, Suikkari A-M, Tiitinen A, Kontula K, Seppala M. Human granulosa cells contain insulin-like growth factor-binding protein (IGF BP-1) mRNA. Clin Endocrinol 1990; 32:635–40.
27 Pekonen F, Laatikainen T, Buyalos R, Rutanen EV. Decreased 34K insulin-like growth factor binding protein in polycystic ovarian disease. Fertil Steril 1989; 51:972–5.
28 Holly JMP, Eden JA, Alaghband-Zadeh J, Carter GD, Jemmott RC, Cianfarani S, Chard T, Wass JAH. Insulin-like growth factor binding proteins in follicular fluid from normal dominant and cohort follicles, polycystic and multicystic ovaries. Clin Endocrinol 1990; 33:53–64.
29 Amirikia H, Savoy-Moore RT, Sundareson AS, Moghissi KS. The effect of long-term androgen treatment on the ovary. Fertil Steril 1986; 45:202–8.
30 Erickson GF, Magoffin DA, Dyer CA, Hofeditz C. The ovarian androgen producing cells: a review of structure/function relationships. Endocr Rev 1985; 6:371–99.
31 Vigersky RA, Loriaux DL. An androgen-binding protein in the cyst fluid of patients with polycystic ovary syndrome. J Clin Endocrinol Metab 1976; 43:817–23.
32 Poretsky L, Kalin MF. The gonadotropic function of insulin. Endocr Rev 1987; 8:132–41.
33 Barbieri RL, Smith S, Ryan KJ. The role of hyperinsulinemia in the pathogenesis of ovarian hyperandrogenism. Fertil Steril 1988; 50:197–212.
34 Magoffin DA, Erickson GF. An improved method for primary culture of ovarian androgen-producing cells in serum free medium; effect of lipoproteins, insulin, and insulin-like growth factor I. In Vitro Cell Dev Biol 1988; 24:862–70.
35 Erickson GF. An analysis of follicle development and ovum maturation. Semin Reprod Endocrinol 1986; 4:233–54.
36 Sanyal MK, Taymor ML, Berger MJ. Cytologic features of oocytes in the adult human ovary. Fertil Steril 1976; 27:501–10.

37 Takeva Z, Kusheva R. *In vitro* cultivation of oocytes from women with proven Stein–Leventhal syndrome. J Reprod Med 1971; 7:195–7.
38 Hubbard GM, Erickson GF. LH-independent luteinization and ovulation in the hypophysectomized rat: a possible role for the oocyte. Biol Reprod 1988; 39:283–94.

Chapter 11
Animal Models for Polycystic Ovary Syndrome

KATRYNA BOGOVICH

Species known to express polycystic ovaries

Polycystic ovary syndrome (PCO) in women involves a peripubertal disruption of the feedback interactions within the hypothalamic–pituitary–gonadal axis, which may arise in the presence or absence of varying degrees of either an adrenal component or insulin resistance [1–3]. Although the serum hormone profiles associated with the established ovarian cystic state in women have been characterized extensively, the marked heterogeneity of these data has confounded, rather than assisted, attempts to determine the fundamental mechanisms involved in the etiology of this syndrome. As a result, reproductive endocrinologists have turned their attention to the development of animal models that are suitable for the elucidation of the fundamental mechanisms involved in the etiology of polycystic ovaries.

Polycystic ovaries arise spontaneously in cows [4,5], cats [6] and aging laboratory rats [7,8], as well as in women. Dogs also can develop cystic ovaries, but do so very rarely. The expression of an anovulatory ovarian cystic state in so many species other than humans suggests that at least one of these species might provide an appropriate model for determining the fundamental hormonally regulated mechanisms that lead to this state in women. At the present time, the expression of PCO appears to be genetically linked in women and cows [1–5] while rats and cats seem to be physiologically predisposed to the development of an anovulatory ovarian cystic state [6–8].

Cows with cystic ovaries have been given the highly descriptive label "nymphomaniac" because of the extremely aggressive sexual behavior they display toward inanimate as well as animate objects [4,5]. Cats are induced ovulators and develop ovarian cysts when they are unable to mate [6]. Unbred cats eventually die from mammary cancer and/or endometrial cancer that develop in association with the ovarian cystic state. This observation is extremely interesting since approximately 25% of women with PCO develop endometrial hyperplasia or endometrial cancer [3].

Aging laboratory rats develop ovarian cysts in association with the onset of constant estrus [7,8]. Constant estrus is an acyclic physiologic state that may result from the rat's hypothalamic–pituitary axis becoming refractory to the constant long-day environment used in most research facilities. Like cats and women, rats also develop endometrial cancer in association with PCO.

Hormonal regulation of ovarian follicular development

At one time the primary role of luteinizing hormone (LH) and androgens during the follicular phase was thought to be the induction of atresia [9,10]. Now, however, we know that preovulatory follicular development requires precisely timed interactions between the ovary, pituitary hormones and gonadal hormones [11–13]. Briefly, follicle-stimulating hormone (FSH) acts specifically at the level of granulosa cell functions, while LH affects both thecal and granulosa cell functions [11–13]. In fact, LH stimulation of thecal androgen production is essential for the healthy, developing follicle to produce sufficient amounts of estradiol to drive follicular growth and ovulation [12,13].

Androgen concentrations reach maximal values in follicular fluid of human follicles early during preovulatory follicular development, while estradiol concentrations rise throughout this process [10]. In contrast, while androgen concentrations in follicles fated to undergo atresia are similar to those observed in healthy follicles, estradiol concentrations never attain preovulatory values [10]. These observations and the competitive inhibition of aromatase activity by 5α-reduced androgens *in vitro* [14] have led to the concept that LH-induced androgens interfere with the ability of FSH to stimulate granulosa cell function and thereby lead to follicular atresia. Together, this concept and the observation of elevated serum concentrations of LH and androgens in the established cystic state of most (if not all) women have led to the hypothesis that LH and elevated serum androgens induce ovarian follicular cysts [1–3]. However, this concept does not explain why follicles become cysts instead of undergoing normal atresia under such conditions.

Early models used to study PCO

Much of what we now know about the hormonal regulation of normal reproductive mechanisms has been obtained from experiments with rats. It is not surprising, therefore, that this species, which displays a natural tendency to express a cystic state, has been used almost exclusively in the design of animal models for PCO. Neonatal, immature, and young adult rats all have been used in attempts to prove a causal relationship between LH and androgens and the induction of follicular cysts [15–18]. Neonatal rats respond to exogenous androgen with the development of cystic ovaries within one week [15,17]. However, these animals also display a complete disruption of normal hypothalamic–pituitary responses and eventually undergo premature ovarian failure. Immature and young adult rats also respond to exogenous androgens and estrogens with the disruption of hypothalamic–pituitary functions, as well as with the development of cystic follicles [16,17]. Therefore, it is not possible to determine if the effects of the steroid treatments lie primarily at the level of the brain, the ovary, or both the ovary and the brain in these models. As a result, it is not possible to determine the mechanisms by which these treatments act to induce ovarian cysts.

In another series of experiments with young adult rats, an attempt was made to determine the role of hypothyroidism in the development of ovarian cysts [18]. However, only 36% of the hypothyroid rats that received 10 IU human chorionic gonadotropin (hCG) developed PCO, while no intact animals treated with 10 IU hCG developed ovarian cysts. Since less than half of the hypothyroid rats developed cystic ovaries in response to such treatment, this model does not appear to address the fundamental hormonal interactions required for the induction of cystic ovaries.

Part of the difficulty encountered in such attempts to understand the etiology of the ovarian cystic state may derive from the tacit assumption that the hormonal milieu associated with the perpetuation of the established cystic state is also involved in the etiology of this state. Each of the previously described models for polycystic ovaries is based on this concept.

New models for studying the etiology of PCO

It is noteworthy that in the steroid-treated rat models for PCO, serum FSH becomes elevated while serum LH becomes suppressed—the reverse of the situation in women and animals with naturally occurring cystic ovaries. Such a reversal of the serum peptide hormone profiles and the LH/FSH ratios normally associated with the ovarian cystic state illustrates an important concept that may help to explain the mechanisms involved in both the naturally occurring and the artificially induced ovarian cystic states. That is, ovarian cysts are induced and are maintained in both women and rats that are undergoing unabated gonadotropin stimulation.

The concept of unabated gonadotropin stimulation may be more important in the etiology of the cystic state than the relative serum concentrations of LH. With this possibility in mind, my group has established three novel models with which to study the hormonal interactions required for the induction of ovarian follicular cysts: (i) the progesterone-synchronized immature rat [19,20]; (ii) the pregnant rat [19]; and (iii) the hypophysectomized rat [19,21].

The progesterone-synchronized immature rat

The progesterone-synchronized immature rat model relies on the ability of elevated, but physiologic, serum progesterone concentrations to suppress both basal and estrogen-induced LH secretion to almost undetectable values while serum FSH and prolactin (PRL) are maintained at basal concentrations [19,20]. In brief, progesterone implants, inserted subcutaneously (s.c.) in 24-day-old rats, produce serum progesterone concentrations between 130–150 ng/ml by day 26 of age. These values, which are similar to those observed in the pregnant rat [12], are maintained throughout the treatment period *in vivo* [20] and have been shown to regulate central mechanisms without inhibiting follicular development at the level of the ovary [13].

Twice-daily s.c. injections of either 0 (control), 0.1, 0.5 or 1.5 IU of hCG were administered to these animals for 9 days beginning on day 27 postpartum. Figure 11.1A shows a typical ovary from a control rat at 36 days of age. Such ovaries have primordial, preantral, and small antral follicles with unstimulated thecal shells and stromal-interstitial tissue. The largest follicles in these ovaries are approximately 450 μm in diameter. In contrast, ovaries from rats treated for 9 days with 0.1 IU hCG (Fig. 11.1B) have very large follicles with large numbers of granulosa cells and stimulated thecal shells. The largest follicles in these ovaries are at least 1 mm in diameter. Rats treated twice daily with just 0.5 IU hCG develop both precystic and cystic follicles by day 36 of age (Fig. 11.1C). These follicles are between 1.5 and 2 mm in diameter. All of these fol-

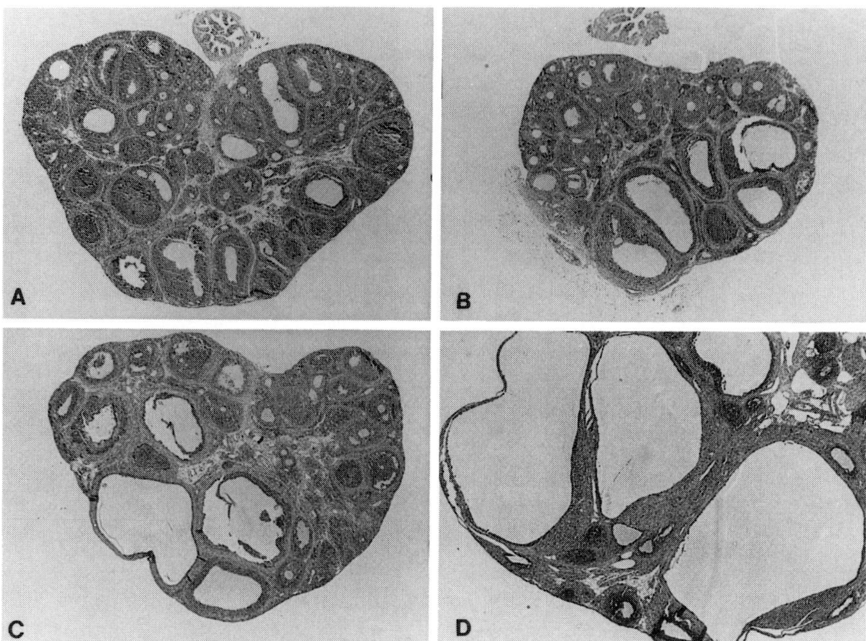

Fig. 11.1 Morphology of the immature rat ovary in response to twice-daily injections of (A) 0 IU hCG; (B) 0.1 IU hCG; (C) 0.5 IU hCG; and (D) 1.5 IU hCG for nine days beginning on day 27 of age.

licles have highly stimulated thecal shells while the number of granulosa cells present varies greatly. In addition, the stromal-interstitial tissue in these ovaries has a "stimulated" appearance. Rats displayed bilateral cystic ovaries after treatment for just 7 days with 1.5 IU hCG (Fig. 11.1D). The fully cystic follicles shown in Fig. 11.1D have stimulated thecal shells and just a remnant of granulosa cells. In addition, these ovaries, like human polycystic ovaries [1–3], have follicles at various stages of development as well as interstitial tissue with signs of collagenization.

The results obtained using this model provide the first direct evidence that unabated stimulation by LH-like activity can induce the development of follicular cysts in a dose- and a time-related manner. Furthermore, these data support the concept that unabated stimulation by LH-like activity may be more important for the induction of follicular cysts than the absolute concentration of LH in serum. An important feature of any model for PCO would be the ability to mimic certain long-term consequences of the disease. Recently, we have demonstrated the induction of endometrial cancer, a significant long-term consequence of the anovulatory cystic state, in a modified version of this model [22].

The pregnant rat

Although the results obtained with the progesterone-synchronized immature rat are intriguing, cystic ovaries occur spontaneously in aging laboratory rats, not immature rats. Therefore, before attempting to correlate the progesterone-synchronized immature rat model for PCO with the naturally occurring induction of follicular cysts in either aging laboratory rats or women, we need to determine if the stage of development or differentiation of the ovary affects the ability of LH/hCG to induce follicular cysts in the rat.

Pregnant rats were used in this series of experiments because they possess ovaries at the highest stage of differentiation as well as naturally elevated serum progesterone concentrations [12]. To adjust for their greater body weight, pregnant rats were treated twice daily for 9 days, from day 13 of pregnancy, with either 0, 1, or 3 IU hCG [19]. Figure 11.2A illustrates that the largest follicles present in the ovaries of control rats on day 22 of pregnancy are preovulatory, and 750 μm in diameter. In contrast, the largest follicles in ovaries from rats treated with 1 IU hCG (Fig. 11.2B) are approximately 1 mm in diameter on day 22 of pregnancy and have at least as many granulosa cells as the preovulatory follicles in the ovaries of the control pregnant rats. However, thecal shells appear much more stimulated in ovaries of pregnant rats treated twice daily with 1 IU hCG than in ovaries of control pregnant rats. Follicular cysts were first observed in rats treated with 3 IU hCG on day 19 of pregnancy (Fig. 11.2C), a time frame similar to that observed with 1.5 IU hCG in the progesterone-synchronized immature rat. This ability of subovulatory doses of LH-like activity to induce follicular cysts in a dose- and a time-dependent manner in both adult and immature ovaries indicates that the fundamental mechanisms required for follicular cyst development do not depend on the differentiated state of the rat ovary.

The hypophysectomized rat

To determine if unabated stimulation by LH-like activity alone were sufficient for the induction of cystic follicles, immature rats, hypophysectomized (HYPOXD) at 21 days of age, were treated with 0.5 IU hCG twice daily for 12 days beginning on day 27 of age [19,21]. Ovaries from control (0 IU hCG) HYPOXD rats were unstimulated (Fig. 11.3A), having only primordial and preantral follicles, many of which were undergoing atresia. In contrast to progesterone-synchronized immature rats, unabated stimulation by hCG fails to induce ovarian cysts in HYPOXD rats (cf. Figs 11.1C and 11.3B). Despite stimulation of the

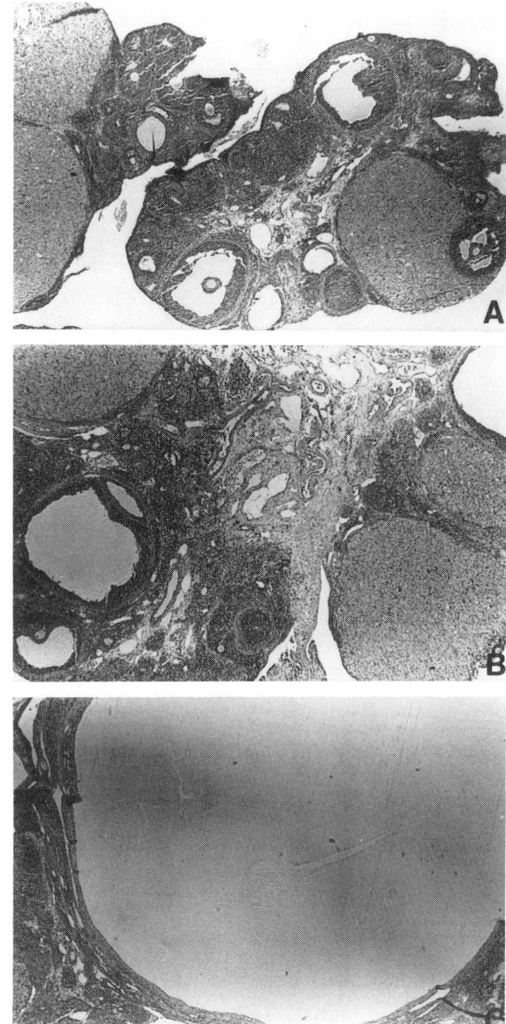

Fig. 11.2 Morphology of pregnant rat ovaries in response to twice-daily injections of (A) 0 IU hCG; (B) 1 IU hCG; and (C) 3 IU hCG for 9 days beginning on day 13 of pregnancy.

thecal and stromal-interstitial tissue, the largest follicles present in hCG-treated HYPOXD rat ovaries are at the preantral stage of development (Fig. 11.3B). These results clearly demonstrate that LH is not the only pituitary hormone needed for the induction of ovarian follicular cysts in the rat.

FSH and PRL seemed the most likely candidates to serve an obligatory role, with LH, in the induction of follicular cysts because of their roles in regulating normal ovarian functions. However, the observation that serum PRL can be either elevated or normal in women and other animals with PCO [1–8,18] seemed to argue against, rather than for, an

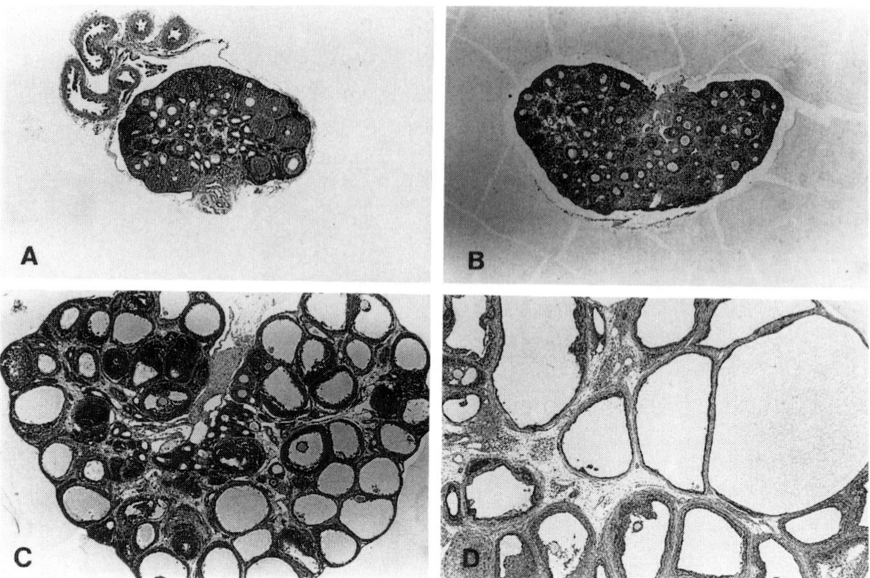

Fig. 11.3 Morphology of hypophysectomized rat ovaries in response to (A) no hormones; (B) 0.5 IU hCG twice daily for 12 days beginning on day 27 of age; (C) 2 μg ovine FSH daily for 13 days beginning on day 26 of age; and (D) 2 μg ovine FSH daily for 13 days plus 0.5 IU hCG twice daily for 12 days beginning on days 26 and 27 of age, respectively.

obligatory role for PRL in the induction of ovarian cysts. In contrast, the observation that serum FSH tends to remain at basal values for both animals and women with cystic ovaries seemed to suggest that FSH might play a role in at least the induction of the ovarian cystic state.

To determine if FSH could play a role in the induction of ovarian cysts, immature HYPOXD rats were given either no hormone (controls); 0.5 IU hCG twice daily for 12 days from day 28 after birth; 2 μg of highly purified ovine FSH daily for 13 days from day 27 after birth, or both FSH and hCG (FSH + hCG) beginning on days 27 and 28, respectively.

The results obtained for control and hCG-treated HYPOXD rats were as described above. By the day after the last FSH injection, ovaries from rats treated only with FSH have many small antral follicles that are undergoing atresia (Fig. 11.3C). Neither the thecal shells nor the stromal-interstitial tissue in these ovaries are stimulated. Therefore, the residual LH activity in this preparation of FSH had little or no effect on ovarian morphology. In contrast, HYPOXD rats treated with FSH + hCG develop ovarian cysts 3 mm in diameter with markedly stimulated thecal shells and a residual layer of granulosa cells (Fig. 11.3D). Cysts were first observed in these ovaries on the eighth day of hCG treatment, an observation that agrees remarkably well with the timing of cyst induction in the progesterone-synchronized immature rat model.

ESTRADIOL PRODUCTION AND AROMATASE ACTIVITY

The ability of unabated stimulation by LH/hCG and FSH to induce follicular cysts in HYPOXD rats raises important questions about the effects of such stimulation on follicular estradiol (E_2) production and aromatase activity. Follicles from control, hCG-treated, and FSH-treated HYPOXD rats possess minimal ability to produce E_2 when incubated for 4 hours in medium alone (Fig. 11.4, left panel). In striking contrast, follicles from HYPOXD rats treated with FSH + hCG produce nanogram amounts of E_2 even on days 9–14 of treatment when the largest follicles in these ovaries are cystic.

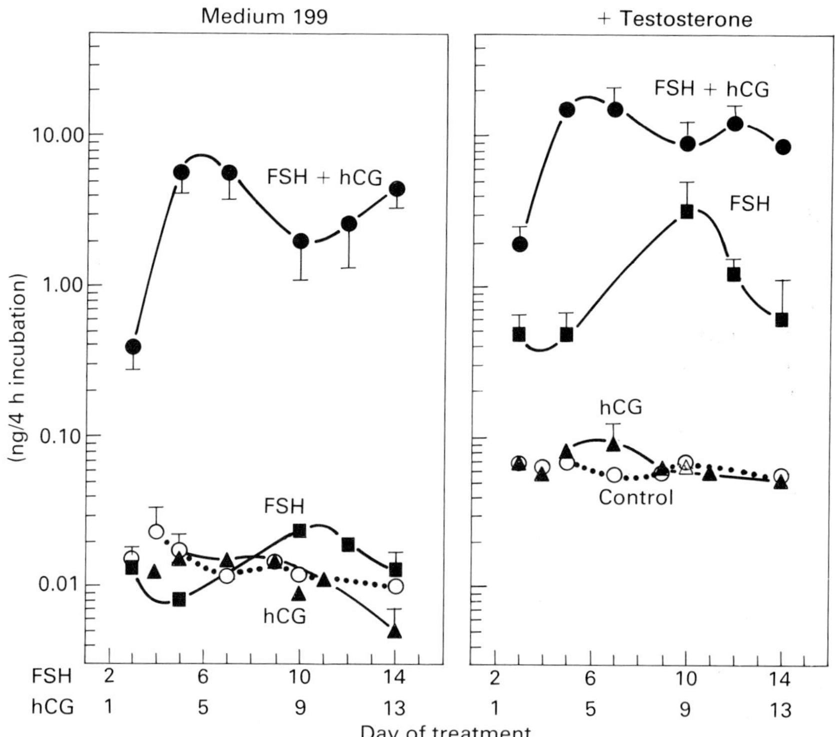

Fig. 11.4 Changes in the ability and capacity of ovarian follicles to produce estradiol in response to unabated gonadotropin stimulation in the HYPOXD rat. The largest follicles were isolated from the ovaries of each treated group on the days indicated and incubated for 4 hours at 37 °C in an atmosphere of $O_2:CO_2$ (95% : 5%) in the presence or absence of either 1 mM 8-bromo cAMP or 300 ng testosterone.

In the presence of exogenous testosterone, follicles from control and hCG-treated HYPOXD rats display equally limited aromatase activity (Fig. 11.4, right panel). Although FSH alone *in vivo* did stimulate follicular aromatase activity, the amount of E_2 produced in 4 hours by follicles from these rats never attains that observed with follicles from animals treated with FSH + hCG.

The data in Figs 11.3 and 11.4 clearly demonstrate two features of the HYPOXD rat model that are extremely important for the interpretation of these results. First, the absence of antral follicles in ovaries from hCG-treated HYPOXD rats (Fig. 11.3B), as well as the control-like values for aromatase activity for follicles from hCG-treated animals (Fig. 11.4, right panel), demonstrates that the hCG used in this model did not possess significant amounts of FSH activity. Second, the unstimulated appearance of the thecal shells and interstitial tissue in ovaries from FSH-treated HYPOXD rats (Fig. 11.3C) and the control-like ability of follicles from these animals to produce E_2 in medium alone (Fig. 11.4, left panel) demonstrate that the residual LH activity in this preparation of ovine FSH was not sufficient to affect the ability of these follicles to produce E_2.

Summary

Our gonadotropin-induced models of PCO demonstrate the following points.

1 Unabated stimulation by gonadotropins may be more important than the relative serum concentrations of these hormones in determining whether or not follicular cysts will develop.

2 The stage of differentiation of the ovary does not seem to play a critical role in the etiology of PCO in the rat.

3 Unabated stimulation by FSH and LH-like activity are sufficient to induce ovarian follicular cysts in the rat.

4 The induction and stimulation of follicular aromatase activity need not be suppressed during the initial induction of ovarian cysts.

Previous models for the induction of ovarian follicular cysts have relied heavily on the hormone profiles associated with the perpetuation of the established cystic state [1–8,16–18]. The data from our new models for the development of ovarian cysts suggest that we may need to consider more carefully the nature of the fundamental hormonal interactions that result in the initial development of the PCO state: perhaps the hormonal milieu associated with the etiology of the cystic ovary is not as complex as the heterogeneous hormonal milieus so often observed in women who have expressed the PCO state for a number of years prior to diagnosis.

References

1 Yen SCC. The polycystic ovary syndrome. Clin Endocrinol 1980; 12:177–208.
2 Coney P-J. Polycystic ovarian disease: current concepts of pathophysiology and therapy. Fertil Steril 1984; 42:667–82.
3 Futterweit W. Polycystic ovary disease. In: Buchsbaum HJ, ed. Clinical Perspectives in Obstetrics and Gynecology. New York: Springer-Verlag, 1984.
4 Roberts SJ. Clinical observations on cystic ovaries in dairy cattle. Cornell Vet J 1955; 45:497–513.
5 Kesler DJ, Garverick HA. Ovarian cysts in dairy cattle: a review. J Anim Sci 1982; 55:1147–59.
6 Stein BS. Genital system. In: Catcott EJ, ed. Feline Medicine and Surgery. Santa Barbara: American Veterinary Publications, Inc., 1975.
7 Peluso JJ, Steger RW, Huang H, Meites J. Pattern of follicular growth and steroidogenesis in the ovary of aging cycling rats. Exp Aging Res 1979; 5:319–33.
8 Peluso JJ, England-Charlesworth C. Formation of ovarian cysts in aged irregularly cycling rats. Biol Reprod 1981; 24:1183–90.
9 Louvet J-P, Harman SM, Schreiber JR, Ross GT. Evidence for a role of androgens in follicular maturation. Endocrinology 1975; 97:366–72.
10 McNatty KP, Hunter WM, McNeilly AS, Sawers RE. Changes in the concentration of pituitary and steroid hormones in the follicular fluid of human Graafian follicles throughout the menstrual cycle. J Endocrinol 1975; 64:555–71.
11 Fortune JE, Armstrong DT. Hormonal control of 17β-estradiol biosynthesis in proestrus rat follicles: estradiol production by isolated theca versus granulosa. Endocrinology 1978; 102:227–35.
12 Bogovich K, Richards JS, Reichert LE Jr. Obligatory role of luteinizing hormone (LH) in the initiation of preovulatory follicular growth in the pregnant rat: specific effects of human chorionic gonadotropin and follicle-stimulating hormone on LH receptors and steroidogenesis in theca, granulosa, and luteal cells. Endocrinology 1981; 109:860–7.
13 Richards JS, Bogovich K. Effects of human chorionic gonadotropin and progesterone on follicular development in the immature rat. Endocrinology 1982; 111:1429–38.
14 Hillier SG, van den Boogaard AJM, Reichert LE Jr, Van Hall EV. Alterations in granulosa cell aromatase activity accompanying preovulatory follicular maturation in the rat ovary with evidence that 5α-reduced C_{19} steroids inhibit the aromatase reaction. J Endocrinol 1980; 84:409–19.
15 Barraclough CS. Modification in the CNS regulation of reproduction after exposure of prepubertal rats to steroid hormones. Recent Prog Horm Res 1966; 22:503–15.
16 Brawer JR, Naftolin F, Martin J, Sonnenschein C. Effects of a single injection of estradiol valerate on the hypothalamic arcuate nucleus and on reproductive function in the female rat. Endocrinology 1978; 103:501–2.
17 Mahesh VB, Mills TM, Bagnell CA, Conway BA. Animal models for study of polycystic ovaries and ovarian atresia. In: Mahesh VB, Dhindsa DS, Anderson E, Kalra SP, eds. Regulation of Ovarian and Testicular Function. New York: Plenum Publishing Corp, 1987, pp. 237–57.
18 Leathem JH. Hormonal influences on the gonadotropin-sensitive hypothyroid rat ovary. Anat Rec 1958; 131:487–500.
19 Bogovich K. Induction of follicular cysts in rat ovaries by prolonged administration of human chorionic gonadotropin. In: Mahesh VB, Dhindsa DS, Anderson E, Kalra SP, eds. Regulation of Ovarian and Testicular Function. New York: Plenum Publishing Corp, 1987, pp. 659–63.

20 Bogovich K. Induction of ovarian cysts in progesterone-synchronized immature rats: evidence that suppression of follicular aromatase activity is not a prerequisite for the induction of cystic follicles. Endocrinology 1989; 124:1646–53.
21 Bogovich K. Luteinizing hormone (LH)-like activity and follicle-stimulating hormone (FSH) are sufficient for the induction of cystic ovaries in hypophysectomized rats. In: Hirshfield AJ, ed. Growth Factors and the Ovary. New York: Plenum Publishing Corp, 1989.
22 Bogovich K. Can an ovarian cystic state induced by human chorionic gonadotropin (hCG) cause abnormal changes in rat endometrial morphology? 72nd Annual Meeting of the Endocrine Society, Atlanta, Ga, 1990, p. 67.

Chapter 12
Ovarian Function in Polycystic Ovary Syndrome: an Overview

GREGORY F. ERICKSON

When it comes to the ovary, the *sine qua non* of polycystic ovary syndrome (PCO) is the failure of a developing follicle within a cohort to regularly undergo the selection process. In this section on folliculogenesis in PCO, the major questions considered are: How does this happen? What is the mechanism? Is there a reliable animal model to study PCO?

Historically, there have been two general theories to explain the absence of follicle selection in PCO. One theory argues that selection does not occur because high circulating levels of luteinizing hormone (LH) evoke a negative growth response causing all follicles within a cohort to undergo atresia. Implicit in this theory is an alteration in the LH signaling pathway in the theca interstitial cells. The other theory argues that the concentration of follicle-stimulating hormone (FSH) in PCO patients is too low to allow the process of selection to proceed. Implicit in this theory is the concept that the concentration of biologically active FSH in the microenvironment is too low to stimulate the growth and development of the granulosa cells. Now, a third theory that growth factors might be involved in the arrest of follicle selection in PCO has emerged. Implicit in the new theory is that an aberrant growth factor response (positive or negative) causes dominant follicles to stop developing in PCO. Indeed data discussed here bring us closer to understanding how the growth factor theory might be involved in the pathogenesis of PCO.

New evidence to support the classical LH theory is put forth by Rosenfield and his colleagues of the University of Chicago. Measuring progestins and androgens in blood of normal and PCO patients, they found that larger than normal quantities of 17-hydroxyprogesterone (17-PROG) are secreted by the theca interstitial cells of PCO follicles. They suggest that the overproduction of 17-PROG in PCO is caused by the high levels of circulating LH, which result in a reduced ability of the P-450$_{17\alpha}$ enzyme to metabolize 17-PROG to androstenedione (Δ^4). This enzyme alteration is thought to be achieved through the desensitization of the LH signaling pathway in the theca interstitial cells. Rosenfield believes that follicle selection stops because the abnormal ratio shuts off estradiol production. A big question in this theory concerns how the alteration in P-450$_{17\alpha}$ activity can have a negative effect in estradiol synthesis, e.g. how can an increase in the ratio of 17-PROG:Δ^4 possess signaling mechanisms that suppress P-450$_{arom}$ expression in the granulosa cells? It is clear that androgen levels (aromatase substrate) are not rate limiting. What then is the mechanism? Until this question is solved, there will remain some concern about its relevance to the pathogenesis of PCO. Consequently, it may be too early to rigorously define functional and clinical implications.

As a causal agent in PCO, FSH has long been the focus of research interests. The seminal experiments supporting this theory were those showing that if one makes multiple injections of FSH into PCO patients, dominant follicles can be selected, e.g. the FSH signal transduction pathway in the granulosa cells is stimulated, which leads to estradiol production and ovulation. These results strongly suggest that it is a lack of FSH activity in the microenvironment that gives rise to aberrant folliculogenesis in PCO. This result is compatible with two possibilities. First, endogenous levels of biologically active FSH in PCO follicular fluid may be too low to affect function. So far, there has been only one report on the concentration of FSH in PCO follicular fluid; it suggests that PCO follicles may contain as much bioactive FSH as that found in the normal dominant follicle. If this finding holds, then a lack of FSH bioactivity in antral fluid would not explain the lack of follicle selection in PCO. Instead, the findings raise the possibility that there may be a block in the FSH signaling pathway. Could molecules like FSH antagonists, FSH agonists, growth factors, or other proteins alter the biologic action of FSH in PCO granulosa cells? Significantly, the results reported recently with epidermal growth factor and the insulin-like growth factor-binding proteins strongly support this idea. Thus, perhaps the most interesting new theory is that the secret of PCO may lie with a local inhibitor of hormone-dependent granulosa differentiation. What will happen to this theory when it is rigorously tested remains to be seen but, if it should prove true, it could be a potential target for therapy.

Section 5
Adrenal Function in Polycystic Ovary Syndrome

Chapter 13
Nonclassical 21-Hydroxylase Deficiency

MARIA I. NEW

Nonclassical steroid 21-hydroxylase deficiency (NC21OHD) is a common hormonal disorder in which the primary metabolic error, a partial reduction in steroid 21-hydroxylation, alters adrenal steroidogenic balance and increases adrenal androgen production. It is a common cause of the excess androgen syndrome. The 21-hydroxylase enzyme, adrenal microsomal cytochrome P-450_{C21}, is coded for by the gene *CYP21*. Gene mutations giving rise to NC21OHD are allelic with the gene mutations causing severely impaired enzyme function and producing the classical endocrine disorder congenital adrenal hyperplasia (CAH); NC21OHD is the most common human autosomal recessive disorder. It occurs with a high frequency in the range 1:100 to 1:1000 in heterogeneous (predominantly caucasoid) populations and with increased frequencies in some ethnic populations, most notably Ashkenazic Jews, among whom the disease occurs with a frequency of 1:30.

There is an overlap in the clinical presentation of nonclassical CAH, either 21-hydroxylase or 3β-hydroxysteroid dehydrogenase (3β-HSD) deficiency, and of polycystic ovary syndrome (PCO) [1,2]. Hirsutism, acne, menstrual abnormalities, and infertility are the clinical manifestations of both. In addition, polycystic ovaries are found on sonography (see Chapter 2) moderately frequently in patients with NC21OHD [3–5], nonclassical 11-hydroxylase deficiency [6] and, more frequently than is generally realized, in nonclassical 3β-HSD deficiency [7]. Furthermore, in cases of classical 21-hydroxylase and classical 3β-HSD, when patients are undertreated, transient PCO may be found on sonography. By sonography and by clinical presentation, PCO and nonclassical forms of CAH sometimes may be indistinguishable. However, the use of an adrenocorticotropic hormone (ACTH) stimulation test will clearly identify CAH. Since low-dose glucocorticoid therapy can reverse in many patients any of the symptoms of hyperandrogenism caused by CAH, as well as the hypothalamic imbalance of luteinizing hormone (LH)/follicle-stimulating hormone (FSH) and the sonographic evidence of ovarian cysts often found in PCO, it is important to be aware of a subset of women with PCO that is secondary to adrenal steroidogenic defect.

Historical comments

From the first understanding of glandular function and steroid imbalance in reproduction, androgen excess of adrenal origin has been postulated as a possible basis of hirsutism, menstrual disturbances, and infertility in women. In gynecological studies in the 1950s, glucocorticoids, then only recently available, were administered to women with elevated urinary 17-oxosteroids. There was a good response in some women, providing empiric support for primary adrenal dysfunction in those cases [8–10]. Biochemical diagnosis of a relative insufficiency of adrenal steroid 21-hydroxylase came in 1957 with a study detailing urinary hormonal measurements in the baseline, following ACTH stimulation, and after hydrocortisone in a eumenorrheic virilized woman [11].

Partial adrenal 21-hydroxylase enzyme deficiencies are variously termed acquired [12,13], adult-onset familial [14], attenuated [15,16], late-onset [17–19], and cryptic adrenal hyperplasia [20,21], from the time when the genetic basis of the nonclassical disorder (NC21OHD) had not yet been established.

Close genetic linkage of classical 21-hydroxylase deficiency (CAH) and HLA and, subsequently, with the HLA-β locus had been reported in 1977 and 1978 [22,23]. Allelism with the classical 21-hydroxylase deficiency trait for NC21OHD was suggested by its strong association with HLA-B14, demonstrated in Ashkenazic Jews [17] and in other ethnic groups [21]. In 1982, Kohn *et al.* [24] presented detailed hormonal and clinical characterization of symptomatic and asymptomatic forms and calculated a peak total log of odds (LOD) score in their study population of 3.575 at $\theta = 0.00$ (θ equals recombinant fraction of 0) for linkage between NC21OHD and the HLA-B locus [24]. Specific HLA-B antigens are found to be in positive linkage disequilibrium with each of the forms of 21-hydroxylase deficiency: salt-wasting (antigens B47 and Bw60 (40)) and simple virilizing classical CAH (antigens B51(5) and B27) [25], and NC21OHD (antigen B14). Decreased associations with NC21OHD are found for the HLA antigen B8.

The landmark study of Speiser *et al.* [26] assessing the population genetics of the nonclassical disorder found it not only to be more common than the classical deficiency causing CAH, but to be the most common human autosomal recessive disease trait. The highest ethnic group-specific frequency is among Ashkenazic Jews. Speiser *et al.* formally demonstrated linkage disequilibrium between NC21OHD and HLA-B14 in Ashkenazic Jewish patients. In other groups with increased NC21OHD frequency, Hispanics and Italians, the B14 association is not as strong, and in another group, Yugoslavs, the B14 antigen is lacking entirely [27,28].

The general high frequency of the NC21OHD disorder is a matter of considerable speculation in genetic research. The phenomenon of genetic drift may be excluded because of the existence of distinct NC21OHD deficiency alleles in different populations and geographic areas. Sex ratio transmission distortion has been disproven (unpublished data). If the NC21OHD trait is being maintained in the human population in the face of the reduced fertility known to be a consequence of the hormonal imbalance, the answer may lie in a selective advantage to the heterozygote. The reduced frequency of HLA-B8,DR3 suggests that autoimmune disorders associated with the HLA-B8,DR3 haplotype may be decreased—a potential advantage.

The highest disease frequency in any ethnic group or population for NC21OHD is seen in Ashkenazic Jews. Almost all Ashkenazic Jews or individuals with Ashkenazic Jewish background affected with NC21OHD are positive on HLA typing for antigen B14 and often for DR1. The recurrence of the B14,DR1 association, noted earlier [17] and shown by Speiser *et al.* to be in positive linkage disequilibrium with NC21OHD [26], suggests the transmission of a single mutation or allelic type in the Ashkenazic population. Since the characteristic Ashkenazic NC21OHD allele and associated B14 antigen are not restricted to any Ashkenazic subgroup and since the frequency of B14 is not as high in Sephardic or Oriental Jews [29], a stem mutation is predicted to have occurred after the Second Diaspora (AD 70) and by the time of consolidation of the major Jewish communities in northern and eastern Europe (probably before AD 1100).

The Roman Jews, a community in continuous existence since the second century BC, have been considered a possible source of DNA sequences branching from the main line of Palestine Jewry before the Second Diaspora and, therefore, antedating the mutational event(s) posited in the generation of the NC21OHD alleles in the Ashkenazic Jewish population. A scientific study of the Roman Jews was initiated to gather data bearing on this. The first DNA typing reports available so far show no new alleles at the test loci for a number of biochemical systems, nor has fixation occurred at any of these loci. Further sampling is needed before the data are sufficient for formal calculation of linkage disequilibrium at the test loci (Kidd K and Kidd JR, unpublished data). Thus, the indications are that the Roman Jews have had a fair degree of outbreeding and it is therefore not highly likely that the original (premutation) DNA sequence types will be identified.

Clinical features

Nonclassical 21-hydroxylase deficiency is variably expressed in individuals with signs of androgen excess appearing alone or in combination at any age. Some patients have had no history of symptoms when identified, but overt hyperandrogenism is expected almost always to develop at some point. Nonclassical 21-hydroxylase deficiency may be the etiology of androgen excess syndromes such as PCO, hirsutism, premature pubarche/adrenarche. Short stature and reduced fertility may also result from NC21OHD.

In childhood, NC21OHD may trigger premature pubarche [30] and has occurred as young as 5 months [24]. Gynecomastia has been identified in a prepubertal boy [31]. Menarche may be advanced in girls.

In adolescent and adult women, hirsutism is a very common manifestation, not infrequently in association with irregular menses or secondary amenorrhea. In different patient series, the prevalence of NC21OHD among hirsute, oligomenorrheic women has ranged from 1.2 to 30% [32–38] (it is significant that ethnic composition was not reported in these studies). Acne [39,40], especially cystic acne resistant to standard therapy [41,42], may be accompanied by hirsutism or irregular menses/amenorrhea. In some young women, male-pattern baldness has been the sole presenting symptom.

Testing of the adrenal axis reveals NC21OHD in a percentage of women with PCO [7,43]. Elevated serum androgens of adrenal origin could act centrally to alter gonadotropin release or could have direct effects on the ovary; once formed, ovarian cysts can autonomously maintain hyperandrogenism. Abnormal responses to luteinizing hormone-releasing hormone (LHRH) have been noted in NC21OHD [44].

Androgens affect the timing of the growth spurt and fusion of the epiphyseal plates of the bones. This results in slightly reduced stature relative to midparental height [45]. Genetic predisposition to short stature may also be a factor since the height of NC21OHD parents is below secular controls.

It is not known how often affected adult men who are otherwise asymptomatic may have disturbed gonadal function [46,47]. Reduced fertility can occur in both sexes.

Basic defect and pathogenesis

Adrenal steroid 21-hydroxylase is a microsomal cytochrome P-450, P-450_{C21}, coded for by the gene *CYP21* (which has a close homolog, pseudogene *CYP21P*). A milder enzyme defect results in the NC21OHD hormonal disorder, which is expressed biochemically, with symptoms of androgen excess appearing at any postnatal stage. Severe enzyme defects result in classical CAH, in which extreme androgen elevations produce virilizing effects *in utero* and result in genital ambiguity or male genital phenotype at birth in genetic females [48–50].

Steroid 21-hydroxylase is a membrane-bound cytochrome P-450 of the adrenal cortex required for synthesis of corticosteroids (i.e. cortisol and aldosterone) from cholesterol. It is one of five enzymes functioning in cortisol biosynthesis (see Fig. 13.1). Congenital adrenal hyperplasia results from defects in any of these, but predominantly (92–95% of cases) from those of 21-hydroxylase. A 21-hydroxylating block in cortisol formation increases levels of proximal steroid intermediates, which then undergo alternate conversion to androgenic steroids. According to the degree of the block and consequent biochemical abnormality, clinical effects range from pseudohermaphroditism in genetic females at birth in classical CAH to the subtle reductions in adult height and fertility in both sexes seen statistically in NC21OHD.

Methodological issues

Identification of NC21OHD is by clinical assessment, hormonal evaluation, HLA typing, DNA analysis, or combinations of these in different cases.

The accepted diagnostic hormonal test is the 60-min ACTH stimulation test. A blood sample is drawn at 0 min (basal) and 60 min after (stimulated) bolus i.v. injection of 0.25 mg Cortrosyn (synthetic ACTH 1–24, Organon, W. Orange, NJ) for basal and stimulated serum 17-hydroxyprogesterone (17-OHP) determined by standard radioimmunoassay (RIA). The values are plotted on a reference nomogram (shown in Fig. 13.2).

Test points for all subjects, with the baseline and ACTH-stimulated serum 17-OHP values as coordinates, form a regression line along which scores aggregate into groups according to the subject 21-hydroxylase

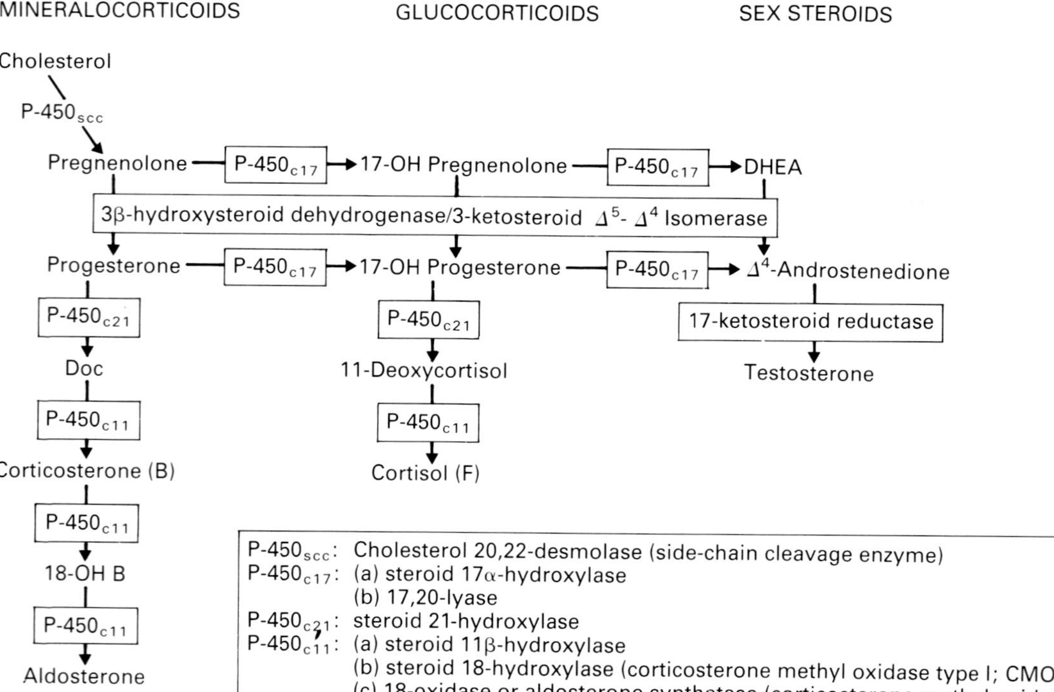
MINERALOCORTICOIDS
GLUCOCORTICOIDS
SEX STEROIDS
Cholesterol
P-450scc
Pregnenolone
P-450c17
17-OH Pregnenolone
P-450c17
DHEA
3β-hydroxysteroid dehydrogenase/3-ketosteroid Δ5- Δ4 Isomerase
Progesterone
P-450c17
17-OH Progesterone
P-450c17
Δ4-Androstenedione
P-450c21
Doc
P-450c11
Corticosterone (B)
P-450c11
18-OH B
P-450c11
Aldosterone
P-450c21
11-Deoxycortisol
P-450c11
Cortisol (F)
17-ketosteroid reductase
Testosterone
P-450scc: Cholesterol 20,22-desmolase (side-chain cleavage enzyme)
P-450c17: (a) steroid 17α-hydroxylase
(b) 17,20-lyase
P-450c21: steroid 21-hydroxylase
P-450c11: (a) steroid 11β-hydroxylase
(b) steroid 18-hydroxylase (corticosterone methyl oxidase type I; CMO I)
(c) 18-oxidase or aldosterone synthetase (corticosterone methyl oxidase type II; CMO II)

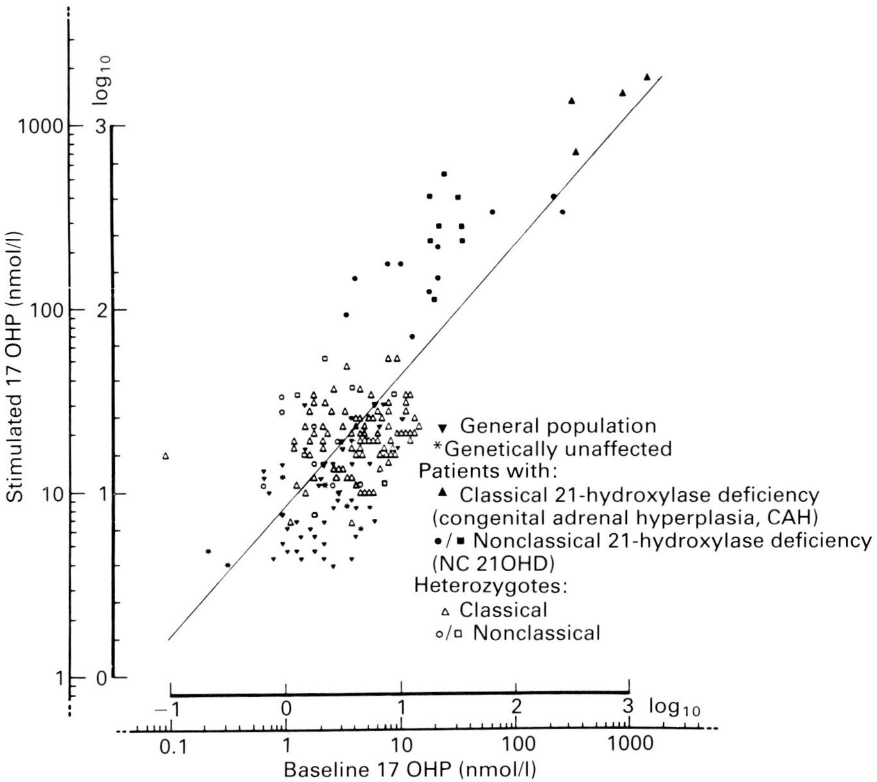

Fig. 13.2 Log–log plot of stimulated (60 min post 25 IU synthetic ACTH i.v. bolus) vs. baseline serum concentration of 17α-hydroxyprogesterone for complete range of genotypes for adrenal steroid 21-hydroxylase enzyme.

Fig. 13.1 (*facing page*) Schematic of steroidogenesis in the adrenal cortex. Major pathways only for unconjugated steroids are shown. There is quasi-independence of the three types of adrenal hormones. (1) Aldosterone synthesis is completed only in the outer histologic zone (zona glomerulosa), which is acutely responsive to the vasoactive peptide angiotensin II and (high) serum potassium concentration. Steroid secretion by this zone is only a few percent of the total and aldosterone is present in serum at 10^{-2} to 10^{-3} times the concentration of cortisol. (2) Cortisol (and sex steroids) are produced by the wide middle zone (zona fasciculata) and inner zone of the mature gland (zona reticularis) under the trophic control of ACTH (corticotropin). 18-Oxidation of steroid intermediates, the third function of P-450_{C11}, is suppressed in these zones and both functions of P-450_{C17} are active. Uncoupling of cortisol and androgen production occurs with certain types of chronic stress. (3) Aromatization (estrogens) not shown.

genotype [51]. Patients with classical CAH have the most severe 21-hydroxylase deficiency and show the greatest elevations of serum 17-OHP. Symptomatic and asymptomatic patients with NC21OHD show comparable, less extreme serum 17-OHP elevations. Heterozygotes for a

21-hydroxylase deficiency of any degree of severity have a still milder abnormality, which is unmasked only by ACTH stimulation testing. The best controls for normal 21-hydroxylase activity are provided by families in which 21-hydroxylase deficiency has been identified: scores for family members who are unaffected and who are predicted by HLA typing not to carry the HLA-associated 21-hydroxylase deficiency gene fall at the lowest point of the regression line. The distribution of hormonal responses from the general population suggests a certain number of unidentified heterozygotes in this group.

Since association of 21-hydroxylase deficiency with HLA was established in 1977, HLA genotyping has been used in family studies as a genetic marker for the enzyme defect in family members.

Gene structure and expression

The gene for cytochrome P-450_{C21} normally exists in two copies in the haploid chromosome, as an active gene (*CYP21*) and a pseudogene (*CYP21P*). On the chromosome, these two genes alternate with the genes for the two isotypes of the component C4 of serum complement, *C4A* and *C4B*, apparently the result of tandem duplication in evolution of an adjacent single 21-hydroxylase/C4 gene pair. These gene pairs have retained a remarkable degree of homology: *C4A* and *C4B* are greater than 99% identical, and the deduced amino acid sequence of *CYP21P* is 98% identical to that of *CYP21* (reviewed in White [52]). Duplications of the *CYP21/CYP21P* and *C4* genes have been observed in NC21OHD [53]. Deletions of the pseudogene produce no endocrinopathy.

Genetic analysis

In 1984, White *et al.* [54] reported localization of the 21-hydroxylase gene to the C4 region of the HLA supergene on chromosome 6. Hybridization analysis of this region revealed two genes each located immediately 3′ to one of two C4 genes (*C4A* and *C4B*) and thus termed 21OHA or the *A* gene (a pseudogene, now termed *CYP21P*) and 21OHB or the *B* gene (the active coding sequence, now termed *CYP21*). Status of this gene pair as one active and one pseudogene was deduced from the hormonal type of individuals with half-deletions of the *C4A-CYP21P–C4B-CYP21* tandem paired arrangement. Sample DNA digested with enzyme TaqI and probed with a 21-hydroxylase sequence showed two bands in normal subjects, one at 3.7 kb and one at 3.2 kb. A subject with null expression of protein C4B and missing the 3.7 kb fragment (called

B) suffered from salt-wasting 21-hydroxylase deficiency. The contrary anomaly was found in subjects with null expression of C4A and lacking the other, 3.2 kb band (called A). The *C4A*-null/*CYP21A*-deleted hormonal type is normal. The *A* gene is thus not essential and, not being able to code for enzyme activity (in the *C4B*-null/*CYP21B*-deleted type), is therefore a pseudogene. The cDNA derived from the *B* gene mRNA transcript predicted a polypeptide of 494 amino acid residues, molecular weight approximately 55 000 Da [55].

Recurring association of NC21OHD with HLA-B14,DR1 suggests a particular allele traveling on this partial haplotype. Molecular characterization of the B14,DR1-associated *CYP21* mutation(s) was performed [56].

Analysis of a *CYP21* gene cloned from a HLA-B14,DR1 homozygous NC21OHD patient identified three deviations from the normal active gene sequence possibly affecting function: (i) single base change (GTC→CTG) in codon 211 causing conservative substitution valine to leucine (both nonpolar amino acids); (ii) three base changes between positions 8 and 13 of intron 6 (CTGTAC→ATGTGT); (iii) a single base change (GTC→TTG) in codon 281 resulting in a second valine to leucine substitution.

Mutation (ii) was excluded from consideration because intronic base changes known to affect 5′-end splicing have all started before position 5 of the intron. Mutations (i) and (iii) cause the same (conservative) substitution, but the significance depends on the environment: amino acids other than valine occur at the residue 211-corresponding position in the P-450 protein of other species, whereas valine-281 is uniformly conserved, suggesting a more critical requirement (perhaps molecular volume). The val_{281}→leu mutation was thus selected as of likely significance, and a 21-mer oligonucleotide probe synthesized to recognize the change in the base sequence. Ten individuals were screened: nine NC21OHD patients (not related) and one normal control. Eight of the NC21OHD patients were of Ashkenazic Jewish extraction and B14,DR1-positive (3 homozygotes and 5 heterozygotes). The ninth patient, who was Yugoslav, typed negative for B14,DR1 as did the control. DNA analysis with the probe identified the mutation in all eight Ashkenazic Jewish patients and not in the B14-negative patient nor the unaffected control (see Fig. 13.3). A second probe specific for the active gene (the *B* gene) was used to screen the positive samples to confirm that the extra (third) *C4-CYP21* sequence known to be carried on the B14,DR1 haplotype is a duplicated *CYP21P* or a *CYP21P*-like pseudogene.

Since altered protein structure might not be the only change causing expression of the NC21OHD phenotype, transcription assays were per-

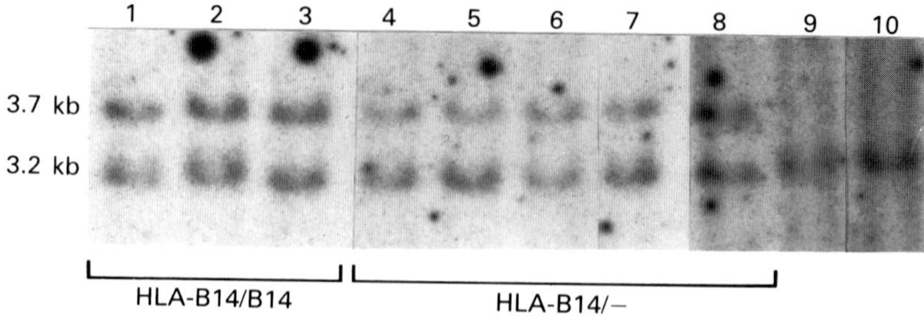

Fig. 13.3 DNA from 10 individuals probed for presence of *CYP21* point mutation $G_{1689}{\rightarrow}T$ (1st position of coding triplet: $val_{281}{\rightarrow}leu$) with oligonucleotide synthesized to correspond with the surrounding base sequence. Samples digested with restriction endonuclease Taq I, which cuts typical fragment 3.7 kb in length from *CYP21* (*B* gene) and 3.2 kb fragment from pseudogene *CYP21P* (*A* gene). Normal haploid type has one *A* and one *B* gene, each with companion serum C4 protein. NC21OHD haplotype positive for HLA-B14 has additional *A* or *A*-like gene and three forms of C4. Lanes 1–3, NC21OHD patients with mutation in *B* gene on both haplotypes as well as on *A* genes. Lanes 4–8, NC21OHD patients with mutation on *B* gene on one haplotype as well as on *A* genes. Lane 9, Yugoslav NC21OHD patient, and lane 10, normal control, both lacking the mutation in question. No hybridization of probe is evident at the 3.7-kb banding position. (Reprinted, with permission of The New England Journal of Medicine, from Speiser *et al.* [56].)

formed using mouse Y1 adrenal cells transfected with the mutant *CYP21*. It was determined that the gene sequence is transcribed to mRNA and a protein synthesized that exhibits reduced enzymatic activity. Stability of mRNA transcripts cannot be assessed in this cell expression system nor can changes in the rate of transcription be detected (the possible result of an undetected mutation in a regulatory DNA region). The single-base change causing missense mutation $val_{281}{\rightarrow}leu$ appears to be a consistent molecular genetic marker for the NC21OHD allele associated with HLA-B14,DR1 (illustrated in Fig. 13.4 as occurring by nonreciprocal intragenic transfer, or gene conversion, from the *A* pseudogene, which carries this changed DNA sequence).

Heterogeneity

According to the enzyme function provided by the alleles present, different allelic pairs have characteristic expression in serum/urinary biochemical values, and depending on other individual factors, in the clinical manifestations. Classical alleles may be correlated with either clinical form of the classical 21-hydroxylase deficiency, that is salt-wasting classical, and simple virilizing classical. It also has been noted, however, that family members presumed to carry the same 21-hydroxylase muta-

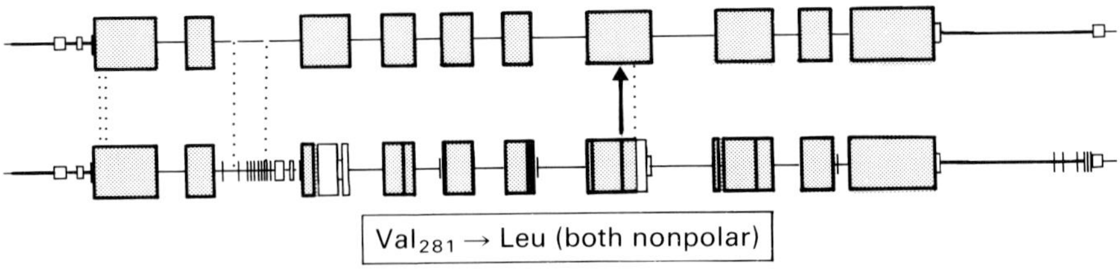

CYP21 mutations

$Val_{281} \rightarrow$ Leu (both nonpolar)

Fig. 13.4 Diagram to scale of approximately 3350 bases encompassing coding, intervening and certain regulatory sequences of the cytochrome P-450_{C21} gene *CYP21* (upper) and pseudogene *CYP21P* (lower) with resident noncorrespondences marked (half-width vertical lines, single-base changes; full-width vertical lines, base changes causing amino acid substitutions; unshaded section in a pseudogene "exon" indicates a termination codon—relative to the reading frame of the active gene—has immediately preceded). Heavy arrow indicates position of point mutation, presumed to occur by nonreciprocal recombination, or gene conversion, from the pseudogene sequence. This mutation causes replacement of amino acid residue 281, valine, with leucine. Although leucine is also hydrophobic, its differing molecular volume may affect what appears to be a critical protein folding region and thus disturb enzyme function.

tions (that is, who are HLA identical) may be discordant for clinical expression. In the nonclassical deficiency it is found that affected individuals may be symptomatic or asymptomatic and show the same biochemical characteristics.

Nonclassically affected individuals are one of two basic genotypes: they may have a partially defective (nonclassical) gene on both chromosomes, or may have a partially defective gene on one haplotype and a classical on the other haplotype (compound heterozygote). Table 13.1 is a glossary of terms outlining the clinical and hormonal features of the two gene types.

There is statistical separation of the hormonal phenotype in NC21OHD caused by two mild defects occurring together as opposed to the phenotype caused by mild in conjunction with a severe defect [57].

Frequencies in Jewish and non-Jewish populations

Estimates of incidence and gene frequencies for allelic forms of NC21OHD in the study population of Speiser *et al.* [26] were 3.7% in Ashkenazic Jews, 1.9% in Hispanics, 1.6% in Yugoslavs, 0.3% in Italians, and 0.1% in the diverse Caucasian population. Ashkenazic Jews had the highest gene frequency for the B14 allele in affecteds compared with controls (69% vs. 12%). A computer-assisted study using more elaborate statistical analytic methods to examine the same test popula-

Table 13.1 Glossary of terms in 21-hydroxylase deficiency (terms after Kohn *et al.* [24]).

Clinical phenotype	Hormonotype	Genotype*
Classical		
SW and SV: prenatal virilization; fully symptomatic	Marked elevation of precursors	$\frac{\text{21-OH def}^{\text{SEVERE}}}{\text{21-OH def}^{\text{SEVERE}}}$
Nonclassical		
Symptomatic: later development of virilization; milder symptoms or Asymptomatic: no virilization or other symptoms	Moderate elevation of precursors	$\frac{\text{21-OH def}^{\text{SEVERE}}}{\text{21-OH def}^{\text{MILD}}}$ or $\frac{\text{21-OH def}^{\text{MILD}}}{\text{21-OH def}^{\text{MILD}}}$
Carrier		
Asymptomatic	Precursor levels greater than normal	$\frac{\text{21-OH def}^{\text{SEVERE}}}{\text{21-OH Normal}}$ or $\frac{\text{21-OH def}^{\text{MILD}}}{\text{21-OH Normal}}$
Normal		
Asymptomatic	Lowest levels: some overlap seen with carriers	$\frac{\text{21-OH Normal}}{\text{21-OH Normal}}$

* Gene types 21-OH def^{SEVERE} and 21-OH def^{MILD} correspond with 21-OH^{CAH} and 21-OH^{CRYPTIC}, respectively, of Levine *et al.* [20] and 21-OH^{0} (= null) and 21-OH^{S} (= susceptibility), respectively, of Kauschansky *et al.* [18].

tion data obtained corresponding results [58], as has a recent pilot project screening for NC21OHD within this (New York) hospital community by assay for 17-OHP in 8 a.m. salivary samples [59].

Polycystic ovary syndrome is characterized by a dysfunction in ovarian steroidogenesis [60]. Although adrenal enzymatic defects leading to androgen overproduction have been associated with PCO, a causative relationship has not yet been demonstrated [61–63]. Several interesting reports have attempted to provide a scheme for the development of PCO [64–66], but the subject remains controversial.

Whatever the additional role of adrenal steroidogenesis in the etiology of PCO, primary adrenal disorders that can present with PCO, steroid 21-hydroxylase deficiency should be looked for in any woman presenting with symptoms of hyperandrogenism (most commonly, hirsutism, acne, or menstrual disorders) or enlarged ovaries on sonography. Although the androgen profile in serum and urine in both the basal and ACTH-stimulated states may not be markedly different from that of women with PCO, the 17-OHP response to ACTH clearly differentiates the patients with an adrenal 21-hydroxylase defect [26], or 3β-HSD [7]. Tests with ACTH are required for the differential diagnosis. Sonograms of the ovary do not distinguish women with excess androgens due to PCO from those with NC21OHD. The use of ACTH tests is also necessary to differentiate PCO from NC21OHD on the basis of LHRH testing of pituitary gonadotropin secretion. The response to LHRH is variably abnormal in virilized women with NC21OHD [44,67].

Treatment

Treatment with glucocorticoids suppresses adrenal androgen overproduction and, with time, clinical signs of androgen excess show improvement. Given the 9-month life expectancy of established hair follicles, remission of hirsutism generally takes at least 1–2 years. Reversal of infertility in women has been noted. One study [68] reported five patients with postmenarchial onset of 21-hydroxylase deficiency who resumed regular menses and demonstrated adequate suppression of 17-ketosteroids and pregnanetriol within 2 months of glucocorticoid therapy alone. Another study [69] found that, of 18 infertile women with acne and/or facial hirsutism and hormonal criteria consistent with 21-hydroxylase deficiency, five conceived after 2–7 months of prednisone treatment alone; four more women conceived within 2 months of the addition of clomiphene to the therapeutic regimen. Hormonal profiles after initiation of therapy were not reported in this study. In a recent review of patients in our clinic, two of three infertile NC21OHD women became pregnant after 1–1.5 years of glucocorticoid therapy [70].

Summary

The syndrome of PCO includes a subgroup of women with NC21OHD which can be treated by low-dose glucocorticoids. Preliminary data indicate that (i) the size of cystic changes of ovaries on sonography and (ii) LH:FSH ratios may improve with dexamethasone treatment. Identification of these disorders by ACTH testing is cost-effective in patients with symptoms of androgen excess as well as in patients with reduced fertility and in asymptomatic family members of patients with proven adrenal steroidogenic defects.

References

1 Featherweight W. Polycystic Ovarian Disease. New York: Springer-Verlag, 1984, p. 120.

2 Lobo RA, Goebelsmann U. Adult manifestations of congenital adrenal hyperplasia due to incomplete 21-hydroxylase deficiency mimicking polycystic ovarian disease. Am J Obstet Gynecol 1980; 138:720–6.

3 Levine LS, Korth-Schutz S, Saenger P, *et al.* Disordered puberty in treated congenital adrenal hyperplasia. In: Lee PA *et al.*, eds. Congenital Adrenal Hyperplasia. Baltimore: University Park Press, 1977, pp. 511–26.

4 Cox RI, Shearman RP. Abnormal excretion of pregnanetriolone and Δ^5-pregnanetriol in the Stein–Leventhal syndrome. J Clin Endocrinol Metab 1961; 21:586–90.

5 Pang S, Levine LS, New MI. Puberty in congenital adrenal hyperplasia. In: Grumbach M, ed. *Control of the Onset of Puberty II.* Williams & Wilkins, Baltimore, 1990, pp. 669–89.

6 Gabrilove JL, Sharma DC, Dorfman RI. Adrenocortical 11β-hydroxylase deficiency and virilism first manifest in the adult woman. N Engl J Med 1965; 272:1189–94.

7 Pang S, Lerner A, Stoner E, *et al.* Late-onset 3β-hydroxysteroid dehydrogenase deficiency. I. A cause of hirsutism in pubertal and postpubertal women. J Clin Endocrinol Metab 1985; 60:428–36.

8 Jones GES, Howard JE, Langford H. The use of cortisone in follicular-phase disturbances. Fertil Steril 1953; 4:49–62.

9 Greenblatt RB. Cortisone in treatment of hirsute woman. Am J Obstet Gynecol 1953; 66:700–10.

10 Jones HW Jr, Jones GES. The gynecological aspects of adrenal hyperplasia and allied disorders. Am J Obstet Gynecol 1954; 68:1330–65.

11 Decourt J, Jayle MF, Baulieu E. Virilisme cliniquement tardif avec excrétion de pregnanetriol et insuffisance de la production du cortisol. Ann Endocrinol 1957; 18:416–22.

12 Newmark S, Dluhy R, Williams G, Pochi P, Rose L. Partial 11- and 21-hydroxylase deficiencies in hirsute women. Am J Obstet Gynecol 1976; 127:594–8.

13 New MI, Lorenzen F, Pang S, Gunczler P, Dupont B, Levine LS. "Acquired" adrenal hyperplasia with 21-hydroxylase deficiency is not the same genetic disorder as congenital adrenal hyperplasia. J Clin Endocrinol Metab 1979; 48:356–9.

14 Blankstein J, Faiman C, Reyes FI, Schroeder ML, Winter JSD. Adult-onset familial adrenal 21-hydroxylase deficiency. Am J Med 1980; 68:441–8.

15 Rosenwaks Z, Lee PA, Jones GS, Migeon CJ, Wentz AC. An attenuated form of congenital virilizing adrenal hyperplasia. J Clin Endocrinol Metab 1979; 49:335–9.

16 Migeon CJ, Rosenwaks Z, Lee PA, Urban MD, Bias WB. The attenuated form of congenital adrenal hyperplasia as an allelic form of 21-hydroxylase deficiency. J Clin Endocrinol Metab 1980; 51:647–9.

17 Laron Z, Pollack MS, Zamir R, Roitman A, Dickerman Z, Levine LS, Lorenzen F, O'Neill GD, Pang S, New MI, Dupont B. Late-onset 21-hydroxylase deficiency and HLA in the Ashkenazi population: a new allele at the 21-hydroxylase locus. Hum Immunol 1980; 1:55–66.

18 Kauschansky A, Kaufman H, Zamir R, Elian E. Late onset adrenal hyperplasia (21-hydroxylase deficiency): 17-OH progesterone response to ACTH stimulation and HLA typing. Horm Res 1981; 14:73–8.

19 Chrousos GP, Loriaux DL, Mann D, Cutler GB Jr. Late-onset 21-hydroxylase deficiency is an allelic variant of congenital adrenal hyperplasia characterized by attenuated clinical expression and different HLA haplotype associations. Horm Res 1982; 16:193–200.

20 Levine LS, Dupont B, Lorenzen F, *et al.* Cryptic 21-hydroxylase deficiency in families of

patients with classical congenital adrenal hyperplasia. J Clin Endocrinol Metab 1980; 51:1316–24.

21 Pollack MS, Levine LS, O'Neill GJ, Pang S, Lorenzen F, Kohn B, Rondanini GF, Chiumello G, New MI, Dupont B. HLA linkage and B14,DR1,BfS haplotype association with the genes for late onset and cryptic 21-hydroxylase deficiency. Am J Hum Genet 1981; 33:540–50.

22 Dupont B, Oberfield SE, Smithwick EM, Lee TD, Levine LS. Close genetic linkage between HLA and congenital adrenal hyperplasia (21-hydroxylase deficiency). Lancet 1977; ii:1309–11.

23 Levine LS, Zachmann M, New MI, Prader A, Pollack MS, O'Neill GJ, Yang S-Y, Oberfield SE, Dupont B. Genetic mapping of the 21-hydroxylase deficiency gene within the HLA linkage group. N Engl J Med 1978; 299:911–15.

24 Kohn B, Levine LS, Pollack MS, Pang S, Lorenzen F, Levy D, Lerner AJ, Rondanini GF, Dupont B, New MI. Late-onset steroid 21-hydroxylase deficiency: a variant of classical congenital adrenal hyperplasia. J Clin Endocrinol Metab 1982; 55:817–27.

25 Dupont B, Virdis R, Lerner AJ, Nelson C, Pollack MS, New MI. Distinct HLA-B antigen associations for the salt-wasting and simple virilizing forms of congenital adrenal hyperplasia due to 21-hydroxylase deficiency. In: Albert ED *et al.*, eds. Histocompatibility Testing 1984. New York: Springer-Verlag, 1984, p. 660.

26 Speiser PW, Dupont B, Rubinstein P, Piazza A, Kastelan A, New MI. High frequency of nonclassical steroid 21-hydroxylase deficiency. Am J Hum Genet 1985; 37:650–67.

27 Dumić M, Brkljačić L, Mardešić D, Plašić V, Lukenda M, Kaštelan A. "Cryptic" form of congenital adrenal hyperplasia due to 21-hydroxylase deficiency in the Yugoslav population. Acta Endocrinol 1985; 109:386–92.

28 Dumić M, Brkljačić L, Speiser PW, Wood E, Crawford C, Plašić V, Baničević M, Radmanović S, Radica A, Kastělan A, New MI. An update on the frequency of nonclassical deficiency of adrenal 21-hydroxylase in the Yugoslav population. Acta Endocrinol 1990; 122:703–10.

29 Bonné-Tamir B, Bodmer JG, Bodmer WF, Pickbourne P, Brautbar C, Gazit E, Nevo S, Zamir R. HLA polymorphism in Israel: an overall comparative analysis. Tissue Antigens 1978; 11:235–50.

30 Temeck JW, Pang S, Nelson C, New MI. Genetic defects of steroidogenesis in premature pubarche. J Clin Endocrinol Metab 1987; 64:609–17.

31 Auchterlonie IA, Cameron J, Wallace AM, Rudd BT, Hudson M, Smith PJ. Prepubertal gynaecomastia as the presenting feature of late-onset 21-hydroxylase deficiency. Horm Res 1985; 22:94–9.

32 Child DF, Bu'lock DE, Anderson DC. Adrenal steroidogenesis in hirsute women. Clin Endocrinol 1980; 12:595–601.

33 Gibson M, Lackritz R, Schiff I, Tulchinsky D. Abnormal adrenal responses to adrenocorticotropic hormone in hyperandrogenic women. Fertil Steril 1980; 33:43–8.

34 Lobo RA, Goebelsmann U. Adult manifestation of congenital adrenal hyperplasia due to incomplete 21-hydroxylase deficiency mimicking polycystic ovarian disease. Am J Obstet Gynecol 1980; 138:720–6.

35 Chrousos GP, Loriaux DL, Mann DL, Cutler GB. Late-onset 21-hydroxylase deficiency mimicking idiopathic hirsutism or polycystic ovarian disease. An allelic variant of congenital virilizing adrenal hyperplasia with a milder enzymatic defect. Ann Intern Med 1982; 96:143–8.

36 Chetkowski R, DeFazio J, Shamonki I, Judd HL, Chang RJ. The incidence of late-onset congenital adrenal hyperplasia due to 21-hydroxylase deficiency among hirsute women. J Clin Endocrinol Metab 1984; 58:595–8.

37 Pang S, Lerner AJ, Stoner E, Levine LS, Oberfield SE, Engel I, New MI. Late-onset adrenal steroid 3β-hydroxysteroid dehydrogenase deficiency. A cause of hirsutism in pubertal and postpubertal women. J Clin Endocrinol Metab 1985; 60:426–38.

38 Kuttenn F, Couillin P, Girard F, *et al.* Late-onset adrenal hyperplasia in hirsutism. N

Engl J Med 1985; 313:224–31.
39 Pekkarinen A, Sonck CE. Adrenocortical reserves in acne vulgaris: the urinary excretion of 17-ketosteroids and total 17-hydroxycorticosteroids. Acta Derm Venereol 1962; 42:200–10.
40 Rose LI, Newmark SR, Strauss JS, Pochi PE. Adrenocortical hydroxylase deficiencies in acne vulgaris. J Invest Dermatol 1976; 66:324–6.
41 Rose LI, Birnbaum MD. Therapy of adrenocortical hydroxylase deficiencies in acne vulgaris. Int J Dermatol 1979; 18:386–9.
42 Marynick SP, Chakmakjian ZH, McCaffree DL, Herndon JH Jr. Androgen excess in cystic acne. N Engl J Med 1983; 308:981–6.
43 Dewailly D, Vantyghem-Haudiquet M-C, Sainsard C, *et al.* Clinical and biological phenotypes in late-onset 21-hydroxylase deficiency. J Clin Endocrinol Metab 1986; 63:418–23.
44 Gangemi M, Benato M, Guacci AM, Menghetti G. Stimulation tests in adrenogenital syndrome induced by 21-hydroxylase deficit. Clin Exp Obstet Gynecol 1983; 10:127–30.
45 New MI, Gertner JM, Speiser PW, del Balzo P. Growth and final height in classical and nonclassical 21-hydroxylase deficiency. J Endocrinol Invest 1989; 12(suppl. 3):91–5.
46 Gerhard I, Eggert-Kruse W, Runnebaum B, Vecsei P. Adrenal function in infertile women. Acta Endocrinol 1987; 283(suppl.): 109–10 (Abstract).
47 Milewicz A, Medras M. 21-Deoxycortisol (21-DF) and 17-hydroxyprogesterone (17-OHP) responses to adrenal-corticotropic hormone in males with idiopathic oligozoospermia. Andrologia 1987; 19:393–7.
48 Bongiovanni AM, Eberlein WR, Goldman AS, New MI. Disorders of adrenal steroid biogenesis. Recent Prog Horm Res 1967; 23:375–449.
49 New MI, Dupont B, Grumbach K, Levine LS. Congenital adrenal hyperplasia. In: Stanbury JB, Wyngarden JB, Fredrickson OS, Goldstein JL, Brown MS, eds. The Metabolic Basis of Inherited Disease, 5th edn. New York: McGraw-Hill, 1983, pp. 9973–1000.
50 New MI, White PC, Pang S, Dupont B, Speiser PW. The adrenal hyperplasias. In: Scriver CR, Beaudet AL, Sly WS, Valle D, eds. The Metabolic Basis of Inherited Disease, 6th edn. New York: McGraw-Hill, 1989, pp. 1881–917.
51 New MI, Lorenzen F, Lerner AJ, *et al.* Genotyping steroid 21-hydroxylase deficiency: hormonal reference data. J Clin Endocrinol Metab 1983; 57:320–6.
52 White PC. Molecular genetics of the class III region of the HLA complex. In: Dupont B, ed. Immunobiology of HLA, Vol. 2; Immunogenetics and Histocompatibility. New York: Springer-Verlag, 1989, pp. 62–9.
53 Werkmeister JW, New MI, Dupont B, White PC. Frequent deletion and duplication of the steroid 21-hydroxylase genes. Am J Hum Genet 1986; 39:461–9.
54 White PC, New MI, Dupont B. HLA-linked congenital adrenal hyperplasia results from a defective gene encoding a cytochrome P-450 specific for steroid 21-hydroxylation. Proc Natl Acad Sci USA 1984; 81:1986–90.
55 White PC, New MI, Dupont B. Structure of human steroid 21-hydroxylase genes. Proc Natl Acad Sci USA 1986; 83:5111–15.
56 Speiser PW, New MI, White PC. Molecular genetic analysis of nonclassic steroid 21-hydroxylase deficiency associated with HLA-B14,DR1. N Engl J Med 1988; 319:19–23.
57 Speiser PW, New MI. Genotype and hormonal phenotype in nonclassical 21-hydroxylase deficiency. J Clin Endocrinol Metab 1987; 64:86–91.
58 Sherman SL, Aston CE, Morton NE, Speiser PW, New MI. A segregation and linkage study of classical and nonclassical 21-hydroxylase deficiency. Am J Hum Genet 1988; 42:830–8.
59 Zerah M, Ueshiba H, Wood E, Speiser PW, Crawford C, McDonald T, Pareira J, Gruen D, New MI. Prevalence of neoclassical steroid 21-hydroxylase deficiency based on a

morning salivary 17-hydroxyprogesterone screening test: a small sample study. J Clin Endocrinol Metab 1990; 70:1662–7.

60 New MI. Polycystic ovarian disease and congenital and late-onset adrenal hyperplasia. Endocrinol Metab Clin North Am 1988; 17:637–48.

61 Loughlin T, Cunningham S, Moore A, Culliton M, Smyth PP, McKenna TJ. Abnormalities in polycystic ovary syndrome. J Clin Endocrinol Metab 1986; 62:142–7.

62 Givens JR, Andersen RN, Ragland JB, *et al.* Adrenal function in hirsutism. I. Diurnal change and response of plasma androstenedione, testosterone, 17-hydroxyprogesterone, cortisol, LH, and FSH to dexamethasone and $\frac{1}{2}$ unit of ACTH. J Clin Endocrinol Metab 1975; 40:988–1000.

63 Goldzieher JW, Axelrod LR. Adrenal and ovarian steroidogenesis in sclerotic ovarian syndrome. Acta Endocrinol 1960; 51(suppl.):617.

64 McKenna TJ. Pathogenesis and treatment of polycystic ovary syndrome. N Engl J Med 1988; 318:558–62.

65 Barnes R, Rosenfield RL. The polycystic ovary syndrome: pathogenesis and treatment. Ann Intern Med 1989; 110:386–99.

66 Ericksen GF, Yen SSC. New data on follicle cells in polycystic ovaries: a proposed mechanism for the genesis of cystic follicles. Semin Reprod Endocrinol 1984; 2:231–43.

67 Speiser PW, Drucker S, New MI. Hypothalamic–pituitary–gonadal axis in nonclassical 21-hydroxylase deficiency. Endocrinology 1987; 120(suppl.):171/A602.

68 Riddick DH, Hammond CB. Adrenal virilism due to 21-hydroxylase deficiency in the post-menarchial female. Obstet Gynecol 1975; 45:15–20.

69 Birnbaum MD, Rose LI. The partial adrenocortical hydroxylase deficiency syndrome in infertile women. Fertil Steril 1979; 32:536–41.

70 Zerah M, Mani P, Mercado AB, New MI. Infertility in females with nonclassical 21-hydroxylase deficiency (NC21-OHD). 72nd Annual Meeting of The Endocrine Society, Atlanta, 1990, 989/272.

Chapter 14
Adrenarche: the Maturing of the Adrenal Cortex

BARRY D. ALBERTSON, GORDON B. CUTLER, JR
& D. LYNN LORIAUX

Almost five decades ago Fuller Albright first recognized that the adrenal gland secretes increasing amounts of androgenic steroids during sexual development. He termed this process "adrenarche." This thesis was published in the *American Journal of the Medical Sciences*, in which Albright described 11 cases of Turner's syndrome and correctly predicted the adrenal origin of public and axillary hair in these subjects [1]. Since that time much has been learned about the endocrinology of the adrenal cortex and the variety of steroid hormones it produces.

This review of adrenarche will address: (i) basic adrenal cortical structure/function relationship; (ii) changing levels of circulating hormones, adrenal histology, and adrenal enzyme activities during adrenarche; (iii) the relationship between gonadal maturation and adrenarche; (iv) animal models of adrenarche; and (v) proposed mechanisms for the initiation and maintenance of the adrenal secretion of sex steroids.

Adrenal histology and steroidogenesis

In adult humans the adrenal cortex can be divided histologically into three distinct regions (Fig. 14.1). Beginning at the outside of the adrenal is the zona glomerulosa, distinguished by small clusters of cells arranged relatively symmetrically along the inner 15–20% of the cortex. Immediately below the glomerulosa is the zona fasciculata, named from the Latin "fasciculus," which means "bundle." Cells in this, the thickest of the three zones, are arranged in long rows or columns, separated by venous spaces. Finally, below the zona fasciculata and above the medullary capsule is the zona reticularis, composed of large eosinophilic staining cells arranged in continuous clusters but distributed less symmetrically through this inner layer.

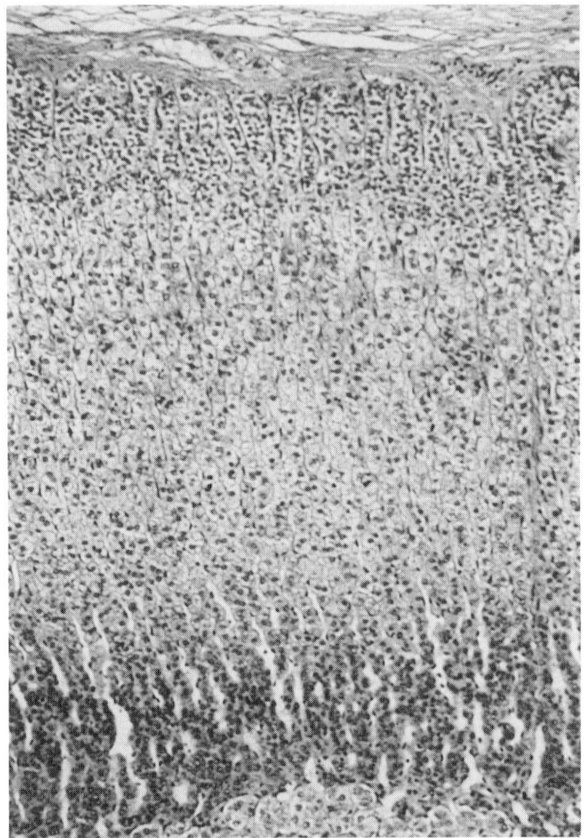

Fig. 14.1 Cross-section from a human adult adrenal cortex. The three cortical zones can easily be distinguished (from outside to inside): zona glomerulosa, zona fasciculata, and the zona reticularis in the deepest cortical compartment.

From work in the 1940s and 1950s, it was established that the adrenal cortex produces three types of steroid hormones: glucocorticoids, mineralocorticoids, and androgens. Thus, it appeared reasonable to hypothesize that each cortical zone produced a distinct sub-class of adrenal steroid (Fig. 14.2). However, the data to support this hypothesis were indirect and linked to the overproduction of certain types of steroid hormones by specific adrenal tumors localized in specific adrenal zones. This basic premise is probably correct (Table 14.1), i.e. the zona glomerulosa predominantly produces mineralocorticoids, the zona fasciculata produces glucocorticoids, and the zona reticularis produces adrenal androgens. However, each zone of the adrenal cortex appears to contain all of the steroidogenic enzymes necessary to produce all of the steroid

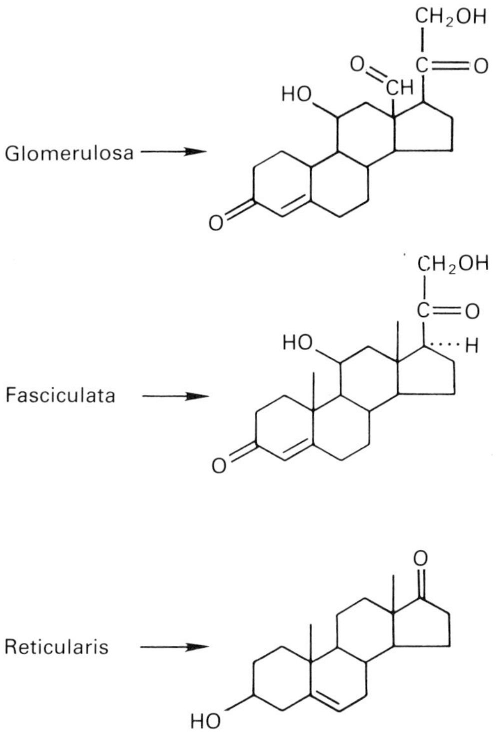

Glomerulosa → [aldosterone structure: CH_2OH, C=O, O=CH, HO, O]

Fasciculata → [cortisol structure: CH_2OH, C=O, H, HO, O]

Reticularis → [dehydroepiandrosterone structure: O, HO]

Fig. 14.2 The three adrenal cortical zones and the proposed groups of steroid hormones secreted by each: zona glomerulosa (aldosterone), zona fasciculata (cortisol), zona reticularis (dehydroepiandrosterone).

hormones, and fine control of the adrenal cortex by extra- and intra-adrenal factors may ultimately determine the unique pattern of hormone secretion from each zone.

Adrenarche is associated with an increase in the adrenal production and secretion of dehydroepiandrosterone (DHEA), DHEA sulfate (DHEAS), Δ^5-androstenediol, Δ^4-androstenedione (Δ4A), testosterone (T), estrone, and their prohormones, pregnenolone and 17-hydroxypregnenolone [2]. However, DHEA and DHEAS are the most useful biochemical markers of adrenarche because their plasma levels derive almost exclusively from adrenal secretion [3–5]. Plasma levels of DHEA and DHEAS increase about 20-fold during adrenarche, which begins at about the age of 7 years (with a range from 5 to 9 years), several years before gonadal activation (Fig. 14.3). Furthermore, there is little or no sex-related differences in the concentrations of DHEA and DHEAS [2].

While DHEA and DHEAS are closely related to the active androgens (as evidenced by their C19 structures), they have little if any intrinsic

Table 14.1 (a) Steroid hormone produced from punch biopsies taken from slices of adrenal cortex from a patient with ectopic ACTH producing Cushing's syndrome. Ratios of adrenal androgens to cortisol are highest in the containing media of cultures that combine the zona reticularis after stimulation with ACTH (cortrosyn 1–24). (b) Steroidogenic enzyme activity in human cortical zones dissected from adrenals of a patient with ectopic ACTH producing Cushing's syndrome.

(a)

Adrenal zone	Androstenedione/Cortisol	DHEA/Cortisol
Fasciculata	43.5 ± 16.7	34.1 ± 25.2
Reticularis	98.0 ± 37.7*	122.5 ± 80.8†

Ratios are mean ± SD of 5 or 6 cultures.
* $P < 0.025$, † $P < 0.05$.

(b)

	3β-HSD	21-OHase	11-OHase	17-OHase	17, 20 D
Total adrenal	13091 ± 284	4376 ± 319	166 ± 8	5386 ± 614	84 ± 13
Fasciculata/ glomerulosa enriched	18139 ± 886	4805 ± 240	83 ± 7	5782 ± 614	64 ± 15
Reticularis enriched	9829 ± 363*	4812 ± 151	50 ± 5†	5296 ± 356	138 ± 22‡

Enzyme activities are expressed as mean ± SEM of four measurements in picomoles product/min/mg mitochondrial or microsomal protein
* $P < 0.005$, † $P < 0.025$, and ‡ $P < 0.005$ are for comparisons made between fasciculata/glomerulosa and reticularis.

androgenic activity. These steroids appear to be prohormones for other androgens (T and dihydrotestosterone, DHT) and thus they derive their androgenic action from peripheral conversion to the active androgens.

The adrenarchal rise in levels of DHEA and DHEAS can produce secondary sexual changes. Thus, in patients with gonadal dysgenesis or prepubertal castration [1] and premature adrenarche [6], adrenal androgens cause the development of both pubic and axillary hair. Also DHEA and DHEAS can have small effects in increasing bone age and skeletal growth in children [2].

Data further supporting the fact that the adrenal reticular zone is the source of increased adrenal androgen at adrenarche have come from Dohm [7] and Grumbach *et al.* [18] (Fig. 14.4), who noted the close temporal relationship between plasma levels of DHEAS and the appearance of the zona reticularis. In newborn infants (Fig. 14.5), there is no reticular zone between the fasciculata and adrenal medulla, while adults have a well-developed reticular zone that consists of compact eosinophilic

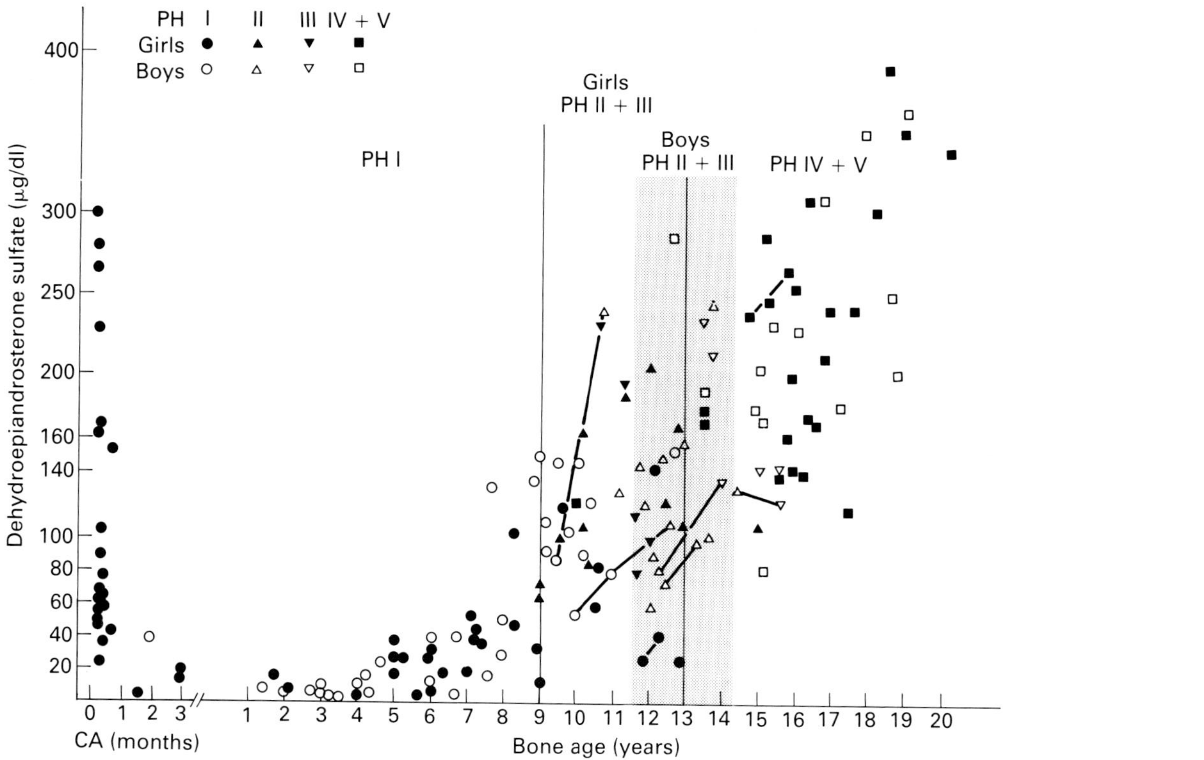

Fig. 14.3 Serum levels of DHEAS in normal boys and girls. Each symbol represents a single value for DHEAS; serial values in individual children are connected by lines. Staging of pubic hair was performed according to Tanner (PH I–IV/V) [62]. The area between the two vertical lines encompasses the normal age of onset of puberty in girls and the shaded/stippled bar encompasses the age of onset of puberty in boys. The pattern of changing DHEA levels in normal boys and girls (not shown) is quantitatively similar to the pattern for DHEAS. (Reprinted, with permission, from Korth-Schutz *et al.* [23], © by The Endocrine Society.)

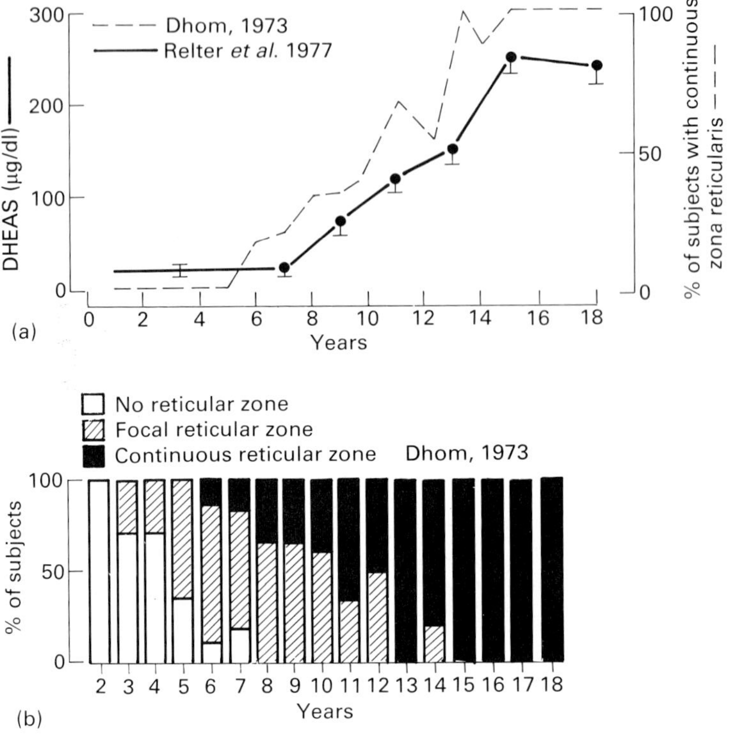

Fig. 14.4 Relationship of growth of the zona reticularis to serum DHEAS levels. Top panel illustrates the temporal relationship between the adrenarchal increase in serum levels of DHEAS and the development of a continuous reticular zone. Bottom panel shows the percentage of adrenal glands from children between the ages of 2 and 18 who suffered sudden death with no antecedent illness, in which there was no reticular zone, some focal islands of reticular tissue, or a continuous reticular zone. (Reprinted, with permission, from Grumbach *et al.* [53].)

cells. The reticular zone, as it develops, first appears as clusters of cells and later becomes a continuous zone. The German pathologist, George Dhom, carefully studied development of the reticular zone in the adrenals of children who suffered sudden death with no antecedent illness (Fig. 14.4, bottom panel). Some children showed areas of focal reticularis by age 3; by age 8, all children had either focal or continuous reticularis; and by age 15, all children had a continuous reticular zone [7].

Adrenocorticotropic hormone (ACTH) stimulates an acute rise in levels of DHEA and DHEAS both before and after adrenarche [4,5]. However, the basal levels and the ACTH-stimulated increases are much greater after adrenarche [8,9]. This observation suggests that a shift in the adrenal steroidogenic pathway that would favor the secretion

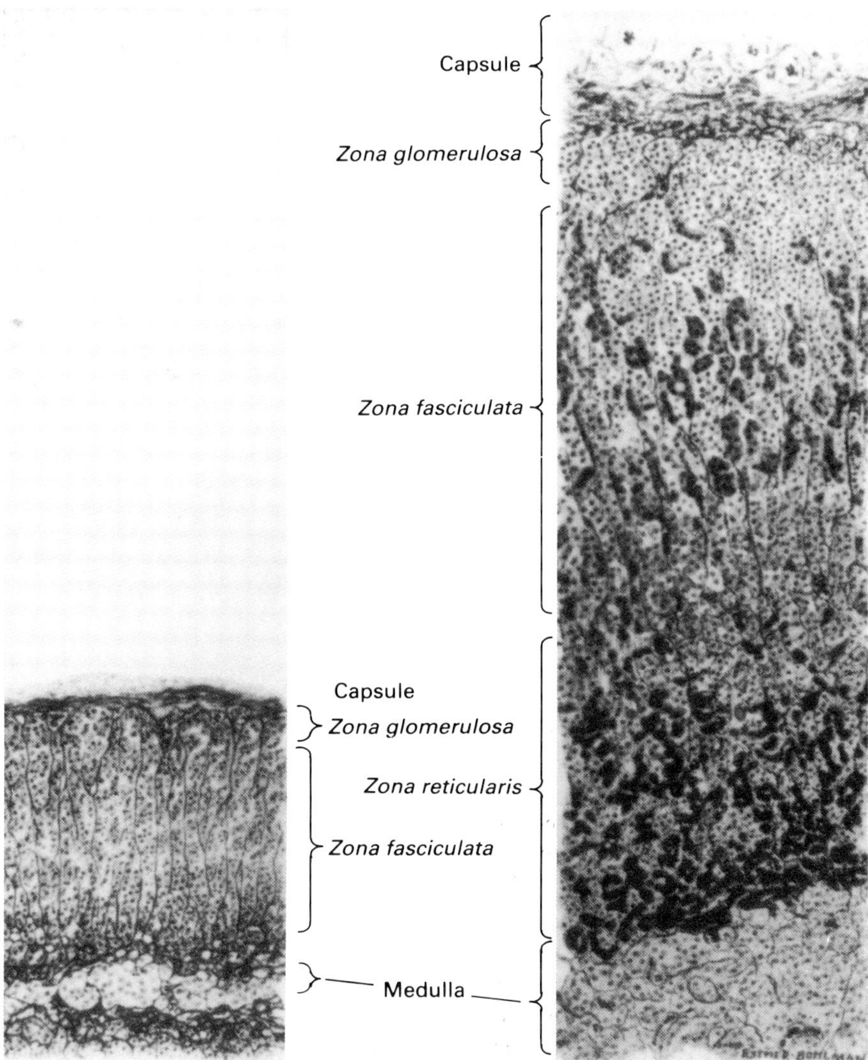

Fig. 14.5 Histology of human infant and adult adrenal cortex showing differences in structural configuration. Left panel shows the cortex of a 6-month-old child. The well-defined zona glomerulosa and the "fetal zone" beneath, which accounts for almost all of the adrenal cortical structure, can be seen. No reticular elements are apparent. The right panel shows an adult adrenal cortex with the differentiated zona glomerulosa, fasciculata and well-defined zona reticularis. (Reprinted, with permission, from Bloom W, Fawcett DW. A Textbook of Histology, 10th edn. Philadelphia: W.B. Saunders, 1975, pp. 540–55.

of DHEA and DHEAS relative to the mineralocorticoids and glucocorticoids might play a key role in adrenarche. Two explanations have been proposed for this shift: (i) a decrease in 3β-hydroxysteroid dehydrogenase-isomerase (3β-HSD) activity (9–11) and (ii) an increase

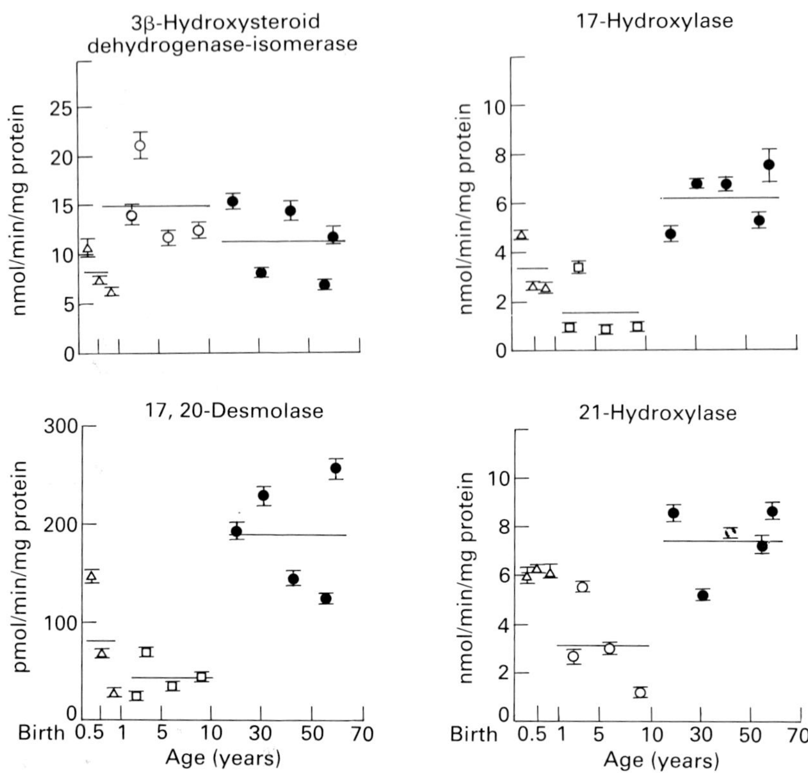

Fig. 14.6 Activity of human adrenal microsomal enzymes as a function of age. Horizontal lines in each graph represent the mean enzymatic activity for each of the three age groups. Moving from left to right in each panel: infants aged 3–8 months ($n = 3$); preadrenarchal or early adrenarchal children aged 2–9 years ($n = 4$); adults aged 20–60 years ($n = 5$). (Reprinted from Schiebinger *et al.* [14], by copyright permission of the American Society for Clinical Investigation)

in 17,20-desmolase activity [9]. Recent studies measuring activities have suggested that adrenarche is associated more with increasing 17-hydroxylase and 17,20-desmolase activities [14], although diminished 3β-HSD activity during this time may play a small role (Fig. 14.6). Data obtained *in vivo* also support this conclusion since, after adrenarche, the ACTH-stimulated products of 17,20-desmolase are enhanced relative to the increments in levels of precursors [9]. While all of the above proposals seem quite plausible, the actual mechanism causing these shifts in adrenal steroidogenic enzymes remains controversial.

Adrenarche and gonadal maturation

Although adrenarche and gonadal maturation (gonadarche) often overlap temporally, clinical studies suggest that adrenarche and gonadarche are independent events, either of which can be activated without the other. The development of adrenarche in the absence of puberty occurs in premature adrenarche, gonadal dysgenesis [1,12,13], and hypogonadotropic hypogonadism [15–17,59,60]. Conversely, gonadarche can occur without adrenarche in cases of true precocious puberty that occurs before the normal age of onset of adrenarche [16,59]. It also appears that normal or physiologic levels of adrenal androgens do not exert a major effect on the onset of puberty. This issue has been studied by Grumbach [18] who examined the time of pubertal onset in girls with premature adrenarche who exhibited an early rise in adrenal sex steroids, and in boys and girls with Addison's disease who were deficient in adrenal androgens. In cases of premature adrenarche in which pubic hair appeared between the ages of 4 and 7, the onset of puberty, as indicated by breast budding, occurred between the ages of 9½ and 11½, i.e. within the normal range of girls (9–14 years). Menarche also occurred within the normal range of 11–15 years. In Addison's disease, puberty in boys, as reflected by genital enlargement, occurs within the normal range of 10–14 years. In girls, breast budding also appeared within the normal range of 9–14 years. Although these observations do not exclude minor changes in the timing of puberty in these disorders, they support the contention that physiologic levels of adrenal androgens and estrogens do not exert a major influence on the timing of puberty.

Animal models of adrenarche

Non-primates

Levels of adrenal androgens vary greatly among most animal species [19] and, in general, non-primate species do not provide a model comparable to human adrenarche because their DHEA and DHEAS levels are quite low (Fig. 14.7). The castrate dexamethasone-suppressed dog does, however, secrete measurable levels of DHEA and androstenedione [20]. It has been established that, during sexual maturation, the dog adrenal develops a zona reticularis, increases its 17-hydroxylase activity, and produces more 17-hydroxyprogesterone [21]. However, the level of adrenal 17,20-desmolase activity in dogs is only about 2% of that observed in humans and does not appear to change during development. Levels of DHEA in castrate dogs were <25 μg/dl (0.88 nM) as compared to 500 μg/dl (17.5 nM) in humans.

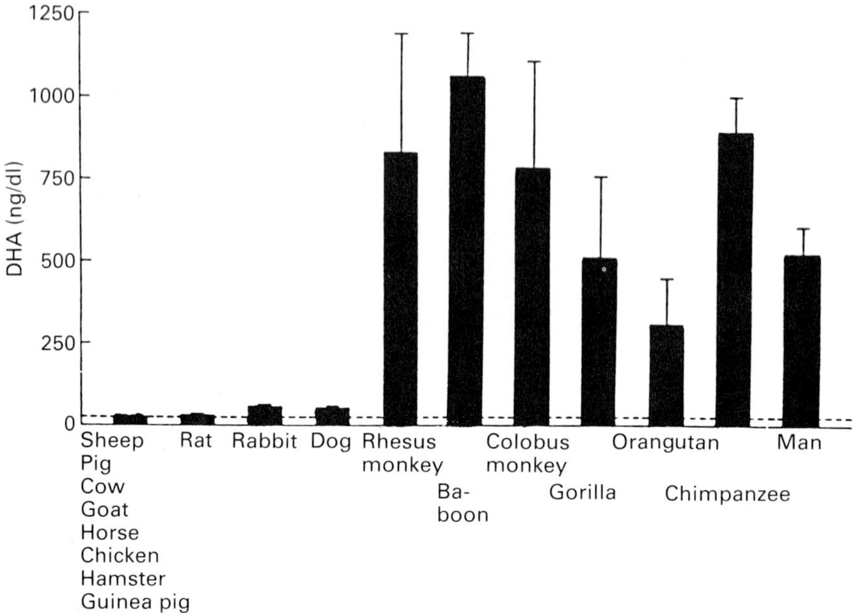

Fig. 14.7 Concentration of DHEA (mean ± SE) in plasma from sexually mature animals representative of various primate and non-primate species. (Reprinted, with permission, from Cutler and Loriaux [63].)

Primates

Old World primates have been examined and found to have similar concentrations of adrenal androgens to those of human beings, but the developmental patterns of adrenal androgens differ markedly. Humans have high DHEA and DHEAS levels at birth [21–24] due to secretion by the fetal adrenal zone [25]. These levels decline rapidly during the first several months of life as the fetal zone regresses, and they remain low until adrenarche. The chimpanzee also has low levels of adrenal androgens prior to the onset of adrenarche, at around the age of 4–5 years, with puberty occurring at approximately age 7 (Fig. 14.8). Rhesus and cynomolgus monkeys and baboons enter puberty at age 3–4 years and have adrenal androgen levels throughout development that are as high or higher than adult levels. These persistent elevations in levels of adrenal androgens may reflect fundamental differences in the regulation of these primates' adrenal androgen secretion. Thus, it appears that the chimpanzee is the best animal to use in investigations of the regulation of adrenarche as it occurs in humans.

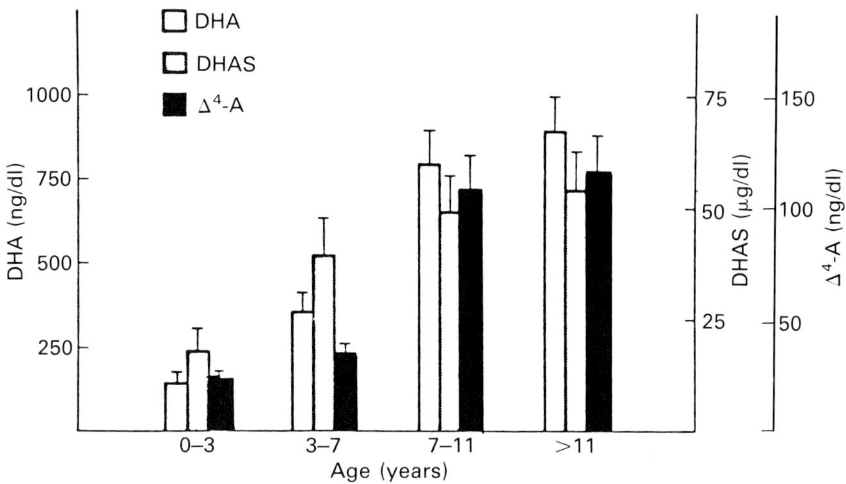

Fig. 14.8 Concentration of DHEA (DHA), DHEAS (DHAS), and Δ4A (mean ± SE) in plasma of chimpanzees as a function of age. Gonadal maturation occurs in chimpanzees between the ages of 7 and 9 years. (Reprinted, with permission, from Cutler *et al.* [19], © by The Endocrine Society.)

Mechanisms controlling adrenarche

Extrapituitary factors

In 1942 Fuller Albright postulated that estrogen may be the hormone that initiates adrenarche because of the increased pubic hair seen in patients with gonadal dysgenesis treated with estrogens [1]. The literature is inconclusive in so far as estrogens have been reported to be able either to stimulate adrenal androgen secretion [12,13,26–28] or to inhibit 3β-HSD activity *in vivo* [10,29–33]. Moreover, adrenarche occurs normally in untreated patients with gonadal dysgenesis and with hypogonadotropic hypogonadism [12,13,15,28,34,35].

Cortisol paracrine hypothesis

The premise that there is a gradual increase in responsiveness of the inner adrenocortical cells to high intra-adrenal levels of cortisol, which was first advanced by Anderson in 1980 [36], can explain the reversal of adrenarche in patients with hypopituitarism or after exogenous administration of glucocorticoid, in which intra-adrenal cortisol levels would be predicted to be low [2]. It would also explain the low DHEA and DHEAS levels sometimes seen in cases of congenital adrenal hyperplasia due to

21-hydroxylase deficiency, since this enzymatic lesion would lead to low intra-adrenal levels of cortisol and thus lowered production of adrenal androgens [37]. Unfortunately, no experimental studies have been carried out to provide support for or to refute this hypothesis and it therefore remains only a hypothesis.

Pituitary factors

GROWTH HORMONE

In some cases of an excess of growth hormone (GH), for example acromegaly, ACTH-stimulation tests produce exaggerated responses in terms of levels of 17-ketosteroid but normal responses for 17-hydroxysteroids [38]. Patients with isolated GH deficiency typically have low plasma DHEAS levels [17]. Growth hormone has been shown to stimulate DHEAS secretion by human fetal adrenal tissue [39]. Furthermore, levels of the principal mediator of GH action, insulin-like growth factor 1, rise in serum during the years of adrenarche [40]. However, as in the case of the "cortisol paracrine hypothesis," no direct evidence exists that proves GH to be "the" adrenarche factor.

PROLACTIN

Prolactin has been extensively studied as a stimulus of adrenal androgen secretion. First, specific receptors for prolactin have been found in the adrenal [41]. Prolactin has also been shown to block 21-hydroxylase activity [42], and such blockage could lead to both decreased production of cortisol (cortisol paracrine hypothesis) and to increased production of Δ^5 steroids. Hyperprolactinemic patients often have elevated plasma levels of DHEA or DHEAS that return to normal when prolactin levels are normalized after pituitary surgery or bromocriptine therapy [43–46]. However, sometimes this effect of prolactin on adrenal androgen secretion is not seen [47–49]. Explanations for these discrepancies have been reviewed by Cutler *et al.* [2] and include the large episodic, diurnal, and age-dependent variations in serum levels of prolactin, and the apparent small magnitude (often between a 50% and 100% increase) of the effect of prolactin on adrenal androgens. Suppression of prolactin in adults using bromocriptine decreases plasma DHEAS levels and the rate of its production [43]. However, it remains to be demonstrated whether or not prolactin regulates adrenal synthesis of androgens and is a factor during adrenarche. Levels of prolactin do not appear to change during adrenarche [50].

PRO-OPIOMELANOCORTIN-DERIVED PEPTIDES: EVIDENCE FOR AN ADRENAL ANDROGEN-STIMULATING HORMONE

Adrenocorticotropic hormone is synthesized in the pituitary corticotroph as part of a larger molecule called pro-opiomelanocortin (Fig. 14.9). It has been suggested that the non-ACTH portions of this precursor may be important regulators of adrenal androgen secretion and may possibly include the adrenal androgen-stimulating factor or hormone [51,52]. α-Melanocyte-stimulating hormone (α-MSH) at high concentrations can stimulate DHEAS secretion by human fetal adrenal tissue [53,54]. However, until recently, little other evidence existed in support of this hypothesis. Albertson *et al.* [55] used the castrate hypophysectomized, ACTH-replaced, adult male chimpanzee as an animal model to test for the presence of an adrenal androgen-stimulating hormone of pituitary origin. Chronic ACTH was administered by single daily injections, beginning the morning after hypophysectomy, with the dose being adjusted to maintain the same 24-hour urinary level of cortisol as before hypophysectomy. Thyroxine was administered orally to prevent hypothyroidism. Despite maintenance of normal secretion of cortisol, as reflected by 24-hour urinary levels of free cortisol, adrenal androgen secretion (assessed by ratios of DHEA to cortisol and of DHEAS to cortisol during a 3-hour infusion of ACTH) decreased significantly in comparison to that of sham-hypophysectomized, control chimpanzees (Fig. 14.10). Cutler *et al.* [56] observed that a 48-hour infusion of ACTH in patients with long-standing panhypopituitarism caused a prompt release of plasma cortisol (which reached 30 μg/dl) at 48 hours, but it also led to a marked decrease in the secretion of DHEA, with result-

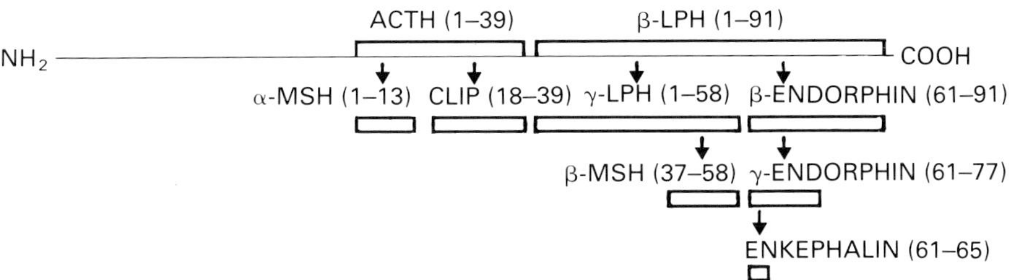

Fig. 14.9 Schematic diagram of pro-opiomelanocortin. The arrows represent potential sites of cleavage, which may or may not occur in humans, that would yield smaller biologically active peptides contained within the structure of ACTH and β-lipotropic hormone (β-LPH). CLIP, corticotropin-like intermediate lobe peptide; α-MSH and β-MSH, α and β melanocyte-stimulating hormone, respectively. The region between NH_2 and ACTH is the amino-terminal portion of pro-opiomelanocortin where the putative adrenal androgen-stimulating activity may be located. (Reprinted, with permission, from Cutler *et al.* [2], © 1990, the Williams & Wilkins Co., Baltimore.)

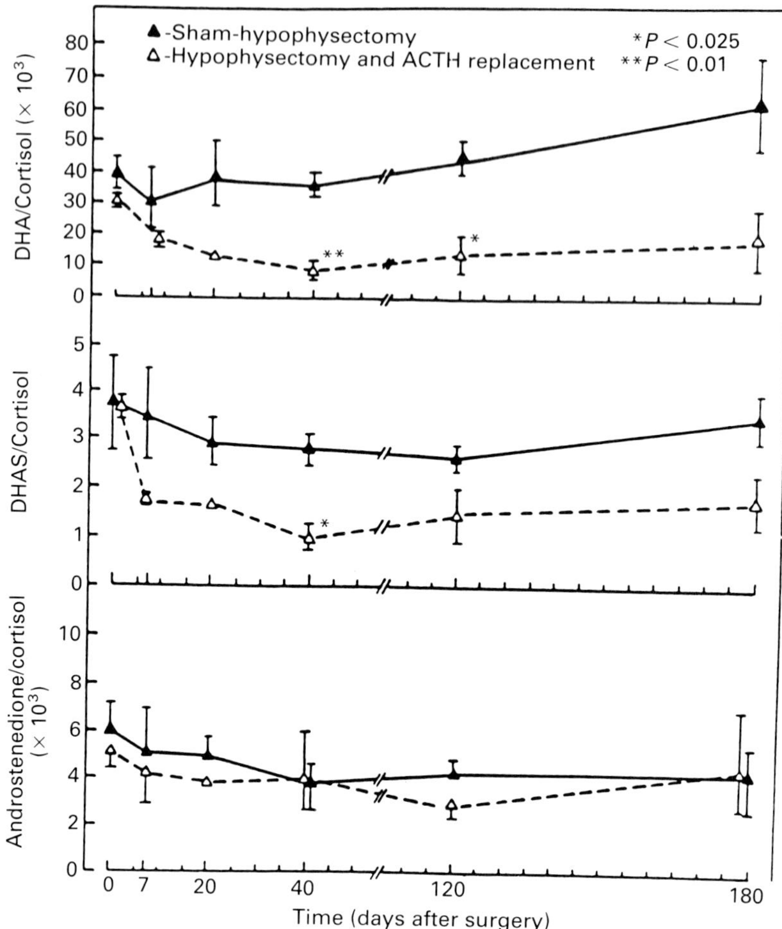

Fig. 14.10 Ratios of plasma levels of DHEA to cortisol, DHEAS to cortisol, and androstenedione to cortisol during 3-hour infusions of ACTH in castrate, hypophysectomized, ACTH-replaced chimpanzees and castrate, sham-hypophysectomized controls. $^{*}P < 0.025$; $^{**}P < 0.01$ (compared to control animals). (Reprinted, with permission, from Albertson *et al.* [55], © by The Endocrine Society.)

ant decreased ratios of DHEA to cortisol and of DHEAS to cortisol, which were similar to those seen before adrenarche. Patients receiving long-term treatment with glucocorticoids had an identical pattern. These observations are consistent with adrenal regulation of androgens through a non-ACTH, pro-opiomelanocortin-derived peptide.

Parker and Odell [20] have examined this issue using dexamethasone-suppressed, castrated dogs that received an infusion of an extract of bovine pituitary gland. Their data showed that the pituitary extract caused a greater increase in DHEA secretion for a given increase in

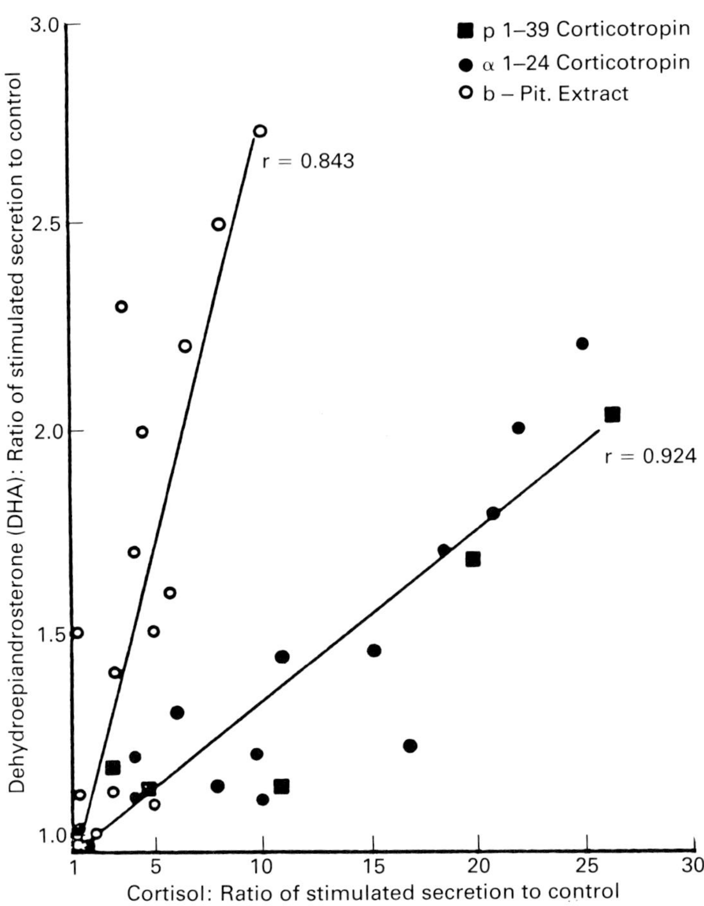

Fig. 14.11 Ratio of stimulated levels of DHEA to controls as a function of the ratio of stimulated levels of cortisol to controls (measured in the same samples) in dogs infused with an extract of bovine pituitary gland. The bovine extract produced greater stimulation of levels of DHEA for a given increase in levels of cortisol than did synthetic ACTH 1–24 or porcine ACTH 1–39. (Reprinted, with permission, from Parker and Odell [20].)

plasma levels of cortisol than an infusion of synthetic ACTH 1–24 or porcine ACTH 1–39 (Fig. 14.11). Moreover, this effect could not be duplicated by infusions of lutenizing hormone-releasing hormone, bovine GH, bovine prolactin, bovine thyroid-stimulating hormone or synthetic arginine vasopressin. Recently, Parker has isolated this putative cortical androgen-stimulating hormone from human pituitary glands [57] and has determined the amino acid sequence of this peptide [58] (Fig. 14.12). The peptide has a molecular weight of 1758 and is composed of 18 amino acids. The sequence is identical to that of a

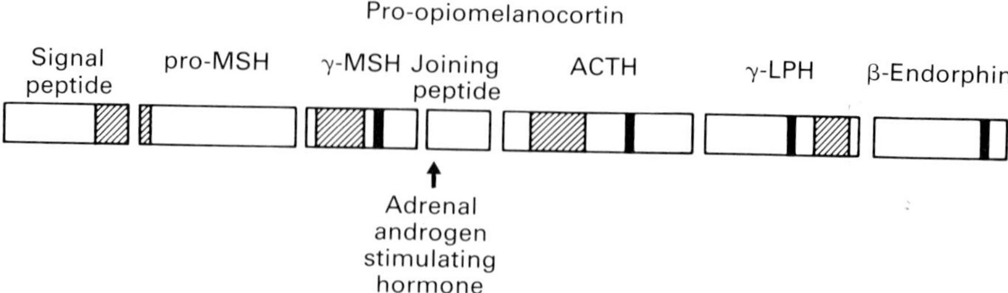

- 18AA, mol. wt 1758: N-Glu-Asp-Val-Ser-Ala-Gly-Glu-Asp-Cys-Gly-Pro-Leu-Pro-Glu-Gly-Gly-Pro-Glu-C
- 18AA-18AA dimer (disulfide linked)
- naturally occurring peptide and synthetic peptide active *in vitro* in adrenal cells from dog, human, human fetal adrenal

Fig. 14.12 Proposed amino acid sequence and characteristics of the putative adrenal androgen-stimulating hormone, showing its location within the pro-opiomelanocortin molecule. (Reprinted, with permission, from Parker *et al.* [58].)

small fragment of the pro-opiomelanocortin molecule, situated just N-terminally to the ACTH portion. This fragment of 18 amino acids can selectively stimulate DHEA production by cultured adrenal cortical cells without affecting the production of cortisol. However, the extent of the stimulation by this factor is not sufficiently large to account clearly for the magnitude of changes observed at adrenarche. Nonetheless, this breakthrough represents the only isolation, purification, and testing of an adrenal androgen-stimulating hormone and the subsequent production of a synthetic molecule. Further experiments should permit elucidation of the mechanisms of action of this peptide and allow us to assess whether it is the bona fide stimulator of the secretion of adrenal androgens at adrenarche.

Summary

Adrenarche is a maturational change in adrenal cortical function that leads to increased adrenal production and secretion of androgens and estrogens. The process begins several years before the onset of gonadal maturation and is closely correlated with the appearance of reticular elements and a continuous reticular zone within the adrenal cortex. While most of the adrenal androgens probably arise from the zona reticularis, evidence suggests that the steroidogenic enzymatic machinery for production of adrenal androgens exists throughout the adrenal cortex. Increased synthesis of adrenal 17-hydroxylase and 17,20-desmolase probably accounts for the major alteration in steroidogenesis during adrenarche.

Although normal puberty can be considered a combination of both adrenal and gonadal maturation, each of these processes can occur independently of the other in pathologic situations. The timing of gonadal maturation does not seem to be influenced by adrenal sex steroids, nor does absence of adrenal androgens cause delayed puberty.

Several animal models are currently being used to study adrenarche, in particular the dog and chimpanzee. The chimpanzee probably provides the closest model, but unfortunately it is a difficult species to utilize because of competing research needs and its inclusion on the list of endangered species.

Several hormones have been shown to influence adrenal androgen secretion, including prolactin, GH, MSH, and derivatives of the proopiomelanocortin prohormone. A peptide of 18 amino acids has been isolated from human pituitary glands and produced synthetically that can stimulate adrenal production of androgens while having little or no effect on glucocorticoid or mineralocorticoid secretion in adrenal cell cultures. Further work is needed to determine whether this molecule is the adrenal androgen-stimulating hormone responsible for adrenarche, whether it has any other physiologic significance, and whether it might represent a possible cause of inappropriate production of androgens in other steroidogenic tissues.

References

1 Albright F, Smith PH, Fraser R. A syndrome characterized by primary ovarian insufficiency and decreased stature. Report of 11 cases with a digression on hormonal control of axillary and pubic hair. Am J Med Sci 1942; 204:625–648.

2 Cutler GB Jr, Schiebinger RJ, Albertson BD, *et al.* The adrenarche (human and animal). In: Grumbach NN, Sizomenke PC, Aubert ML, eds. Control of the Onset of Puberty. Baltimore: Williams and Wilkins, 1990, pp. 506–33.

3 Abraham GE. Ovarian and adrenal contribution to peripheral steroids during the menstrual cycle in two hirsute women. Obstet Gynecol 1975; 46(1):29–36.

4 dePeretti E, Forest MG. Pattern of plasma dehydroepiandrosterone sulfate levels in humans from birth to adulthood. Evidence for testicular production. J Clin Endocrinol Metab 1978; 47:572–8.

5 Nieschlag E, Loriaux DL, Ruder HJ, Zucker IR, Kirschner MA, Lipsett MB. The secretion of dehydroepiandrosterone and dehydroepiandrosterone sulfate in man. J Endocrinol 1973; 57:123–34.

6 Rosenfield RL. Plasma 17-ketosteroids and 17-beta-hydroxysteroids in girls with premature development of sexual hair. J Pediatr 1971; 85:260–6.

7 Dhom G. Prepubertal and pubertal growth of the adrenal (adrenarche). Bietr Pathol 1973; 150:357–77.

8 Genazzani AR, Pintor C, Facchinetti F, Inanudi P, Maci D, Corda R. Changes throughout puberty in adrenal secretion after ACTH. J Steroid Biochem 1979; 11:571–7.

9 Rich BH, Rosenfield RL, Lucky AW, Helke JC, Otto P. Adrenarche: changing adrenal response to adrenocorticotropin. J Clin Endocrinol Metab 1981; 52:1129–37.

10 Sobrinho LG, Kase NG, Grunt JA. Changes in adrenocortical function in patients with

gonadal dysgenesis after treatment with estrogen. J Clin Endocrinol Metab 1971; 33:110–15.

11 Warne GL, Carter JN, Faiman C, Reyes FD, Winter JSD. Hormonal changes in girls with precocious adrenarche: a possible role for estradiol or prolactin. J Pediatr 1979; 92:743–7.

12 Lucky AW, Marynick SP, Rebar RW, *et al.* Replacement oral ethyl estradiol therapy for gonadal dysgenesis: growth and adrenal androgen studies. Acta Endocrinol 1979; 91:519–28.

13 Rosenfield RL, Fang VS. Effects of prolonged physiologic estradiol therapy on the maturation of hypogonadal teenagers. J Pediatr 1974; 85:830–7.

14 Schiebinger RJ, Albertson BD, Cassorla FG, *et al.* Developmental changes in plasma adrenal androgens during infancy and adrenarche are associated with changing activities of adrenal microsomal 17-hydroxylase and 17,20 desmolase. J Clin Invest 1981; 67:1177–82.

15 Copeland KC, Paunier L, Sizonenko PC. The secretion of adrenal androgens and growth patterns of patients with hypogonadotrophic hypogonadism and idiopathic delayed puberty. J Pediatr 1977; 91:985–90.

16 Sklar CA, Kaplan SL, Grumbach MM. Evidence for dissociation between adrenarche and gonadarche: studies in patients with idiopathic precocious puberty, gonadal dysgenesis, isolated gonadotropin deficiency and constitutional delayed growth and adolescence. J Clin Endocrinol Metab 1980; 51:548–57.

17 Cohen HN, Wallace AM, Beastall GH, Fogelman I, Thompson JA. Clinical value of adrenal androgen measurement in the diagnosis of delayed puberty. Lancet 1981; i: 689–92.

18 Grumbach MM, Richards GE, Conte FA, Kaplan SL. Clinical disorders of adrenal function and puberty: an assessment of the role of the adrenal cortex in normal and abnormal puberty in man and evidence for an ACTH-like pituitary adrenal androgen-stimulating hormone. In: James VHT, Serio M, Giusti G, Martini L, eds. The Endocrine Function of the Human Adrenal Cortex. London: Academic Press, 1978, pp. 583–612.

19 Cutler GB Jr, Glenn M, Bush M, Hodgen GD, Graham CE, Loriaux DL. Adrenarche: a survey of rodents, domestic animals and primates. Endocrinology 1978; 103:2112–18.

20 Parker LN, Odell WD. Evidence for the existence of cortical androgen-stimulating hormone. Am J Physiol 1979; 236:E616–E620.

21 Schiebinger RJ, Albertson BD, Barnes KM, Cutler GB Jr, Loriaux DL. Developmental changes in rabbit and dog adrenal function: a possible homologue of adrenarche in the dog. Am J Physiol 1981; 240:E694–E699.

22 Korth-Shutz S, Levine LS, New MI. Dehydroepiandrosterone sulfate (DS) levels, a rapid test for abnormal adrenal androgen secretion. J Clin Endocrinol Metab 1976; 42:1005–13.

23 Korth-Shutz S, Levine LS, New MI. Serum androgens in normal prepubertal and pubertal children and in children with precocious adrenarche. J Clin Endocrinol Metab 1976; 42:117–27.

24 Korth-Schutz S, Levine LS, New MI. Evidence for the adrenal source of androgens in precocious adrenarche. Acta Endocrinol 1976; 82:342–52.

25 Serón-Ferré M, Lawrence C, Siiteri P, Jaffe R. Steroid production by definitive and fetal zones of the human fetal adrenal gland. J Clin Endocrinol Metab 1978; 46:834–8.

26 Migeon CJ, Espiner EA, Donald RA. Lack of effect of prolactin suppression on plasma dehydroepiandrosterone sulfate. Clin Endocrinol 1979; 10:539–44.

27 Madden JP, Milewich L, Parker CR Jr, Carr BC, Boyar RM, MacDonald PC. Effect of oral contraceptive treatment on the serum concentration of dehydroepiandrosterone sulfate. Am J Obstet Gynecol 1978; 132:380–4.

28 Sklar CA, Kaplan SL, Grumbach MM. Lack of effect of estrogens on adrenal androgen secretion in children and adolescents with a comment on estrogens and pubic hair growth. Clin Endocrinol 1981; 14:311–20.

29 Anderson DC, Yen SSC. Effects of estrogens on adrenal 3-beta-hydroxysteroid dehydrogenase in ovariectomized women. J Clin Endocrinol Metab 1976; 43:561–70.
30 Bongiovanni AM, Eberlein WR, Goldman AS, New MI. Disorders of adrenal steroid biogenesis. Recent Prog Horm Res 1967; 23:375–439.
31 Yates J, Deshpande N. Kinetic studies on the enzymes catalyzing the conversion of 17-alpha-hydroxyprogesterone and dehydroepiandrosterone and androstenedione in the human adrenal gland *in vitro*. J Endocrinol 1974; 60:27–35.
32 Winter JSD, Fujieda K, Faiman C, Reyes FI, Thliveris J. Control of steroidogenesis by human fetal adrenal cells in tissue culture. In: Genazzani AR, Thijssen JHH, Siiteri PK, eds. Adrenal Androgens. New York: Raven Press, 1980, pp. 55–62.
33 Abraham GP, Maroulis GB. Effect of exogenous estrogen on serum pregnenolone, cortisol and androgens in postmenopausal women. Obstet Gynecol 1975; 45:271–4.
34 Forest MG, Saez JM, Bertraud J. Present concepts of initiation of puberty. Neonatal and prepubertal hormone influences. In: Franchimont P, ed. Some Aspects of Hypothalamic Regulation of Endocrine Functions. Stuttgart: FK Shattauer Verlag, 1975, pp. 339–66.
35 Lee PA, Kowarski A, Migeon CJ, Blizzard RM. Lack of correlation between gonadotropins (LH, FSH) and adrenal androgen levels in agonadal children. J Clin Endocrinol Metab 1975; 40:664–9.
36 Anderson DC. The adrenal androgen-stimulating hormone does not exist. Lancet 1980; ii: 454–6.
37 Korth-Shutz S, Virdis R, Saenger P, Chow PM, Levine LS, New MI. Serum androgens as a continuing index of adequacy of treatment of congenital adrenal hyperplasia. J Clin Endocrinol Metab 1978; 46:452–9.
38 Lim NY, Dingman JF. Androgenic adrenal hyperfunction in acromegaly. N Engl J Med 1964; 271:1189–94.
39 Brown TJ, Ginz B, Oakey RE. Effects of polypeptide hormone preparations on steroid production by the human fetal adrenal gland during superfusion. J Endocrinol 1978; 79:60–1.
40 Bala RM, Lopatka J, Leung A, McCoy E, McArthur RG. Serum immunoreactive somatomedin levels in normal adults, pregnant women at term, children at various ages and children with constitutionally delayed growth. J Clin Endocrinol Metab 1981; 52:508–13.
41 Posner BL, Kelly PA, Shiu RPC, Friesen HG. Studies of insulin, growth hormone and prolactin-binding tissue distribution, species variation, and characterization. Endocrinology 1974; 95:521–31.
42 Albertson BD, Sienkiewicz ML, Kimball D, Munabi A, Cassorla FC, Loriaux DL. New evidence for a direct effect of prolactin on adrenal steroidogenic enzyme activity in the rat. Endocr Res 1987; 13:317–33.
43 Schiebinger RJ, Chrousos GP, Cutler GB Jr, Loriaux DL. The effect of serum prolactin on plasma adrenal androgens and the production and metabolic clearance rate of DHAS in normal and hyperprolactinemic subjects. J Clin Endocrinol Metab 1986; 62:202–9.
44 Pepi GJ, Albrecht ED. Program of the 63th Annual Meeting of the Endocrine Society, Cincinnati, Ohio, Abstract 605.
45 Lobo RA, Kletzky OA, Kaptein EM, Goebelsimann U. Prolactin modulation of dehydroepiandrosterone sulfate secretion. Am J Obstet Gynecol 1980; 138:632–6.
46 Boccuzzi G, Gaidano GD, Fossati D, Tamagnone C, Angelo A. Plasma dehydroepiandrosterone sulfate after acute sulpiride injection in chronic hyperprolactinemia. In: Genazzini AR, Thijssen THH, Siiteri PK, eds. Adrenal Androgens. New York: Raven Press, 1980, pp. 103–7.
47 Parker LN, Chang S, Odell WD. Adrenal androgens in patients with chronic marked elevation of prolactin. Clin Endocrinol 1978; 8:1–5.
48 Metcalf MC, Espiner EA, Donald RA. Lack of effect of prolactin suppression on plasma DHEA-sulfate. Clin Endocrinol 1979; 10:539–44.

49 Belisle S, Menard J. Adrenal androgen production in hyperprolactinemic states. Fertil Steril 1980; 33:396–400.
50 Parker LN, Sack J, Fisher DA, Odell WD. The adrenarche: prolactin, gonadotropins, adrenal androgens and cortisol. J Clin Endocrinol Metab 1978; 46:396–401.
51 Eipper BA, Mains RP. Structure and biosynthesis of pro-adrenocortin/endorphin and related peptides. Endocr Rev 1980; 1:1–27.
52 Grumbach MM, Richards GE, Conte FA, Kaplan SL. Clinical disorders of adrenal function and puberty: an assessment of the role of the adrenal cortex in normal and abnormal puberty in man and evidence for an ACTH-like pituitary adrenal stimulating hormone. In: James VHT, Serio M, Giusti G, Martini L, eds. The Endocrine Function of the Human Adrenal Cortex. New York: Academic Press, 1978, pp. 583–612.
53 Silman RE, Chard T, Lowry PJ, Smith I, Young IM. Human fetal pituitary peptides and parturition. Nature 1976; 260:716–18.
54 Silman RE, Holland D, Chard T, Lowry PJ, Hope J, Robinson JS, Thornburn GD. ACTH "family tree" of the rhesus monkey changes with development. Nature 1978; 276:526–8.
55 Albertson BD, Hobson WC, Burnett BS, *et al.* Dissociation of cortisol and adrenal androgen secretion in the hypophysectomized, adrenocorticotropin-replaced chimpanzee. J Clin Endocrinol Metab 1984; 59:13–18.
56 Cutler GB Jr, Davis SE, Johnsonbaugh RE, Loriaux DL. Dissociation of cortisol and adrenal androgen secretion in patients with secondary adrenal insufficiency. J Clin Endocrinol Metab 1979; 49:604–9.
57 Parker LN, Lifrak ET, Odell WD. A 60 000 molecular weight human pituitary glycoprotein stimulates adrenal androgen secretion. Endocrinology 1983; 113:2092–6.
58 Parker LN, Lifrak E, Shively J, *et al.* Human adrenal gland cortical androgen-stimulating hormone (CASH) is identical with a portion of the joining peptide of pituitary pro-opiomelanocortin (POMC). National Endocrine Society, Seattle, Washington, 1989, Abstract 299.
59 Counts DR, Pescovitz OH, Barnes KM, *et al.* Dissociation of adrenarche and gonadarche in precocious puberty and in isolated hypogonadotropic hypogonadism. J Clin Endocrinol Metab 1987; 64:1174–8.
60 Cutler GB Jr, Loriaux DL. Adrenarche and its relationship to the onset of puberty. Fed Proc 1988; 39:2384–90.

Chapter 15
Adrenal Abnormalities in Polycystic Ovary Syndrome and the Impact of their Correction

T. JOSEPH McKENNA & SEAN K. CUNNINGHAM

The possibility that a primary abnormality of the adrenal gland plays a fundamental role in the development of polycystic ovary syndrome (PCO) is suggested by a number of related observations. It may develop secondary to florid and well-established, although relatively rare, adrenal abnormalities, for example androgen-secreting adrenal tumor [1], congential adrenal hyperplasia [2], Cushing's syndrome [3]. Furthermore, dehydroepiandrostrone sulfate (DHEAS), the most plentiful steroid normally present in the adult woman, is uniquely of adrenal origin and is found to be elevated in many patients with PCO [4]. In addition, when rats were treated with adrenal androgens, they developed ovarian abnormalities analagous to PCO [5] (see Chapter 11). Prompted by these observations, we have examined adrenal function in patients with idiopathic hirsutism (IH) and PCO by comparing glucocorticoid and androgen responses to endogenous and exogenous stimulation. Furthermore, we examined the possibility that all the hormonal abnormalities of PCO could be corrected by adrenal suppression.

Idiopathic hirsutism and PCO are related disorders both associated with chronic hyperandrogenemia [6,7]. The disorders are distinguished by the development of more profound hyperandrogenemia in PCO and the consequent occurrence of hyperestronemia and the characteristic abnormalities in gonadotropins, for example elevated luteinizing hormone (LH)/follicle-stimulating hormone (FSH) ratio in blood and an exaggerated LH response to luteinizing hormone-releasing hormone (LHRH). In the majority of PCO patients the precise sequence of events leading to the endocrine abnormalities in PCO is the subject of ongoing debate [7–9].

Materials and methods

In the studies reported here, the data were obtained from 40 normal women, 34 patients with IH [10] and 19 patients with PCO [11]. Blood was obtained during the early follicular phase of the menstrual cycle in women with regular ovulation. Hormonal and sex hormone-binding globulin levels were measured under random conditions, before and after α1–24 adrenocorticotropic hormone (ACTH), 250 μg i.v., between 8 and 10 hours and on the morning following metyrapone, 2–3 g by mouth, at midnight with a snack. Metyrapone inhibits 11β-hydroxylase and thereby impairs the final step in cortisol biosynthesis. As a result, plasma cortisol levels fall and ACTH and related pro-opiomelanocortin (POMC) fragments, e.g. β-lipotropin, β-endorphin, the 16k-fragment, are secreted in an attempt to overcome the block in cortisol biosynthesis [12]. However, stimulated adrenal androgen biosynthesis is not perturbed by metyrapone and provides an index of adrenal androgen responsiveness to endogenous stimulation. In addition, the plasma concentration of the cortisol precursor, 11-deoxycortisol, can be used as an index of activity in the cortisol biosynthetic pathway [13]. Both LH and FSH were measured in blood samples obtained prior to and 10, 20, 30, 45 and 60 min after administration of LHRH 200 μg i.v. Dexamethasone was administered in low dose, 0.5 mg by mouth, on retiring each night for at least 3 months.

Results

Basal hormonal profiles in IH and PCO

The hormonal findings in the two disorders are summarized in Table 15.1. These findings confirm elevated androgen levels in IH and PCO; estradiol is similar to normal in both disorders but estrone is elevated in PCO. While the LH response to LHRH is significantly greater in PCO than in normal women, the response in IH was intermediate between the two other groups although not statistically different from normal.

Steroid responses to ACTH and to metyrapone

In patients with IH the androstenedione, dehydroepiandrosterone (DHEA), 17-hydroxyprogesterone and cortisol increments following stimulation with ACTH were significantly higher than increments occurring in normal women (Table 15.2). Furthermore, 8 hours following the administration of metyrapone the mean testosterone increment in plasma of women with IH was significantly higher than that occurring in normal women [10]. When the metyrapone-induced plasma steroid responses were examined in PCO patients, the increments achieved in testosterone, androstenedione and 11-deoxycortisol were excessive [11]. These observations indicate the presence of adrenal hyperresponsiveness of both androgen and glucocorticoid pathways in patients with IH or PCO (see Chapter 9). The pattern achieved does not conform to any of the classical enzymatic defects occurring in congenital adrenal hyperplasia [14]. Although 17-hydroxyprogesterone increments following ACTH were higher than in normal women, the levels achieved were much lower than those seen in patients with 21-hydroxylase deficiency. When plotted on the nomogram described by New and coworkers [14], the levels achieved fall within the range of the general population. The possibility of Cushing's syndrome had been excluded in all subjects using the overnight dexamethasone suppression test [15].

Hormonal and clinical response to dexamethasone

Following treatment with dexamethasone, previously elevated testosterone and androstenedione levels were similar to those occurring in normal women. The sex hormone-binding globulin levels rose significantly and, as a result of these changes, the testosterone/sex hormone-binding globulin ratio was significantly suppressed (Table 15.1). In addition, DHEA and DHEAS levels were suppressed to values significantly lower than those seen in normal women [10,11]. The mean estrone level fell in women with PCO following treatment with dexamethasone but was still significantly higher than that seen in normal women. While basal LH levels were similar prior to and following treatment with dexamethasone in PCO, the maximum LH increment induced by LHRH, which was significantly higher in PCO than in normal women prior to treatment, was no longer significantly different although the mean level achieved was still higher than that seen in normal women (Table 15.1).

The excessive testosterone, androstenedione and 11-deoxycortisol responsiveness to metyrapone seen in PCO was markedly suppressed following treatment with dexamethasone so that the increments noted were significantly lower than those seen in untreated normal women (Table 15.2). While the mean 11-deoxycortisol response to metyrapone was suppressed following treatment with dexamethasone, 12 of 16 patients maintained a normal glucocorticoid response [13]. This observation is important when considering the possibility of glucocorticoid excess during treatment, or of adrenal suppression following the withdrawal of dexamethasone. Indeed, the excessive cortisol response to

Table 15.1 Hormonal profiles (mean ± SD) in IH and PCO and the impact of dexamethasone treatment.

	Normal women	IH	PCO	PCO-treated dexamethasone
Testosterone (nmol/l)	1.2 ± 0.34	1.6 ± 0.55*	1.9 ± 0.6*	1.3 ± 0.7
SHBG[‡] (nmol/l)	42 ± 13.5	31.0 ± 11.8*	26.9 ± 12.8*	30.0 ± 15.2*†
Testosterone/SHBG	3.09 ± 1.25	5.55 ± 2.9*	9.05 ± 6.75*	4.8 ± 2.6*†
Androstenedione (A_1) (pmol/l)	6.0 ± 1.7	7.7 ± 2.6*	9.8 ± 3.3*	6.6 ± 3.5†
Estradiol (pmol/l)	200.9 ± 135	171 ± 85	182.5 ± 117	159.6 ± 62.8
Estrone (E_1) (pmol/l)	178.1 ± 70.8	175 ± 87	293.2 ± 136*	237.8 ± 112.8*
E_1/Δ^4	33.7 ± 15.7	25.7 ± 15.2	31.0 ± 12.7	41.3 ± 12.5†
Basal LH (IU/l)	4.6 ± 2.5	4.4 ± 1.5	5.3 ± 3.1	6.3 ± 6.2
LHRH-stimulated LH (IU/l)	12.3 ± 11.3	30.0 ± 55	50.9 ± 39.1*	37.9 ± 45.2
Basal FSH (IU/l)	4.1 ± 1.5	3.7 ± 1.1	2.7 ± 1.3*	2.8 ± 1.5*
LHRH-stimulated FSH (IU/l)	3.0 ± 1.8	2.6 ± 1.8	4.5 ± 4.8	2.0 ± 1.3†
Basal LH/FSH	1.1 ± 0.5	1.3 ± 0.7	2.7 ± 1.3*	—

* $P < 0.05–0.001$, significantly different from normal women.

† $P < 0.05–0.005$, significantly different from pretreatment values.

‡ Assumes that 1 mole dihydrotestosterone (DHT) binds 1 mole SHBG; more accurately nmol DHT bound to SHBG per litre.

Table 15.2 Incremental steroid responses (nmol/l; mean ± SD) to ACTH and metyrapone in IH and PCO.

	Normal women untreated	PCO/IH untreated	PCO/IH dex-treated
ACTH			
Androstenedione	2.0 ± 1.5	4.5 ± 3.8*	1.2 ± 1.3†
DHEA	18 ± 25	39 ± 23*	15 ± 13*
17-OH-Progesterone	1.8 ± 1.1	3.2 ± 1.8*	2.3 ± 2.5
Cortisol	252 ± 122	511 ± 329*	473 ± 225*
Metyrapone			
Testosterone	1.1 ± 0.4	1.5 ± 0.6*	0.6 ± 0.6†
Androstenedione	10.8 ± 3.0	16.2 ± 5.7*	8.4 ± 90†
11-Deoxycortisol	353 ± 101	453 ± 136*	192 ± 130*†

ACTH data from McKenna *et al.* [6].
Metyrapone data from McKenna [7].
* $P < 0.05$, significantly different from normal women.
† $P < 0.05$, significantly different from untreated PCO/IH.

ACTH was still present following treatment with dexamethasone in IH [10]. This suggests that an adrenal abnormality persisted following suppression of adrenal stimulation.

In our original study, 10 of 15 patients who were submitted to extensive evaluation resumed regular ovulatory menstrual bleeding [11]. In a much more extensive clinical experience, the response rate of approximately two-thirds has been maintained. Approximately 50% of patients in whom ovulation is induced using dexamethasone treatment continue to ovulate regularly when the dose of dexamethasone is reduced from 0.5 to 0.25 mg each night. In addition, approximately 50% of patients treated with dexamethasone for 6 months demonstrate improvement in hirsutism [10]. Occasional patients, particularly those who are significantly overweight at the initiation of treatment, tend to gain more weight while taking dexamethasone. Only very rarely do patients complain of gastrointestinal upset or depression on the dosage used.

POMC fragment levels in plasma and responses to metyrapone prior to and following treatment with dexamethasone

The ACTH, β-endorphin, β-lipotropin and 16k-fragment levels were similar in normal women and women with IH/PCO [12]. Furthermore, values achieved in normal women and patients were similar 8 hours following the administration of metyrapone. Following at least 3 months' treatment with dexamethasone, both basal and stimulated values for

ACTH appeared to be relatively less suppressed than the values of other POMC fragments measured [12]. In order to examine this possibility, we used a sensitive index, β-lipotropin, β-endorphin and 16k-fragment values obtained 8 hours following the ingestion of metyrapone expressed as a ratio of simultaneous ACTH values, both before and following treatment with dexamethasone. The results obtained are shown in Fig. 15.1. While there was a tendency for the ratios to fall for each of the three comparisons when treated with dexamethasone, statistical significance was achieved only in the case of the 16k-fragment : ACTH ratio [12]. Therefore, treatment with dexamethasone appears to preferentially suppress blood levels of POMC fragments other than ACTH.

Discussion

In this paper we have summarized clear findings of excessive adrenal androgen and glucocorticoid responsiveness to both the stimulation of the adrenal gland by α1–24 ACTH [10] and, more importantly, in the response to endogenous ACTH and possibly other POMC fragments released in response to metyrapone-induced hypocortisolemia. Since the responses of ACTH and other POMC fragments were similar in

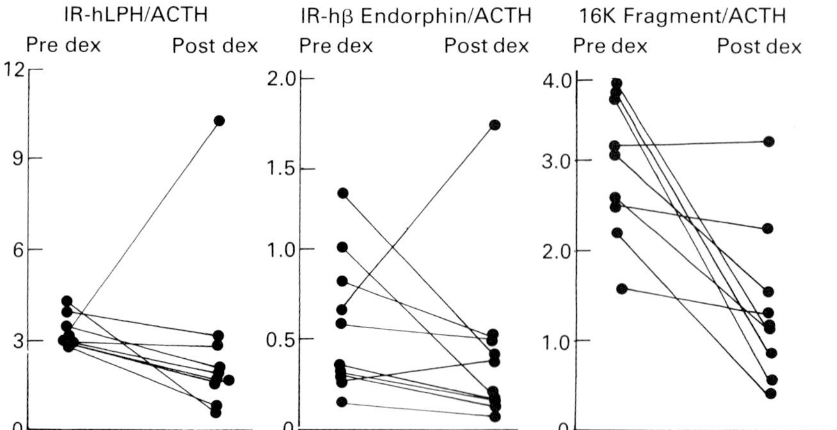

Fig. 15.1 β-Lipotropin (IR-hLPH), β-endorphin, and 16k-fragment expressed as a function of simultaneous ACTH levels obtained 8 hours after the administration of metyrapone, prior to treatment with dexamethasone (Pre dex) and following at least 3 months of treatment with dexamethasone (Post dex). While the mean ratios were lower following dexamethasone than prior to treatment, statistical significance was achieved only in the case of the 16k-fragment/ACTH ratio ($P < 0.05$). (Reprinted, with permission, from Cunningham *et al.* [12].)

normal women and in IH/PCO patients, the abnormality could be one of increased adrenal sensitivity rather than excessive adrenal stimulation. However, these abnormalities are clearly dependent on hypothalamic–pituitary secretion since the abnormalities were largely corrected following treatment with dexamethasone. As previously noted, the basal pattern of steroid precursors or products, or that seen following stimulation with ACTH or metyrapone, does not indicate an adrenal abnormality involving one of the classical enzymatic defects occurring in congenital adrenal hyperplasia [14]. Rather, there appears to be a generalized hyperresponsiveness of the adrenal glands, the mechanism of which awaits elucidation since Cushing's syndrome was specifically excluded in all of these patients.

Dexamethasone was administered at night only to blunt the early morning surge in ACTH and related peptides that occurs prior to waking [16]. Dexamethasone is ideal for this purpose because of its prolonged biological half-life relative to other glucocorticoids available for this purpose [17]. We have previously demonstrated that this dosage schedule of dexamethasone was associated simultaneously with the resolution of signs of glucocorticoid excess that had occurred and the control of androgen excess, which had not been achieved in a patient with congenital adrenal hyperplasia using cortisone acetate 37.5 mg per day in divided doses [18]. Furthermore, we have previously demonstrated that this treatment is effective in inducing regular ovulation in women with classical 21-hydroxylase deficiency [19]. Dexamethasone 0.5 mg is equivalent to physiologic glucocorticoid requirement and thus avoids the criticism of potentially suppressing gonadotropin secretion directly as a result of a pharmacologic effect. Whereas glucocorticoid excess is associated with suppression of gonadotropin secretion [20], this dose of dexamethasone supported the occurrence of ovulation in congenital adrenal hyperplasia [19]. Evaluation of the response to treatment was undertaken 3–6 months after the start of dexamethasone administration.

Successful treatment of patients with PCO using dexamethasone, i.e. induction of regular ovulation, was associated with significant suppression of testosterone and testosterone/sex hormone-binding globulin ratios that was not seen in patients who failed to respond clinically [11]. A fall in the mean estrone levels occurred in responders but a small increase was seen in nonresponders. The responsiveness of both testosterone and androstenedione to metyrapone was significantly suppressed in responders but not in the clinical nonresponders [11]. While both responders and nonresponders demonstrated suppression of 11-deoxycortisol increments following metyrapone, this was much greater in responders than in nonresponders. Poor compliance of nonresponders to treatment with dexamethasone is one possible explanation for these differences [11].

We have previously reported the preferential suppression of androgens rather than cortisol or glucocorticoid precursors following treatment with small doses of dexamethasone 0.25–0.5 mg each night in patients with IH [10] and in patients with congenital adrenal hyperplasia [19]. It is for this reason that the apparent dissociation of ACTH and other POMC fragments following treatment with dexamethasone is of particular interest. It is tempting to speculate that one of these POMC fragments other than ACTH has an important role in modifying adrenal androgen production. Indeed, Parker *et al.* [21] have recently suggested that the joining peptide, i.e. the section of POMC adjoining the 16k-fragment, preferentially stimulates androgen production in human adrenal cell suspensions [21] (see Chapter 14). It is possible, therefore, that the primary abnormality occurring in some patients with IH/PCO is an excess of the non-ACTH POMC fragment or fragments, which preferentially stimulates androgen production. However, the mechanism of adrenal androgen excess occurring in PCO awaits definition and a role for POMC fragments other than ACTH remains in the realm of conjecture. We have previously suggested that at least some patients who develop PCO do so as a result of perturbed gonadotropin secretion occurring as a consequence of elevated estrone levels. Estrone is mainly derived in peripheral adipose tissue. Hyperestronemia may occur either as a consequence of excess availability of its precursor, androstenedione, possibly as a result of excessive adrenal secretion, or due to excessive conversion of androstenedione to estrone in obese subjects who have an abundance of aromatase activity in adipose tissue (Fig. 15.2). The theoretical sequence whereby dexamethasone brings about correction of the hormonal and clinical abnormalities of PCO is depicted in Fig. 15.3. Dexamethasone, by inhibiting adrenal androgen secretion, reduces the substrate available for conversion to estrone. In turn, this may bring about a reduction in LH and an increase in FSH secretion and thereby reduced ovarian androgen production, depleting further the circulating androgen pool. As a consequence, another reduction in estrone levels may occur lessening further the stimulus to abnormal gonadotropin secretion. In some patients, this will result in suppression of androgens and estrone to normal and the resumption of regular ovulatory menstrual cycles. However, in some patients, the correction of the initiating abnormality may have little effect on reversing the secondary abnormalities in the hypothalamic–pituitary–ovarian axis, which may have become self-sustaining, no longer dependent on a contribution from the adrenal gland.

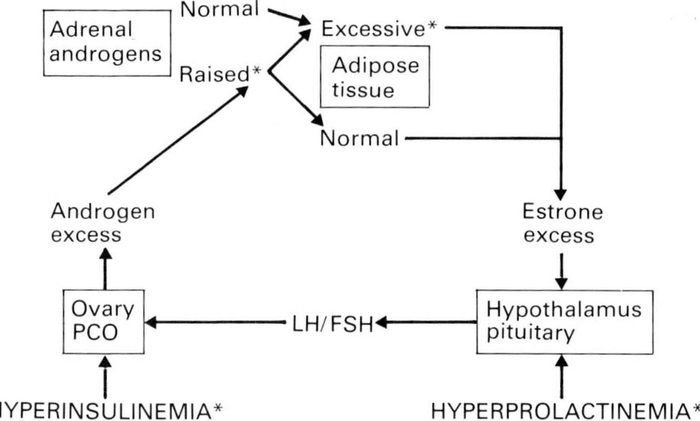

Fig. 15.2 Schematic model proposed for the development of polycystic ovary syndrome. The asterisks indicate potential initiating abnormalities in the cycle of events leading to the development of polycystic ovary syndrome. (Reprinted, with permission of The New England Journal of Medicine, from McKenna [7].)

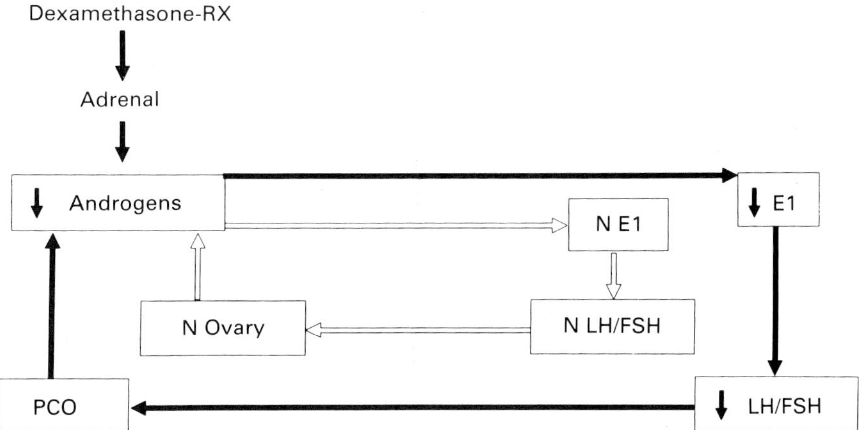

Fig. 15.3 Schematic representation of the mechanism whereby adrenal suppression (Dex-RX) may lead to the correction of the polycystic ovary syndrome (see text for detailed explanation).

In IH and PCO there is excessive adrenal androgen and glucocorticoid responsiveness to stimulation by exogenous ACTH and by endogenous adrenal stimulation induced by metyrapone, indicating either an intrinsic adrenal abnormality or abnormal priming of the adrenal by disturbed stimulatory processes. Furthermore, the adrenal and gonadotropin abnormalities and the clinical manifestations of PCO respond to suppression of the hypothalamic–pituitary–adrenal axis using low-dose nocturnal dexamethasone. It is possible that dexamethasone reduces the production of a POMC fragment other than ACTH that is responsible for androgen secretion. In this way, the cycle initiated by adrenal androgen excess, including its conversion to estrone with consequent abnormal gonadotropin secretion and thereby the development of PCO, can be reversed by treatment with glucocorticoids.

References

1 Kase EN, Kowal J, Perloff W, Soffer LJ. *In vitro* production of androgens by a virilizing adenoma and associated polycystic ovaries. Acta Endocrinol 1963; 44:15–19.

2 Hague WM, Honour JW, Adam J, Vecsei P, Jacobs HS. Steroid responses to ACTH in women with polycystic ovaries. Clin Endocrinol 1989; 30:355–66.

3 Yen SSC. Polycystic ovary syndrome. Clin Endocrinol 1980; 12:177–97.

4 Hoffman DI, Klove K, Lobo RA. Prevalence and significance of elevated dehydroepiandrosterone sulfate levels in anovulatory women. Fertil Steril 1984; 42:76–81.

5 Mahesh VB. Various concepts of pathogenesis of polycystic ovary disease. In: Mahesh VB, Greenblatt RB, eds. Hirsutism and Virilization. Pathogenesis, Diagnosis and Management. Boston: John Wright, Inc., 1983, pp. 247–76.

6 McKenna TJ, Cunningham SK, Loughlin T. The adrenal cortex and virilization. Clin Endocrinol Metab 1985; 14:997–1020.

7 McKenna TJ. Pathogenesis and treatment of polycystic ovary syndrome. N Engl J Med 1988; 318:558–62.

8 Barnes R, Rosenfield RL. The polycystic ovary syndrome: pathogenesis and treatment. Ann Intern Med 1989; 110:386–99.

9 Stewart PM, Shackleton CHL, Beastall GH, Edwards CRW. 5α-Reductase activity in polycystic ovary syndrome. Lancet 1990; 335:431–3.

10 Moore A, Magee F, Cunningham S, Culliton M, McKenna TJ. Adrenal abnormalities in idiopathic hirsutism. Clin Endocrinol 1983; 18:391–9.

11 Loughlin T, Cunningham S, Moore A, Culliton M, Smyth PPA, McKenna TJ. Adrenal abnormalities in polycystic ovary syndrome. J Clin Endocrinol Metab 1986; 62:142–7.

12 Cunningham SK, Loughlin T, Bertagna X, Girard F, McKenna TJ. Plasma pro-opiomelanocortin fragments and adrenal steroids following administration of metyrapone in normal and hirsute women. J Endocrinol Invest 1988; 11:247–53.

13 Cunningham SK, Moore A, McKenna TJ. Normal cortisol response to corticotropin in patients with secondary adrenal failure. Arch Intern Med 1983; 143:2276–9.

14 White PC, New MI, Dupont B. Congenital adrenal hyperplasia. N Engl J Med 1987; 316:1519–24 and 1580–6.

15 Cronin C, Igoe D, Duffy MJ, Cunningham SK, McKenna TJ. The overnight dexamethasone test is a worthwhile screening procedure. Clin Endocrinol 1990; 33:27–33.

16 Imura H. ACTH and related peptides: molecular biology, biochemistry and regulation of secretion. Clin Endocrinol Metab 1985; 14:845–66.

17 Haque N, Thrasher K, Werk EE Jr, Knowles HC Jr, Sholiton LJ. Studies on dexamethasone metabolism in man: effect of diphenylhydantoin. J Clin Endocrinol Metab 1972; 34:44–50.

18 Moore G, Lacroix A, Rabin D, McKenna TJ. Gonadal dysfunction in adult men with congenital adrenal hyperplasia. Acta Endocrinol 1980; 95:185–95.

19 McKenna TJ, Moore G, Orth DN, Burr IM, Liddle GW, Lacroix A. The biosynthsis of androgens in 21-hydroxylase deficiency. In: Genazzani AR, Thijssen JHH, Siiteri PK, eds. Adrenal Androgens. New York: Raven Press, 1980, pp. 135–9.

20 Sakakura M, Takebe K, Nakagawa S. Inhibition of luteinizing hormone secretion induced by synthetic LRH by long-term treatment with glucocorticoids in human subjects. J Clin Endocrinol Metab 1975; 40:774–9.

21 Parker L, Lifrak E, Shively J, Lee T, Kaplan B, Walker P, Calaycay J, Florsheim W, Soon-Shiong P. Human adrenal gland cortical androgen-stimulating hormone (CASH) is identical with a portion of the joining peptide of pituitary pro-opiomelanocortin (POMC). 71st Annual Meeting The Endocrine Society, Seattle, Washington, June 1989, Programme and Abstracts, p. 97.

Chapter 16
The Role of Adrenal Androgens in Polycystic Ovary Syndrome: an Overview

GEORGE R. MERRIAM

Because both the adrenal and the ovary produce androgens, and adrenal suppression with glucocorticoids can reduce androgen production and sometimes produce clinical improvement in hyperandrogenic patients, there has been long-standing interest in the possible role of the adrenal in polycystic ovary syndrome (PCO). These efforts have ranged from the description of a clinical syndrome resembling PCO in patients with attenuated congenital adrenal hyperplasia (CAH), to attempts to define the role of the adrenal and its regulators in idiopathic PCO patients.

In a syndrome as heterogeneous as PCO, CAH has great utility in providing a subgroup of patients with more uniform etiology. Although patients with classical CAH are usually diagnosed in childhood, New and others have described cohorts of patients with attenuated CAH who presented after puberty with symptoms of hyperandrogenism and many of the classical features of PCO. The frequency of this disorder varies widely in different populations. New reported that in New York city this condition was found in as many as 16% of children presenting with precocious adrenarche, while Kirshner described a much lower prevalence in a neighboring population in New Jersey. The validity of this extremely high frequency has been confirmed by Morton's population genetics studies, by screening based on salivary 17-hydroxyprogesterone, and by independent studies of Ashkenazi Jewish populations in New York and Israel.

The high frequency of a gene associated with infertility problems, which would otherwise be expected to extinguish it rapidly, suggests the possibility that the heterozygous state may confer a selective advantage for reproductive success. The Ashkenazi Jewish population, which includes groups that do not practice contraception, provides a base in which this subject could be studied.

The observed prevalence of attenuated 21-hydroxylase deficiency depends not only on the ethnic background of the patients, but also on the symptoms that bring them to medical attention. Although the 16% frequency in patients seen with precocious adrenarche is known, the prevalence in patients presenting with hirsutism or infertility is not. As pointed out by Kissebah, the same genotype and biochemical abnormality may occur even in individuals with no clinical symptoms.

Although patients with CAH can have many of the same clinical abnormalities and gonadotropin changes seen in idiopathic PCO, it is not known how completely these patients mimic the PCO phenotype. Wild noted that half of CAH patients had been reported to have ultrasonographic findings similar to those seen in PCO, although he, New, and Rosenfield noted that no good correlation between these changes and the degree of control of hyperandrogenism had been observed. There are also no good data as to whether the histologic changes of PCO, particularly thecal overgrowth, were seen in patients with CAH.

Merriam noted that earlier investigators had speculated that increased adrenal androgens from an "abnormal adrenarche" might cause secondary ovarian and gonadotropin changes that would reinforce themselves in a vicious circle, and then gradually fade from view as a first cause [1]. He noted that the generally good clinical responses to treatment of attenuated CAH patients with glucocorticoids, and of tumor patients with surgery argued strongly against the existence of such a vicious circle. Albertson inquired whether there was any known association between PCO and precocious adrenarche, but there seemed to be no data on this subject.

The regulation of adrenal androgen secretion was discussed from both the viewpoints of normal physiology and implications for PCO. Buster asked how the very weak adrenal androgens could have clinical effects, and whether they were direct ovarian effects or secondary to perturbation of the hypothalamic–pituitary–ovarian axis. Albertson responded that it was likely that most effects resulted from further metabolism to more potent androgens.

The mechanisms and factors that govern adrenarche are still controversial. There is considerable evidence, reviewed by Albertson (Chapter 14), that pituitary hormones other than adrenocorticotropic hormone (ACTH) may stimulate adrenal androgens, leading to the possibility that abnormal levels or patterns of these factors might be responsible for some patients with PCO. However, McKenna and others have found no difference in plasma levels of several pro-opiomelanocortin (POMC) fragments in PCO patients. Evan Simpson indicated that he remained unconvinced of the need to postulate such a factor, whose effects were only of the order of a 50% stimulation of adrenal androgen secretion. He suggested that the relative production of adrenal androgens was regulated by the relative activities of several enzymes, particularly of 3β-hydroxysteroid dehydrogenase vs. 17-hydroxylase/17,20-desmolase, as they competed for the further metabolism of 17-hydroxypregnenolone. These two enzymes respond very differently to a variety of known growth factors and other regulatory factors, and it seems unnecessary to postulate a novel adrenal androgen-stimulating hormone to explain the changes occurring with adrenarche or small doses of glucocorticoids. However, this still leaves open the question of whether these enzyme and structural changes are primarily due to intra- or extra-adrenal factors.

McKenna's work (see Chapter 15) summarized data that a very high proportion of PCO patients had evidence demonstrating overproduction of adrenal androgens, including exaggerated responses to ACTH, although these increases were much less than those seen in CAH. He indicated that the abnormality appeared to differ fundamentally from CAH, in that they derived not from a block in an enzyme but from a more generalized increase in many enzyme activities. Rosenfield indicated that his data using stimulation with a gonadotropin-releasing hormone (GnRH) agonist analog suggested a similar increase in ovarian androgen-synthesizing activity (cf. Chapter 9). He speculated that patients with idiopathic PCO might have an enhancement in androgen synthesis in both glands due to a common but still unknown mechanism, and suggested that it would be of great interest to study the GnRH agonist responses of patients with attenuated CAH.

Except in the CAH patients, there did not seem to be a general consensus as to how frequently PCO patients respond clinically to partial adrenal suppression with glucocorticoids, a widely used treatment that can carry the risks of adrenal suppression. McKenna indicated his experience that there was evidence for some improvement in hirsutism, acne, or menstrual irregularities in two-thirds of PCO patients given dexamethasone, while others stated that they had found a much lower rate of success. Thus the relative risks and benefits of using glucocorticoids in PCO patients without CAH remain controversial.

Reference

1 Yen SSC. Chronic anovulation caused by peripheral endocrine disorders. In: Yen SSC, Jaffe RB, eds. Reproductive Endocrinology, 2nd ed. Philadelphia: Saunders, 1986, Ch. 16.

Section 6
Growth Factors

Chapter 17
Insulin-like Growth Factors and the Ovary: an Overview

LINDA C. GIUDICE & RON G. ROSENFELD

The insulin-like growth factors (IGFs), or somatomedins, constitute a family of growth hormone (GH)-dependent peptides with structural similarities to insulin and with broad mitogenic and metabolic actions [1]. Originally identified by their ability to stimulate incorporation of sulfate in cartilage, these peptides are believed to mediate many, if not all, of the anabolic actions of GH. In 1978, Rinderknecht and Humbel [2,3] identified, purified and sequenced two somatomedins from human plasma; they named them IGF-I and IGF-II, because of their striking structural homology with insulin. The two peptides themselves exhibit 62% homology. The sequences of cDNAs encoding human preproIGF-I and -II have been determined and the respective 130 and 180 amino acids of these precursors predicted [4–6].

As in the case of insulin, both IGF-I and IGF-II are presumed to stimulate biologic responses by binding with high affinity and specificity to their respective receptors, in addition to their binding to the insulin receptor itself [7,8]. Both receptors for insulin and IGF-I have been found to be heterotetramers, composed of two alpha subunits of M_r 135 000 and two beta subunits of M_r 90 000 linked by interchain disulfide bonds [9–11]. The alpha subunits are entirely extracellular and contain the respective binding sites for insulin and IGF-I. The beta subunits span the cell membrane; the intracellular domains contain an adenosine triphosphate (ATP)-binding site and tyrosine-autophosphorylation sites. Both the receptors for insulin [12,13] and for IGF-I [14] have recently been cloned, the nucleotides sequenced, and the complete primary structures of the proteins deduced. The insulin receptor is 1355 or 1367 amino acids in length, depending upon differential splicing in exon 11. The deduced sequence of the receptor for

IGF-I corresponds to a protein 1337 amino acids in length, with a signal peptide of 30 amino acids that is removed during cellular processing. Cleavage of an Arg-Lys-Arg-Arg sequence results in the generation of an alpha subunit of M_r 80 423 and a beta subunit of M_r 70 866. The fully glycosylated subunits have M_r values of 135 000 and 90 000, respectively. As anticipated from results of structural studies, extensive similarity with the receptor for insulin was observed, including overall structure, subunit size, and primary sequence, with the largest region of homology being in the tyrosine kinase domain of the beta subunit (86% homology). However, the gene for the insulin receptor has been localized to chromosome 19, while the gene for the IGF-I receptor has been identified on the distal long arm of chromosome 15. Thus, the two receptors are products of distinct genes and are presumably subject to different regulatory systems.

The receptor for IGF-II (type II), by contrast to the receptor for IGF-I, is a monomeric glycoprotein which, although it can be phosphorylated, is without intrinsic kinase activity. On polyacrylamide gels it migrates as a protein of M_r 240 000 in its unreduced form, and as a protein of M_r 250 000–260 000 after reduction. This difference in size is believed to reflect the presence of intrachain disulfide bonds, which normally act to compact the molecule. The type II receptor does not bind insulin and binds IGF-I with 100- to 1000-fold lower affinity than the binding of IGF-II [15].

The cDNA for the receptor for IGF-II has recently been cloned and sequenced. The type II receptor is identical to the cation-independent receptor for mannose-6-phosphate, which is believed to be involved in the intracellular transport of lysosomal enzymes to lysosomes [16]. The receptor appears to bind IGF-II and mannose-6-phosphate at two distinct sites, although these sites may interact in as yet undefined ways. The role of the receptor for IGF-II in mediating the potent metabolic and mitogenic effects of IGF-II remains to be established. In cultured rat granulosa cells, for example, IGF-II appears to exert its effects upon follicle-stimulating hormone (FSH)-supported accumulation of progesterone via the type I receptor for IGF-I [17].

In addition to binding to their receptors on the cell membrane, the IGFs also bind with high affinity to a family of structurally related, circulating IGF-binding proteins (IGFBPs) [18]. Although originally identified in serum [19], these IGFBPs have been found in a wide variety of biologic fluids, including amniotic fluid [20,21], cerebrospinal fluid [22,23], seminal plasma [24], and follicular fluid [25–27], as well as in conditioned media from multiple cell lines [18]. The circulating IGFBPs are believed both to prolong the half-life of the IGFs and to regulate the endocrine effects of these growth factors. In cell lines and tissues, by contrast, these IGFBPs are believed to modulate the local actions of the IGFs in an autocrine/paracrine fashion. Some investigators have reported that IGFBPs inhibit the mitogenic effects of the IGFs, presumably by competing with cell-surface receptors for IGFs [28,29]. Under other circumstances, investigators have claimed that the IGFPBs may potentiate the actions of IGF [30]. Whether they augment or attenuate the actions of the IGFs, the IGFBPs probably represent a group of autocrine/paracrine regulatory proteins, the physiologic effects of which depend upon their relative expression in particular type of cell.

Three human IGFBPs have been identified to date: IGFBP-1 is the major binding protein in human amniotic fluid and its molecular weight is 25 000 [31,32]; IGFBP-2 appears to be the major fetal/neonatal IGFBP [33,34], is also found in cerebrospinal fluid and other tissues of the central nervous system [35], and its molecular weight is 31 000; IGFBP-3 is the major binding protein of adult serum [36], is GH dependent, and is glycosylated, with a core protein weight of 31 000. Two additional IGFBPs have been identified, one in cerebrospinal fluid [37] and the other in osteoblast-conditioned media [38]. Figure 17.1 depicts a schematic view of the IGF peptide–binding protein–receptor system.

IGF and the ovary

The human ovary contains a large number of primary follicles, most of which undergo atresia that begins in fetal life and continues until the menopause. A small number of follicles is recruited in each menstrual cycle and, of those, only one is usually selected to undergo further differentiation, maturation and ultimate ovulation as a mature, fertilizable oocyte. Folliculogenesis is dependent on the gonadotropins, FSH and luteinizing hormone (LH). There are clearly other hormonal controls of the process of folliculogenesis, and many substances of ovarian origin have been proposed as regulators of this process, among which are the steroid hormones (estradiol and progesterone), polypeptides (inhibin, activin and follistatin), and growth factors (IGFs) [39].

The liver appears to be the main source of circulating IGF, and hepatic synthesis appears to be mediated by GH [1]. IGF-I is also produced locally in other tissues, and in such tissues its synthesis does not appear to be entirely GH dependent, e.g. rat uterus, where estradiol is the principal modulator of levels of mRNA for IGF-I [40–42]. In rat and porcine ovary, production of IGF-I appears to be dependent upon GH, gonadotropins and estradiol. IGF-II is also synthesized in a wide variety of tissues, especially in the fetus. The function of IGF-II is less well

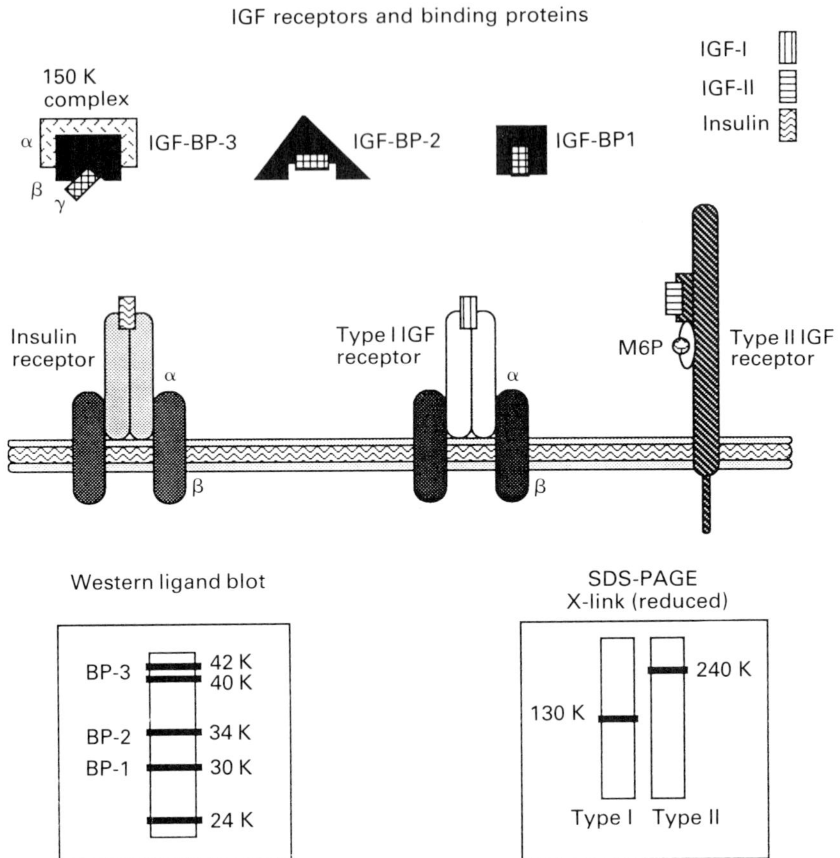

Fig. 17.1 Schematic representation of the family of IGF peptides, binding protein (IGFBPs) and receptors. At the time of writing, two additional IGFBPs have been identified.

understood than that of IGF-I, and it remains unclear which receptor(s) mediate its biologic actions. Nevertheless, data are accumulating in support of its importance in fetal growth and development [43]. In human granulosa cells, levels of IGF-II mRNA are regulated by gonadotropins.

Complementary and genomic DNA for human IGF-I and rat and human IGF-II have been cloned. Multiple transcripts of IGF-I and IGF-II mRNAs have been described in various fetal and adult tissues [44]. It is not currently known which of the mRNAs is (are) actually translated, nor is it known whether levels of several species of mRNA can be differentially regulated in a given tissue.

Studies with rats have shown that expression of the IGF-I gene in the ovary is confined to the granulosa cells of developing follicles [45,46]. *In vivo*, GH increases ovarian levels of immunoreactive IGF-I in rat ovary [47], although a direct effect of GH on isolated rat granulosa cells has not yet been demonstrated. Levels of IGF-I mRNA in immature rat granulosa cells are gonadotropin dependent [46], and experiments *in vivo* have shown that rat ovarian IGF-I mRNA is regulated by estradiol alone and in combination with GH, but not by GH alone [46]. Studies with porcine granulosa cells have shown that IGF-I is synthesized by these cells in culture, and that synthesis of IGF-I is stimulated by gonadotropins, GH and estradiol, as well as by other growth factors [48–51]. In humans, luteinizing granulosa cells have been examined for production of IGF-I and IGF-II. Such cells were harvested from women who were undergoing treatment with LH and FSH for the induction of ovulation and who had received human chorionic gonadotropin prior to follicular aspiration for retrieval of oocytes. Thus, these aspirated granulosa cells were mature and luteinizing, and they differed markedly in their stage of development from the granulosa cells examined in other species described above. Both the mRNA for IGF-II and the peptide itself were detected in these cells but neither IGF-I nor its mRNA was found [52–54]. Furthermore, the expression of IGF-II mRNA in cultured human granulosa cells appears to be regulated by gonadotropins. Levels of IGF in human follicular fluid (FF), derived from patients who were undergoing procedures for *in vitro* fertilization, have not been consistent [27,55–57], probably reflecting interference of IGFBPs in the various assays employed [18]. Nevertheless, both IGF-I and IGF-II have been detected in FF, although the cells from which the IGF-I originates remain to be identified. Indeed, it is unclear at this time whether or not IGF-I is important in human folliculogenesis. In support of a role for IGF-I in the human ovary is the observation that IGF-I regulates the level of the mRNA that encodes aromatase in human granulosa and granulosa-luteal cells [58,59]. In addition, the clinical observation that administration of GH to women who are undergoing induction of ovulation by treatment with LH and FSH decreases the requirement for the gonadotropins suggests that GH may stimulate the production of IGF-I in the developing granulosa cells, and IGF-I then stimulates the action of FSH and follicular development [60].

It has been shown in numerous studies that IGFs have a local effect on the ovary. Receptors of IGF are present in the ovary [39], and IGFs have been shown to stimulate replication and differentiation of cultured granulosa cells [61,62]. In concert with FSH, IGF-I has been shown to stimulate aromatase activity (and hence the synthesis of estradiol) [58,59], as well as the synthesis of progesterone and receptors for LH [60,61]. In addition, IGF-I stimulates the synthesis of proteoglycans [63], which may play a role in follicular antrum formation and follicular atresia [39]. Thus, it is clear that the IGF autocrine/paracrine system is present in the ovary and may play a role in both folliculogenesis and follicular atresia.

As discussed above, the IGFs circulate as complexes of individual IGF peptides and members of a family of structurally related IGFBPs, which appear to modulate actions of IGF. Cultured preovulatory granulosa cells from rats secrete several IGFBPs. The major IGFBP in conditioned media from rat granulosa cells is a 28 kDa IGFBP, as yet unidentified. It is noteworthy that the concentration of this IGFBP in media appears to be sharply reduced after treatment of cells with FSH [64]. The significance of this finding remains uncertain, but it provides a hypothetical explanation for the enhancement by FSH of the action of IGF: reduction of local levels of IGFBPs would increase the availability to free IGF to cell-surface receptors.

IGFBP-3 has been isolated from porcine follicular fluid and inhibits DNA synthesis and FSH-stimulated production of steroids by cultured preovulatory granulosa cells from rats [26]. In humans, IGFBP-1 has been shown by radioimmunoassay to be present in preovulatory follicular fluid, luteal cells of hyperstimulated preovulatory follicles, and corpora lutea [25]. In addition, luteinizing human granulosa cells in culture synthesize IGFBP-1, and the synthesis of IGFBP-I is regulated via protein kinase C and pathways that are dependent on adenylate cyclase [65,66]. In sera of women with polycystic ovarian disease, levels of IGFBP-1 have been shown to be markedly reduced [67]. We have recently shown that human follicular fluid contains IGFBP-2 and IGFBP-3, as well as IGFBP-1 [27]. We have also recently found that luteinizing human granulosa cells contain mRNAs that encode IGFBP-1, IGFBP-2 and IGFBP-3, and that cultured human granulosa cells synthesize and secrete all three IGFBPs into the culture media (unpublished observations).

IGFs and polycystic ovary syndrome

Polycystic ovary syndrome (PCO) is a disorder characterized by anovulation, hyperandrogenemia, relatively increased levels of circulating LH and low levels of FSH, oligomenorrhea or amenorrhea, and infertility. The etiology of this condition is unclear, but the endocrine abnormalities appear to perpetuate themselves unless appropriately treated. The initial stages of folliculogenesis, i.e. recruitment and growth to the small antral stage, are unaffected but the next stage, selection of dominant preovulatory follicles, does not occur in patients with this syndrome. As a result, there is an accumulation of many small antral follicles in the polycystic ovary. The mechanisms responsible for the arrest of folliculogenesis have not been elucidated, although a growing body of evidence suggests that the IGF system may be involved in regulating follicular development in polycystic ovaries. Polycystic ovary syndrome has been associated with resistance to insulin and hyperinsulinemia, and it has been theorized that the excess insulin acts on the ovary via the insulin and type I receptors for IGF to cause overproduction of androgens from the ovarian stroma. IGF-I and LH have been shown to act synergistically in stimulating the production of thecal androgens [68], and the excess of androgens may promote follicular atresia. The polycystic ovary contains numerous small antral follicles, which appear atretic in terms of their ratio of estradiol to androstenedione. Indeed, the granulosa cells from polycystic ovary follicles produce little aromatase *in vitro* in the absence of stimulation by FSH, but the aromatase activity increases when these cells are exposed to FSH *in vitro*. IGF-I can stimulate the production of aromatase by the polycystic ovary granulosa cells in culture, and IGF-I and FSH act synergistically in this regard [69]. The defect in PCO is, thus, not the inability of the granulosa cells to respond to IGF-I. Indeed, it has been postulated that follicular fluid in the small antral follicles contains inhibitors of IGF-I and/or the action of FSH [64]. It is possible that alterations in the IGF autocrine/paracrine system, which result in decreased availability of IGF at the ovarian level, may be responsible for both the failure of follicles to be selected to achieve dominance and the overproduction of androgens by the ovary. These events could lead to the clinical picture of multiple small follicles in the ovary, with no follicle achieving dominance, and, consequently, the development of chronic anovulation.

Acknowledgments

Supported in part by NIH grants HD25220 (to L.C.G.) and DK28229 (to R.G.R.).

References

1 Daughaday WH, Rotwein P. Insulin-like growth factors I and II. Peptide, messenger ribonucleic acid and gene structures, serum and tissue concentrations. Endocr Rev 1989; 10:68–91.

2 Rinderknecht E, Humbel RE. The amino acid sequence of human insulin-like growth factor-I and its structural homology with proinsulin. J Biol Chem 1978; 253:2769–76.

3 Rinderknecht E, Humbel RE. Primary structure of human insulin-like growth factor-II. FEBS Lett 1978; 89:283–6.

4 Jansen M, van Schaik FMA, Ricker AT, *et al.* Sequence of cDNA encoding human insulin-like growth factor-I precursor. Nature 1983; 306:609–11.

5 Bell GI, Merryweather JP, Sanchez-Pescador R, *et al.* Sequence of a cDNA clone encoding human preproinsulin-like growth factor-II. Nature 1984; 310:775–7.
6 Dull TJ, Gray A, Hayflick JS, Ullrich A. Insulin-like growth factor-II precursor gene organization in relation to insulin gene family. Nature 1984; 310:777–81.
7 Rosenfeld RG, Hintz RL. Somatomedin receptors: structure, function and regulation. In: Conn PM, ed. The Receptors, Vol. III. Orlando: Academic Press, 1986, pp. 281–296.
8 Rosenfeld RG. Receptors for insulin-like growth factors I and II. In: Muller EE, Cocchi D, Locatelli V, eds. Advances in Growth Hormone and Growth Factor Research. Roma-Milano: Pythagora Press, 1989, pp. 133–143.
9 Kasuga M, Van Obberghen E, Nissley SP, Rechler MM. Demonstration of two subtypes of insulin-like growth factor receptors by affinity cross-linking. J Biol Chem 1981; 256:5305–8.
10 Chernausek SD, Jacobs S, Van Wyk JJ. Structural similarities between human receptors for somatomedin-C and insulin: analysis by affinity labeling. Biochemistry 1981; 20:7345–50.
11 Massague J, Czech MP. The subunit structures of two distinct receptors for insulin-like growth factors I and II and their relationship to the insulin receptor. J Biol Chem 1982; 257:5038–45.
12 Ullrich A, Bell JR, Chen EY, *et al.* Human insulin receptor and its relationship to the tyrosine kinase family of oncogenes. Nature 1985; 313:756–61.
13 Ebina Y, Ellis L, Jarnagin K, *et al.* The human insulin receptor cDNA: the structural basis for hormone-activated transmembrane signalling. Cell 1985; 40:747–58.
14 Ullrich A, Gray A, Tam AW, *et al.* Insulin-like growth factor-I receptor primary structure: comparison with insulin receptor suggests structural determinants that define structural specificity. EMBO J 1986; 5:2503–12.
15 Rosenfeld RG, Conover CA, Hodges D, *et al.* Heterogeneity of insulin-like growth factor-I affinity for the insulin-like growth factor-II receptor: comparison of natural, synthetic and recombinant DNA-derived insulin-like growth factor I. Biochem Biophys Res Commun 1987; 143:199–205.
16 Morgan DO, Edman JC, Standring DN, *et al.* Insulin-like growth factor II receptor as a multifunctional binding protein. Nature 1987; 329:301–7.
17 Adashi EY, Resnick CE, Rosenfeld RG. Insulin-like growth factor-I (IGF-I) and IGF-II hormonal action in cultured rat granulosa cells: mediation via type I but not type II IGF receptors. Endocrinology 1989; 126:216–22.
18 Rosenfeld RG, Lamson G, Pham H, *et al.* Insulin-like growth factor binding proteins. Recent Prog Horm Res 1990; 46:99–205.
19 Hintz RL, Liu F. Demonstration of specific plasma protein binding sites for somatomedin. J Clin Endocrinol Metab 1977; 45:988–95.
20 Chochinov RH, Mariz IK, Hajek AS, Daughaday WH. Characterization of a protein in mid-term human amniotic fluid which reacts in the somatomedin C radioreceptor assay. J Clin Endocrinol Metab 1977; 44:902–8.
21 Drop SLS, Kortleve DJ, Guyda HJ. Isolation of a somatomedin-binding protein from preterm amniotic fluid: development of a radioimmunoassay. J Clin Endocrinol Metab 1984; 59:899–907.
22 Hossenlopp P, Seurin D, Segovia-Quinson B, Binoux M. Identification of an insulin-like growth factor-binding protein in human cerebrospinal fluid with a selective affinity for IGF-II. FEBS Lett 1986; 208:439–44.
23 Rosenfeld RG, Pham H, Conover CA, Hintz RL, Baxter RB. Structural and immunological comparison of insulin-like growth factor (IGF) binding proteins of cerebrospinal and amniotic fluids. J Clin Endocrinol Metab 1989; 68:638–46.
24 Rosenfeld RG, Pham H, Oh Y, Lamson G, Giudice LC. Identification of insulin-like growth factor-binding protein-2 and a low molecular weight IGF-BP in human seminal plasma. J Clin Endocrinol Metab 1989; 69:963–5.
25 Seppala M, Wahlstrom T, Koskimies AI, *et al.* Human preovulatory follicular fluid,

luteinized cells of hyperstimulated preovulatory follicles, and corpus luteum contain placental protein 12. J Clin Endocrinol Metab 1984; 58:505–10.

26 Ui M, Shimonaka M, Shimasaki S, Ling N. An insulin-like growth factor binding protein in ovarian follicular fluid blocks follicle-stimulating hormone-stimulated steroid production by ovarian granulosa cells. Endocrinology 1989; 125:912–16.

27 Giudice LC, Farrell EM, Pham H, Rosenfeld RG. Identification of insulin-like growth factor binding protein-3 (IGFBP-3) and IGFBP-2 in human follicular fluid. 37th Annual Meeting, Society for Gynecologic Investigation, St Louis, March 1990, Abstract 429.

28 Rutanen E-M, Pekonen F, Makinen T. Soluble 34K binding protein inhibits the binding of insulin-like growth factor I to its receptors in human secretory phase endometrium: evidence for autocrine/paracrine regulation of growth factor action. J Clin Endocrinol Metab 1988; 66:173–80.

29 Ritvos O, Ranta T, Jalkanen J, *et al.* Insulin-like growth factor (IGF) binding protein from human decidua inhibits the binding and biological action of IGF-I in cultured choriocarcinoma cells. Endocrinology 1988; 122:2150–7.

30 Elgin RB, Busby WH, Clemmons DR. An insulin-like growth factor (IGF) binding protein enhances the biologic response to IGF-I. Proc Natl Acad Sci USA 1987; 84:3254–8.

31 Lee Y-L, Hintz RL, James PM, Lee PDK, Shively JE, Powell DR. Insulin-like growth factor (IGF) binding protein complementary deoxyribonucleic acid from human Hep G2 hepatoma cells: predicted protein sequence suggests an IGF binding domain different from those of the IGF-I and IGF-II receptors. Mol Endocrinol 1988; 2:404–11.

32 Brinkman A, Groffen C, Kortleve DJ, Geurts Van Kessel A, Drop SLS. Isolation and characterization of a cDNA encoding the low molecular weight insulin-like growth factor binding protein (IBP-1). EMBO J 1988; 7:2417–23.

33 Binkert C, Landwehr J, Mary J-L, Schwander J, Heinrich G. Cloning, sequence analysis and expression of a cDNA encoding a novel insulin-like growth factor binding protein (IGFBP-2). EMBO J 1989; 8:2497–502.

34 Donovan SM, Oh Y, Pham H, Rosenfeld RG. Ontogeny of serum insulin-like growth factor binding proteins in the rat. Endocrinology 1989; 125:2621–7.

35 Lamson G, Pham H, Oh Y, Schwander J, Rosenfeld RG. Expression of the BRL-3A insulin-like growth factor binding protein (rBP-30) in the rat central nervous system. Endocrinology 1989; 123:1100–2.

36 Wood WJ, Cachianes G, Henzel WJ, *et al.* Cloning and expression of the growth hormone-dependent insulin-like growth factor-binding protein. Mol Endocrinol 1988; 2:1176–85.

37 Roghani M, Hossenlopp P, Lepage P, Balland A, Binoux M. Isolation from human cerebrospinal fluid of a new insulin-like growth factor-binding protein with a selective affinity for IGF-II. FEBS Lett 1989; 255:253–8.

38 Mohan S, Bautista CM, Wergedal J, Baylink DJ. Isolation of an inhibitory insulin-like growth factor (IGF) binding protein from bone cell-conditioned medium: a potential regulator of IGF action. Proc Natl Acad Sci USA 1989; 86:8338–42.

39 Adashi EY, Resnick CE, D'Ercole AJ, Svoboda ME, Van Wyk JJ. Insulin-like growth factors as intraovarian regulators of granulosa cell growth and function. Endocr Rev 1985; 6:400–20.

40 Murphy LJ, Murphy LC, Friesen HG. Estrogen induces insulin-like growth factor-I expression in the rat uterus. Mol Endocrinol 1987; 1:445–50.

41 Murphy LJ, Friesen HG. Differential effects of estrogen and growth hormone on uterine and hepatic insulin-like growth factor I gene expression in the ovariectomized hypophysectomized rat. Endocrinology 1988; 122:325–32.

42 Ghahary A, Chakrabati S, Murphy LJ. Localization of the sites of synthesis and action of insulin-like growth factor-I in the rat uterus. Mol Endocrinol 1990; 4:191–5.

43 Hill DJ, Milner RDG. Somatomedins and fetal growth. In: The Fetus and Independent Life. Ciba Foundation Symposium 86. London: Pitman, 1981, pp. 124–151.
44 Murphy LJ, Bell GI, Friesen HG. Tissue distribution of insulin-like growth factor-I and -II messenger ribonucleic acid in the adult rat. Endocrinology 1987; 120:1279–82.
45 Oliver JE, Altman TJ, Powell JF, Wilson CA, Clayton RN. Insulin-like growth factor I gene expression in rat ovary is confined to the granulosa cells of developing follicles. Endocrinology 1989; 124:267–79.
46 Hernandez ER, Roberts CT, Le Roith D, Adashi EY. Rat ovarian insulin-like growth factor I (IGF-I) gene expression is granulosa cell-selective: 5′-untranslated mRNA variant representation and hormonal regulation. Endocrinology 1989; 125:572–4.
47 Davoren JB, Hsueh AJW. Growth hormone increases ovarian levels of immunoreactive somatomedin C/insulin-like growth factor I *in vivo*. Endocrinology 1986; 118:888–91.
48 Hammond JM, Baranao JLS, Skaleris D, *et al.* Production of insulin-like growth factors by ovarian granulosa cells. Endocrinology 1985; 117:2553–7.
49 Hsu CJ, Hammond JM. Gonadotropins and estradiol stimulate immunoreactive insulin-like growth factor-I production by porcine granulosa cells *in vitro*. Endocrinology 1987; 120:198–203.
50 Hsu CJ, Hammond JM. Concomitant effects of growth hormone on secretion of insulin-like growth factor-I and progesterone by cultured porcine granulosa cells. Endocrinology 1987; 121:1343–6.
51 Mondschein JS, Hammond JM. Growth factors regulate immunoreactive insulin-like growth factor-I by cultured porcine granulosa cells. Endocrinology 1988; 123:463–8.
52 Voutilainen R, Miller WL. Coordinate trophic hormone regulation of mRNAs for insulin-like growth factor II and the cholesterol side-chain cleavage enzyme, P-450_{scc}, in human steroidogenic tissues. Proc Natl Acad Sci USA 1987; 84:1590–4.
53 Ramasharma K, Li CH. Human pituitary and placental hormones control human insulin-like growth factor II secretion in human granulosa cells. Proc Natl Acad Sci USA 1987; 84:2643–7.
54 Geisthovel F, Moretti-Rojas I, Asch RH, Rojas FJ. Expression of insulin-like growth factor-II (IGF-II) messenger ribonucleic acid (mRNA), but not IGF-I mRNA in human preovulatory granulosa cells. Hum Reprod 1989; 4:889–902.
55 Ramasharma K, Cabrera CM, Li CH. Identification of insulin-like growth factor-II in human seminal and follicular fluids. Biochem Biophys Res Commun 1986; 140: 536–42.
56 Geisthovel F, Moretti-Rojas IM, Rojas FJ, Asch RH. Immunoreactive insulin-like growth factor I in human follicular fluid. Hum Reprod 1989; 4:35–8.
57 Rabinovici J, Dandekar P, Bernstein D, Rosenthal S, Kaplan S, Martin M. Insulin-like growth factor in serum and follicular fluid of women undergoing *in vitro* fertilization. 45th Annual Meeting of the American Fertility Society, November 1989, San Francisco, Abstract P-062.
58 Steinkampf MP, Mendelson CR, Simpson ER. Effects of epidermal growth factor and insulin-like growth factor I on the levels of mRNA encoding aromatase cytochrome P-450 of human ovarian granulosa cells. Mol Cell Endocrinol 1988; 59:93–9.
59 Erickson GF, Garzo VG, Magoffin DA. Insulin-like growth factor-I regulates aromatase activity in human granulosa and granulosa-luteal cells. J Clin Endocrinol Metab 1989; 69:716–24.
60 Homburg R, Eshel A, Abdalla HI, Jacobs HS. Growth hormone facilitates ovulation induction by gonadotrophins. Clin Endocrinol 1988; 29:113–17.
61 Baranao JLS, Hammond JM. Comparative effects of insulin and insulin-like growth factors on DNA synthesis and differentiation of porcine granulosa cells. Biochem Biophys Res Commun 1984; 124:484–8.
62 Veldhuis JD, Furlanetto RW, Juchter D, Garmey J, Veldhuis P. Tropic actions of human somatomedin-C/IGF-I on ovarian cells: *in vitro* studies with swine granulosa cells. Endocrinology 1985; 116:1235–41.

63 Adashi EY, Resnick CE, Svoboda ME, Van Wyk JJ. Somatomedin-V synergizes with follicle-stimulating hormone in the acquisition of progestin biosynthetic capacity by cultured rat granulosa cells. Endocrinology 1985; 116:2135–40.

64 Adashi EY, Resnick CE, Hernandez ER, Hurwitz A, Rosenfeld RG. Follicle-stimulating hormone inhibits the constitutive release of insulin-like growth factor binding proteins by cultured rat ovarian granulosa cells. Endocrinology 1990; 126:1305–7.

65 Suikkari A-M, Jalkanen J, Koistinen R, *et al.* Human granulosa cells synthesize low molecular weight insulin-like growth factor binding protein. Endocrinology 1989; 124:1088–90.

66 Jalkanen J, Suikkari A-M, Koistinen R, *et al.* Regulation of insulin-like growth factor binding protein-1 production in human granulosa luteal cells. J Clin Endocrinol Metab 1989; 69:1174–9.

67 Pekonen F, Laatikaninen T, Byualos R, Rutanen E-M. Decreased 34 K insulin-like growth factor binding protein in polycystic ovarian disease. Fertil Steril 1989; 51: 972–5.

68 Cara JF, Rosenfield RL. Insulin-like growth factor I and insulin potentiate luteinizing hormone-induced androgen synthesis by rat ovarian thecal-interstitial cells. Endocrinology 1988; 123:733–9.

69 Erickson GF, Magoffin DA, Cragun JR, Chang RJ. The effects of insulin and insulin-like growth factors-I and -II on estradiol production by granulosa cells of polycystic ovaries. J Clin Endocrinol Metab 1990; 70:894–902.

Chapter 18
The Intraovarian IGF-I System

ELI Y. ADASHI, CAROL E. RESNICK,
ELEUTERIO R. HERNANDEZ, ARYE HURWITZ,
CHARLES T. ROBERTS, DEREK LEROITH
& RON ROSENFELD

As the significance of putative intraovarian regulators becomes increasingly evident, much of the attention is focused on insulin-like growth factors (IGFs). Indeed, a large body of evidence now suggests the existence of an intraovarian IGF system complete with ligands, receptors, and binding proteins. More importantly, IGFs have been shown to exert a variety of significant effects at the level of the somatic ovarian cell, a feature that raises the possibility of a meaningful role *in vivo*. Nonetheless, there is at this time no compelling evidence to indicate that IGFs (or, for that matter, any other putative intraovarian regulator) are indispensable to ovarian function. However, a large body of somewhat indirect evidence strongly suggests such a possibility. The purpose of this chapter is to review and summarize key developments in this area.

Ovarian IGF-I production

Ovarian production of IGF-I was initially suggested by studies which revealed that the level of immunoreactive (i) IGF-I in porcine follicular fluid substantially exceeded that encountered in serum [1]. Further evidence consisted of the demonstration of cycloheximide-inhibitable, gonadotropin- and estradiol-dependent iIGF-I in serum-free medium conditioned by cultured porcine granulosa cells [2,3]. Although the ovarian content of iIGF-I in rats appears to be dependent on growth hormones [4], a direct effect of growth hormone at the level of the rat granulosa cell remains to be demonstrated. Extending such investigations to the transcriptional level, we have recently shown that both the adult and immature rat ovary (as well as the isolated, immature granulosa cell) are sites of IGF-I gene expression and that expression may be subject to gonadotropic regulation [5]. It is significant that of all adult rat organs tested [6], the ovary (O) displays the third highest level of IGF-I gene expression, the uterus (U) and liver (Li) being the most active in this regard. In contrast, human granulosa cells may be a site of IGF-II rather than IGF-I gene expression [7]. These observations and the absence of IGF-II gene expression in the adult rat ovary [6] suggest possible species specificity. However, profound differences in the experimental conditions may favor IGF-II gene expression as a (fetal) marker of dedifferentiation.

We have recently undertaken an assessment of the relative ovarian abundance of IGF-I transcripts with alternative 5′-untranslated (UT) regions, of their cellular localization, and of hormonal regulation in this system (5). To this end, a solution hybridization/RNase protection assay was employed wherein total rat ovarian RNA was hybridized with a 404-base ^{32}P-labelled rat IGF-I riboprobe that corresponded to the Class A 5′-UT variant. As in liver, three protected bands representing fragments of (322 [Class A], 297 [Class B], and 242 [Class C] bases) were noted, in keeping with established alternative 5′-UT transcripts. The ovarian Class C variant (like the hepatic variant) proved the most abundant. The ovarian Class B variant was barely detectable. Cellular localization studies revealed that these ovarian IGF-I transcripts were primarily, if not exclusively, of granulosa but not of theca-interstitial cell origin. Treatment of immature (21–23 days old) hypophysectomized rats with a diethylstilbestrol (DES)-containing subcutaneous silastic implant for a total of 5 days resulted in a twofold increase in the (densitometrically quantified) abundance of ovarian IGF-I transcripts, a diametrically opposite effect (a 2.6-fold decrease) being noted at the level of the liver. Whereas treatment of hypophysectomized rats with ovine growth hormone (oGH) by itself (150 mg, q.d., s.c. × 5 days) resulted in a fivefold increase in hepatic IGF-I gene expression, a limited, albeit distinct, inhibitory effect was observed on the steady-state levels of ovarian IGF-I mRNA. In contrast, combined treatment with oGH and DES yielded a threefold increase in the abundance of ovarian IGF-I transcripts, there being no net alteration in hepatic IGF-I gene expression. Taken together, these findings reveal ovarian expression of the three known 5′-UT IGF-I mRNA variants, document the granulosa cell as the main somatic ovarian cell for IGF-I mRNA generation, and indicate that hepatic and ovarian IGF-I gene expression are differentially regulated in diametrically opposed directions.

The studies described above and related studies have resulted in a tentative consensus as to the regulation of ovarian (or more specifically granulosa cell) IGF-I gene expression. It appears that biosynthesis of granulosa cell-derived IGF-I may well be GH, follicle-stimulating hormone (FSH), and estrogen dependent. It is further presumed that granulosa cell-derived IGF-I is capable of traversing the cellular plasma membrane to enter the extracellular fluid, wherein it may bind to specific cell membrane type-I IGF receptors on its very cell of origin or else on adjacent cells. In this way, granulosa cell-derived IGF-I may exert autocrine or paracrine effects, respectively. These concepts are indeed at the very heart of the intraovarian IGF hypothesis. Stated in a different way, it has been presumed that locally generated IGF-I would, in fact, play a meaningful role *in vivo* by regulating activities of its cell of origin or else that of immediately adjacent cell types. Although an attractive hypothesis, this idea has not yet been rigorously examined experimentally. Preliminary studies suggest, however, that immunoneutralization of granulosa cell-derived IGF-I may inhibit, at least in part, FSH- and GH-mediated granulosa cell differentiation. Nonetheless, much additional work is required before unequivocal conclusions can be reached as to the relevance *in vivo* of IGF-I to ovarian physiology. Indeed, limitations imposed by current experimental approaches may well require that definite proof await more sophisticated experimental paradigms. In particular, it is to be hoped that transgenic technology will develop to a level sufficient to allow selective ablation of IGF-I at the level of the ovary, such that reproductive function can be evaluated in both an experimental group and in controls.

Ovarian receptors for IGF-I

Both porcine [8] and murine [9] granulosa cells have now been shown to display high-affinity, low-capacity binding sites for IGF-I. In our hands [10], binding to FSH-primed rat granulosa cells proved time, temperature, and pH dependent, with optimal steady-state conditions being achieved after an 8-hour incubation at 15 °C at pH 8.0. Although subject to regulation by the cellular density of plating, the binding of ^{125}I-labeled IGF-I to its receptor proved saturable (apparent K_d, 3.3×10^{-9} M) as well as reversible, with complete or partial tracer displacement being effected by competitive inhibition and dilution, respectively. Scatchard and Hill analyses yielded linear plots consistent with the existence of a single class of non-interacting binding sites. Specificity studies revealed that the competition for ^{125}I-labeled IGF-I binding followed a rank order of potency of IGF-I > multiplication stimulating activity (MSA) > insulin, a pattern compatible with a type-I IGF receptor. Limited or zero displacement was observed with a series of chemically related and unrelated polypeptides as well as with an antiserum raised against human insulin receptors in rabbits. Using affinity cross-linking, we have also been able to observe that whole ovarian membranes of untreated (or FSH-treated) immature, hypophysectomized, DES-treated rats are endowed with specific type-I IGF receptors. Similar results have more recently been obtained with isolated granulosa cells from the same experimental model (unpublished).

We recently reported that FSH and luteinizing hormone (LH) are capable of up-regulating the binding of IGF-I by granulosa cells, an effect further augmented by GH but not by prolactin [11]. Specifically, we were able to show that FSH is capable of up-regulating IGF-I binding in a time- and dose-dependent fashion and that cyclic adenosine monophosphate (cAMP), its purported intracellular second messenger, may play an intermediary role in this regard. Indeed, granulosa cell IGF-I binding was enhanced after elevation of the intracellular level of cAMP by a series of cAMP-generating agonists, by inhibition of cAMP-phosphodiesterase activity, or by the provision of nondegradable cAMP analogs. High doses of forskolin (10^{-5} M), like FSH, proved capable of augmenting IGF-I binding by themselves, while an essentially inert dose (10^{-7} M) acted synergistically with FSH in this regard. It is significant that heterologous up-regulation of receptors was not limited to FSH, and similar increments were observed with luteotropic, β_2-adrenergic, but not lactogenic granulosa cell agonists. Related studies *in vivo* using immature, hypophysectomized, DES-treated rats revealed that the ability of FSH to up-regulate granulosa cell IGF-I binding (i) is not strictly a phenomenon observed *in vitro* and that it can be fully reproduced *in vivo*, (ii) is due to enhancement of IGF-I binding capacity rather than of affinity, (iii) may be subject to diametrically opposed modulation by somatogenic and gonadotropin-releasing hormone (GnRH)-like granulosa cell agonists (up- and down-regulation, respectively), and (iv) is best maintained by gonadotropins but not by prolactin. Inasmuch as gonadotropin dependence constitutes a unique attribute of the ovarian granulosa cell, our findings further suggest that the granulosa cell IGF-I receptor may have thoroughly adapted to its unique environment, thus providing the first example of a cell type for which the complement of IGF-I receptors may be cAMP dependent. Given the pivotal role of FSH in the induction of granulosa cell receptors for luteotropic and lactogenic ligands, this finding strongly suggests that the acquisition of IGF-I responsiveness may be part and parcel of granulosa cell ontogeny. Accordingly, gonadotropins may condition the cell to respond optimally to IGF-I, thereby conferring selective advantage upon follicles that are so endowed.

Both IGF-I and IGF-II have been shown to promote the differentiation and proliferation of granulosa cells. While both type-I and type-II

IGF receptors have been observed in rat granulosa cells, the nature of the IGF receptor that mediates reception of IGF cannot be completely evaluated at this time because of the lack of specific reagents. However, the availability of antibodies specific for the rat type-II IGF receptor (R-II-PAB1) has made studies of this type of receptor possible. To validate the utility of the R-II-PAB1 antiserum at the level of the rat granulosa cell, its ability to immunoneutralize the granulosa cell type-II IGF receptor was examined [12]. Significantly, R-II-PAB1 (10–100 mg/ml) proved a potent inhibitor of ^{125}I-labeled IGF-II (but not of ^{125}I-labeled IGF-I) binding to preparations of granulosa cell membranes. Substantial, albeit finite, R-II-PAB1-mediated inhibition of the cross-linking of ^{125}I-labeled IGF-II was also observed. Moreover, R-II-PAB1 proved highly potent in immunoprecipitating the type-II IGF receptor from rat granulosa cells. In light of these observations, we have proceeded to use R-II-PAB1 to assess the functional role of the rat granulosa cell type-II IGF receptor in the hormonal action of IGF-I and IGF-II. To this end, granulosa cells primed with FSH (20 ng/ml) were cultured for 72 hours in the absence or presence of IGF-I or IGF-II (50 ng/ml), with or without increasing (receptor-active) concentrations of R-II-PAB1 (10–100 mg/ml). Control incubations were carried out with an ammonium sulfate precipitate of nonimmune rabbit serum dialyzed against phosphate-buffered saline. Both R-II-PAB1 and nonimmune rabbit serum were without effect on the cytodifferentiative action of IGF-I and IGF-II. Subject to the limitations inherent in the immunoneutralizing potency of R-II-PAB1, these findings are in keeping with the hypothesis that (inasmuch as the conventional cytodifferentiative process is concerned) the granulosa cell type-II IGF receptor does not appear to participate in transmembrane signaling upon binding of IGF. These findings also suggest that the hormonal action of IGF-I and IGF-II at the level of the granulosa cell may be exerted largely, if not exclusively, via the type-I IGF receptor. Thus, the potential relevance and the functional role(s), if any, of the granulosa cell type-II IGF receptor remain to be determined.

The granulosa cell as a site of IGF-I action

Studies carried out in the last several years have clearly established the granulosa cell as a site of IGF-I action. The action of IGF-I at the level of the rat, but not porcine, granulosa cell appears largely (but not exclusively) contingent upon its ability to synergize with pituitary gonadotropins. These effects can be explained by enhanced cellular viability, plating efficiency or DNA synthesis. Thus, this ability of IGF-I to augment the differentiated phenotypic expression of the developing granulosa cell may be distinct from its established, growth-promoting property and is thus considered a novel biologic effect of this polypeptide [13]. In this connection, we have been able to show that IGF-I is capable of augmenting FSH-supported (but not basal) biosynthesis of progesterone and estrogen, as well as the FSH-mediated acquisition of LH receptors. More recently, IGF-I was also found to augment basal as well as FSH-supported biosynthesis of proteoglycans [14]. In this respect, IGF-I appears to exert its classic "sulfation factor" activity at the level of the granulosa cell, manifesting the very chondrotropic effect that led to its discovery. Fractionation of the major extracellular proteoglycan species revealed that FSH favored the exclusive production of dermatan sulfate, whereas IGF-I supported the simultaneous biosynthesis of both heparin and dermatan sulfate. These findings suggest that IGF-I may effect marked quantitative as well as qualitative alterations in proteoglycan economy. Given the possible role of proteoglycans in follicular antrum formation and follicular atresia, these findings raise the possibility that IGF-I of granulosa cell origin may participate in the growth as well as demise of the developing ovarian follicle.

The granulosa cell as a site of IGF-binding protein generation

Insulin-like growth factor binding protein(s) (IBPs) are multifunctional proteins that regulate not only the transport of IGFs but also their presentation to cell-surface receptors. The latter function is thought to be carried out by GH-independent low-molecular-weight IBPs capable of binding IGFs (but not insulin) with affinities in the 10^{-10}–10^{-9} M range [15,16]. One such binding moiety (IBP2) from mouse hepatocytes (cell line BRL 3A) has recently been purified [17,18] and its gene cloned [18,19]. It is a 270-residue (29.5-kDa) mature, non-glycosylated protein endowed with the RGD adhesion (cell-attachment) sequence [20], which is commonly (but not exclusively) observed in matrix proteins. Although the precise role(s) of tissue-derived IBPs remains a matter of study, both stimulation [21,22] and inhibition [23,24] of IGF binding and action have been reported. Thus, the synthesis and secretion of IBPs may play a major role in the regulation of IGF hormonal action at the level of the target cell even at a time when the extracellular concentrations of IGFs remain constant. As such, this development adds a new level of complexity to the interaction of IGFs at the cellular level.

Although the relevance of IBPs to ovarian physiology remains unknown, immunoreactive IBP1 (previously referred to as placental protein 12) has been found in abundance in human ovarian follicular [25] and cyst [26] fluid. Although not detected in unstimulated ovarian tissue or in non-luteinized granulosa cells, IBP1 was detectable in luteinized granulosa cells as well as in corpora lutea [25]. Moreover, metabolically labeled (highly luteinized) human granulosa cells derived from ovaries subjected to gonadotropic hyperstimulation have been found capable of synthesis *de novo* of an IBP1-related species, as assessed by immunoisolation [27]. In related experiments, acid-chromatographed extracts of whole ovaries of murine origin [28], as well as media conditioned by porcine granulosa cells [2,3], were found to contain hormonally dependent, low-molecular-weight IGF-I binding activity. Most recently, IBP3 from porcine follicular fluid was found to suppress FSH hormonal action at the level of the murine granulosa cell [28].

To explore the possibility that the granulosa cell is also capable of hormonally controlled elaboration of IBPs, granulosa cells from immature, DES-primed rats were cultured for up to 72 hours under serum-free conditions in the absence or presence of FSH [29]. Media conditioned by untreated granulosa cells manifested constitutively released polyethylene glycol-precipitable, ^{125}I-labeled IGF-I binding activity, the daily elaboration of which proved constant throughout the 72-hour experimental period. However, treatment of granulosa cells with FSH resulted in dramatic inhibition of the accumulation of IGF-I binding activity (89% at a dose of 100 ng/ml). Systemic administration of FSH(10 mg/rat/day for 2 days) revealed that this gonadotropic action is not strictly a phenomenon observed *in vitro* but that it can be fully reproduced under certain circumstances *in vivo*. Western ligand blotting of gels after SDS-PAGE of media conditioned by untreated granulosa cells revealed three species of IBPs that formed a major doublet band (28–29 kDa) as well as a single minor band (23 kDa). Treatment with FSH virtually eliminated the 23-kDa species and substantially reduced the relative representation of the 28- and 29-kDa species of IBP (82 and 74% inhibition, respectively). Taken together, these observations disclose the multiplicity of granulosa cell-derived IBPs and reveal the striking ability of FSH to suppress their constitutive release both *in vitro* and *in vivo*. This FSH action is all the more noteworthy in light of the generally stimulatory effect exerted by FSH at the level of the granulosa cell. Inasmuch as FSH may be concerned with the promotion of granulosa cell development, its ability to attenuate the release of (presumptively inhibitory) IBPs may enhance the access of endogenously produced IGF-I to its cognate cell-surface receptors and hence its hormonal action on cells.

Summary

Although much remains to be learned with respect to the possible relevance of IGF-I to ovarian physiology, it is possible at this time to suggest tentatively some possible functions of IGF-I in this connection.

1 *Amplification* of gonadotropin hormonal action: a key requirement given the exponential nature of follicular development.

2 *Integration* of follicular development: an essential facet concerned with the coordination of granulosa–theca cooperation.

3 *Selection* of dominant follicle(s): a speculative proposition, assuming the timely and selective activation of the IGF-I system in "chosen" follicles.

Aside from its possible role(s) in the course of established follicular cycles, IGF-I (and/or IGF-II) may also participate in the actual formation of the follicular apparatus during the late fetal/early neonatal period. Although the ovary is gonadotropin independent at that time, we have shown previously that IGF-I may well interact with vasoactive intestinal peptide (VIP)-like ligands input now implicated in the morphodifferentiation of the follicular apparatus. Similarly, IGF-I may be concerned with the promotion of juvenile and early pubertal levels of follicular gonadotropin (FSH), and ovarian IGF-I may have a bearing on the puberty-promoting effect of GH. Indeed, an association appears to exist between isolated GH deficiency and delayed puberty both in rodents and in human subjects, a process reversed by systemic GH replacement therapy. Given that ovarian IGF-I and its receptor may be GH dependent, it is tempting to speculate that the ability of GH to accelerate pubertal maturation may be due, at least in part, to the promotion of ovarian IGF-I production and reception, with the consequent local potentiation of gonadotropin action [30].

Acknowledgments

Supported in part by NIH Research Grant HD-19998 and USPHS, E.Y.A. the recipient of Research Career Development Award 1-K04-HD-00697 from the NICHHD, NIH.

References

1 Hammond JM. Peptide regulators in the ovarian follicle. Aust J Biol Sci 1981; 34:491–504.

2 Hammond JM, Baranao JLS, Skaleris D, Knight AB, Romanus JA, Rechler MM. Production of insulin-like growth factors by ovarian granulosa cells. Endocrinology 1985; 117:2553–5.

3 Hsu C-J, Hammond JM. Gonadotropins and estradiol stimulate immunoreactive insulin-like growth factor-I production by porcine granulosa cells *in vitro*. Endocrinology 1987; 120:198–207.
4 Davoren JB, Hsueh AJW. Growth hormone increases ovarian levels of immunoreactive somatomedin-C/insulin-like growth factor I *in vivo*. Endocrinology 1986; 118:888–90.
5 Hernandez ER, Roberts CT, LeRoith D, Adashi EY. Rat ovarian insulin-like growth factor (IGF-I) gene expression is granulosa cell-selective: 5′-untranslated mRNA variant representation and hormonal regulation. Endocrinology 1989; 125:572–4.
6 Murphy LJ, Bell GI, Friesen HB. Tissue distribution of insulin-like growth factor I and II messenger ribonucleic acid in the adult rat. Endocrinology 1987; 120:1279–82.
7 Voutilainen R, Miller WL. Coordinate tropic hormone regulation of mRNAs for insulin-like growth factor II and the cholesterol side-chain-cleavage enzyme, $P450_{scc}$, in human steroidogenic tissues. Proc Natl Acad Sci USA 1987; 84:1590–4.
8 Veldhuis JD, Furlanetto RW, Juchter D, Garmey J, Veldhuis P. Trophic actions of human somatomedin-C/insulin-like growth factor I on ovarian cells: *in vitro* studies with swine granulosa cells. Endocrinology 1985; 116:1235–42.
9 Davoren JB, Kasson BG, Li CH, Hsueh AJW. Specific insulin-like growth factor (IGF) I- and II-binding sites on rat granulosa cells: relation to IGF action. Endocrinology 1986; 119:2155–62.
10 Adashi EY, Resnick CE, Hernandez ER, Svoboda ME, Van Wyk JJ. Characterization and regulation of a specific cell membrane receptor for somatomedin C/insulin-like growth factor I in cultured rat granulosa cells. Endocrinology 1986; 122:194–201.
11 Adashi EY, Resnick CE, Svoboda ME, Van Wyk JJ. Follicle-stimulating hormone enhances somatomedin-C binding to cultured rat granulosa cells: evidence for cAMP-dependence. J Biol Chem 1986; 261:3923–6.
12 Adashi EY, Resnick CE, Rosenfeld RG. Insulin-like growth factor-I (IGF-I) and IGF-II hormonal action in cultured rat granulosa cells: mediation via type I but not type II IGF receptors. Endocrinology 1990; 126:216–22.
13 Adashi EY, Resnick CE, D'Ercole AJ, Svoboda ME, Van Wyk JJ. Insulin-like growth factors as intraovarian regulators of granulosa cell growth and function. Endocr Rev 1985; 6:400–20.
14 Adashi EY, Resnick CE, Svoboda ME, Van Wyk JJ, Hascall VC, Yanagishita M. Independent and synergistic actions of somatomedin-C in the stimulation of proteoglycan biosynthesis by cultured rat granulosa cells. Endocrinology 1986; 118:456–9.
15 Binoux M, Hossenlopp P, Hardouin S, Seurin D, Lassarre C, Gourmelen M. Somatomedin (insulin-like growth factors)-binding proteins: molecular forms and regulation. Horm Res 1986; 24:141–51.
16 Baxter RC. The insulin-like growth factors and their binding proteins. Comp Biochem Physiol 1988; 91B:229–35.
17 Mottola C, MacDonald RG, Brackett JL, Mole JE, Anderson JK, Czech MP. Purification and amino-terminal sequence of an insulin-like growth factor-binding protein secreted by rat liver BRL-3A cells. J Biol Chem 1986; 261:11180–8.
18 Brown AL, Chiariotti L, Orlowski CC, Mehlman T, Burgess WH, Ackerman EJ, Bruni CB, Rechler MM. Nucleotide sequence and expression of a cDNA clone encoding a fetal rat binding protein for insulin-like growth factors. J Biol Chem 1989; 264:5148–54.
19 Margot JB, Binkert C, Mary J-L, Landwehr J, Heinrich G, Schwander J. A low-molecular-weight insulin-like growth factor-binding protein from rat: cDNA cloning and tissue distribution of its messenger RNA. Mol Endocrinol 1989; 3:1053–66.
20 Ruoslahti E, Pierschbacher MD. New perspectives in cell adhesion: RGD and integrins. Science 1987; 238:491–7.
21 De Vroede MA, Tseng LY-H, Katsoyannis PG, Nissley SP, Rechler MM. Modulation of insulin-like growth factor I binding to human fibroblast monolayer cultures by insulin-

like growth factor I binding to human fibroblast monolayer cultures by insulin-like growth factor carrier proteins released to the incubation media. J Clin Invest 1986; 77:602–13.

22 Elgin RG, Busby WJ Jr, Clemmons DR. An insulin-like growth factor (IGF) binding protein enhances the biologic response to IGF-I. Proc Natl Acad Sci USA 1987; 84:3254–8.

23 Drop SLS, Valiquette G, Guyda HJ, Corvol MT, Posner BI. Partial purification and characterization of a binding protein for insulin-like activity (ILAs) in human amniotic fluid: a possible inhibitor of insulin-like activity. Acta Endocrinol 1979; 90:505–18.

24 Ritvos O, Ranta T, Jalkanen J, Suilkhari AM, Voutilainen R, Bohn H, Rutanen E-M. Insulin-like growth factor (IGF) binding protein from human decidua inhibits the binding and biological action of IGF-I in cultured choriocarcinoma cells. Endocrinology 1988; 122:2150–7.

25 Seppala M, Wahlstrom T, Koskimies AI, Tenhunen A, Rutanen E-M, Koistinen R, Huhtoniemi I, Bohn H, Stenman U-H. Human preovulatory follicular fluid, luteinized cells of hyperstimulated preovulatory follicles, and corpus luteum contain placental protein 12. J Clin Endocrinol Metab 1984; 58:505–10.

26 Seppala M, Than G. Insulin-like growth factor binding protein PP12 in ovarian cyst fluid. Arch Gynecol Obstet 1987; 241:33–5.

27 Suikkari AM, Jalkanen J, Koistinen R, Butzow R, Ritvos O, Ranta T, Seppala M. Human granulosa cells synthesize low molecular weight insulin-like growth factor-binding protein. Endocrinology 1989; 124:1088–90.

28 Ui M, Shimonaka M, Shimasaki S, Ling N. An insulin-like growth factor-binding protein in ovarian follicular fluid blocks follicle-stimulating steroid production by ovarian granulosa cells. Endocrinology 1989; 125:912–16.

29 Adashi EY, Resnick CE, Hernandez ER, Hurwitz A, Rosenfeld RG. Follicle-stimulating hormone inhibits the constitutive release of insulin-like growth factor binding proteins by cultured rat ovarian granulosa cells. Endocrinology 1990; 126:1305–7.

30 Homburg R, Eshel A, Abdalla HI, Jacobs HS. Growth hormone facilitates ovulation induction by gonadotropins. Clin Endocrinol 1988; 29:113–17.

Chapter 19
Growth Factors: an Overview

STEPHEN FRANKS

A lively and wide-ranging discussion focused predominantly on the role of insulin-like growth factors (IGFs) and their binding proteins in the physiology and disorders of ovarian function.

Insulin-like growth factors and their binding proteins

Production and action of IGF-I in the human ovary

Erickson posed the question, "Is IGF-I synthesized in the human ovary?" Data from experiments in the rat suggest that IGF-I gene expression occurs in both interstitial cells and granulosa cells [1,2] but, interestingly, there is, as yet, no evidence for IGF-I gene expression in human granulosa cells. Data from two groups have shown the presence of mRNA for IGF-II, but not for IGF-I, in human granulosa cells obtained after superovulation therapy [3,4].

Adashi referred to recent data from his own group, which appeared to support these findings in that IGF-I gene expression in unstimulated human ovaries was evident in theca and stromal tissue but not in granulosa cells [5]. Thus, the source of IGF-I in human follicular fluid [6] remains to be defined. It is likely that the IGF-I is derived from circulating IGF-I, but the interstitial cells of the ovary could contribute to the intrafollicular pool.

The possible role of IGF-I in stimulating abnormal steroidogenesis in the polycystic ovary was discussed in answer to a point raised by Merriam. Erickson suggested that IGF-I could directly stimulate the activity of 17α-hydroxylase/17,20-lyase (GF Erickson, pers. comm.). This possibility might help to explain abnormal production of androgens by the ovary but would not account for the impaired function of granulosa cells observed in anovulatory women with polycystic ovary syndrome (PCO). Erickson further suggested that there might be a counter-regulatory factor (as yet undefined) that prevents the expression of IGF-I action in the granulosa cells.

A further comment on the action of IGF-I in theca cells was made by Cara. Using rat theca cells, he had observed that IGF-I increased the binding of luteinizing hormone (LH) to its receptor and postulated that the effect of IGF-I was to overcome the down-regulation of the LH receptor by LH itself [7]. This effect might be of relevance to increased production of androgens in PCO since it would provide a mechanism for enhanced steroidogenesis even in the absence of high circulating levels of LH.

There was an extensive discussion of the effects of the various binding proteins for IGFs on ovarian steroidogenesis. Interest was expressed in recent data that suggested that IGF binding-proteins (in particular, IGFBP-3) were able to inhibit the action of follicle-stimulating hormone (FSH) on the granulosa cell by a mechanism that did not involve binding to IGFs [8].

However, the interaction of IGF-I and its binding proteins in the ovary were also discussed. Rosenfeld commented that there was a large volume of data to suggest an inhibitory effect of IGF-binding proteins on the action of IGF-I. A fascinating example of this interaction is to be found in recent experiments from Adashi's laboratory that indicate that the addition of IGFBP-1 to rat granulosa cells in culture inhibits not only the effect of IGF-I itself but also that of FSH, i.e. the data suggest an obligatory role for IGF-I in FSH-induced production of estrogen [9].

IGF-binding proteins and polycystic ovary syndrome

Givens raised the issue of the relevance of circulating and follicular-fluid levels of IGFBP-1 in patients with PCO. Seppala and colleagues had reported low circulating concentrations of IGFBP-1 in women with PCO [10] but closer analysis of their data revealed that the low levels were found in obese women with PCO and were consistent with the observed effects of insulin on hepatic production of IGFBP-1 [11,12]. It was pointed out that follicular-fluid IGFBP-1 is likely both to be derived from circulating (hepatic) IGFBP-1 and to be produced locally by granulosa cells. Recent data from a collaborative study from the laboratories of Franks and Seppala show that concentrations of IGFBP-1 in follicular fluid and in medium conditioned by granulosa cells obtained from polycystic ovaries were similar to those observed in follicular fluid and medium from cultures of normal granulosa cells (HD Mason, R Koistinen, M Seppala, S Franks, unpublished results). Rosenfeld pointed out that other IGF-binding proteins may be just as, if not more, important, than IGFBP-1 in the functions of human granulosa cells, a suggestion borne out by the recent studies of Holly *et al.* [13].

Rosenfeld summarized the possible role of IGF-binding proteins in the ovary as follows: the binding proteins are paracrine and autocrine factors (just like IGFs themselves); they are produced by many types of cell, in concert with IGFs; and they (in the context of the ovary) may lead to differential expression of steroidogenic enzymes in either theca or granulosa cells.

Epidermal growth factor, transforming growth factor α and ovarian function

Dunaif asked about the effects of epidermal growth factor (EFG) and transforming growth factor α (TGFα) on the function of human granulosa cells. Franks cited data from the work of Simpson and colleagues [14] and from his own laboratory [15] that indicate an inhibitory action of EGF and TGF on aromatase activity in human granulosa cells. Mason and colleagues [15] have also shown that EGF is a potent inhibitor of estradiol production in granulosa cells obtained from polycystic as well as normal ovaries.

Growth factors and the adrenal gland

Morris raised the issue of regulation by growth factors of steroidogenesis in the adrenal gland. McAllister commented on her own studies of human adrenal cells in culture that indicated that 17α-hydroxylase and 3β-hydroxysteroid dehydrogenase (3β-HSD) were regulated in opposite directions by different growth factors (JA McAllister, ER Simpson, pers. comm.). IGF-I appeared to stimulate 17α-hydroxylase activity and inhibit that of 3β-HSD, whereas TGF-α and EGF inhibited 17α-hydroxylase and stimulated 3β-HSD. A similar relationship between growth factors and these key steroidogenic enzymes was also observed in the ovary, namely whatever stimulated 17α-hydroxylase activity inhibited that of 3β-HSD and vice versa.

Givens wondered whether the apparently biphasic effect of insulin on circulating concentrations of dehydroepiandrosterone sulfate could be explained by cross-reaction of insulin with the IGF-I receptor. Rosenfield replied that the affinity of insulin for the IGF-I receptor was about 0.1% of that of IGF-I itself, i.e. very high circulating levels of insulin would be required to activate the IGF-I receptor. However, such levels may, of course, be present in insulin-resistant states.

The above discussion was evidence of the interest and excitement generated by the study of the action of growth factors on the ovary. There seems little doubt that locally produced growth factors, both stimulatory and inhibitory, can modulate the action of gonadotropins on ovarian steroidogenesis. A further level of complexity is introduced by the study of the actions of proteins that bind IGFs. These proteins appear to be generated within both the theca and granulosa cell compartments of the ovary and can modulate the effects of IGF-I, but they may themselves have direct effects on FSH-induced production of estradiol. The possibility that binding proteins may differentially affect the expression of the action of IGF-I in theca and granulosa cells is intriguing and deserves further study as efforts are continued to understand the abnormalities of ovarian steroidogenesis that characterize PCO.

References

1 Oliver JE, Aitman TJ, Wilson CA, Clayton RN. Insulin-like growth factor I gene expression in the rat ovary is confined to the granulosa cells of developing follicles. Endocrinology 1989; 124:2671–9.

2 Hernandez ER, Roberts CT, Leroith D, Adashi EY. Rat insulin-like growth factor I gene expression is granulosa cell selective: 5′-untranslated mRNA variant representation and hormonal regulation. Endocrinology 1989; 125:572–4.

3 Ramashara K, Li CH. Human pituitary and placental hormones control human insulin-like growth factor II secretion in human granulosa cells. Proc Natl Acad Sci USA 1987; 84:2643–7.

4 Voutilainen R, Miller WL. Coordinate trophic hormone regulation of mRNA's for insulin-like growth factor II and cholesterol side-chain-cleavage enzyme P450 seen in human steroidogenic tissues. Proc Natl Acad Sci USA 1987; 84:1590–4.

5 Hurwitz A, Hernandez ER. IGF-I mRNAs with divergent 5′ and 3′ regions are expressed in the premenopausal human ovary. Proceedings of the Endocrine Society, 72nd Annual Meeting, Atlanta, Ga, 1990, Abstract 680.

6 Eden JA, Jones J, Carter GD, Alaghband-Zadeh J. A comparison of follicular fluid levels of insulin-like growth factor-I in normal dominant and cohort follicles, polycystic and multicystic ovaries. Clin Endocrinol 1988; 79:327–36.

7 Cara JF, Azzarello J. Insulin-like growth factor I stimulates androgen synthesis and increases LH-binding capacity in rat ovarian theca-interstitial cells by separate transcriptional and translational mechanisms. Proceedings of the Endocrine Society, 72nd Annual Meeting, Atlanta, Ga, 1990, Abstract 607.

8 Bicsak TA, Shimonaka M, Malkowski M, Ling N. Insulin-like growth factor-binding protein (IGF-BP) inhibition of granulosa cell function. Endocrinology 1990; 126:2184–9.

9 Adashi EY, Resnick CE, Hernandez ER. Insulin-like growth factor I as an intraovarian regulator: basic and clinical implications. Proceedings of VII World Congress on Human Reproduction, Helsinki, June 1990. Ann N Y Acad Sci 1991; 626:161–8.

10 Suikkari AM, Ruutiainen K, Erkolla R, Seppala M. Low levels of low-molecular-weight

plasma insulin-like growth factor-binding protein in women with polycystic ovarian disease. Hum Reprod 1989; 4:136–9.

11 Kiddy DS, Hamilton-Fairley D, Seppala M, Koistinen R, James VHT, Reed MJ, Franks S. Diet-induced changes in sex hormone-binding globulin and free testosterone in women with normal or polycystic ovaries, correlation with serum insulin and insulin-like growth factor I. Clin Endocrinol 1989; 31:757–63.

12 Singh A, Hamilton-Fairley D, Koistinen R, Seppala M, James VHT, Franks S, Reed MJ. Effect of insulin-like growth factor type I and insulin on the secretion of sex hormone-binding globulin and IGF-I-binding protein by human hepatoma cells. J Endocrinol 1990; 124:R1–R3.

13 Holly JMP, Eden JA, Alaghband-Zadeh J, Carter GD, Jemmott RC, Cianfarani S, Chard T, Wass JAH. Insulin-like growth factor-binding protein in follicular fluid from normal dominant and cohort follicles, polycystic and multicystic ovaries. Clin Endocrinol 1990; 33:53–64.

14 Steinkampf MP, Mendelson CR, Simpson ER. Effects of epidermal growth factor and insulin-like growth factor I on the levels of mRNA encoding aromatase cytochrome P-450 of human granulosa cells. Mol Cell Endocrinol 1988; 59:93–9.

15 Mason HD, Margara R, Winston RML, Beard RW, Reed MJ, Franks S. Inhibition of oestradiol production by epidermal growth factor in human granulosa cells of normal polycystic ovaries. Clin Endocrinol 1991; 33:511–17.

Section 7
Insulin

Chapter 20

Molecular Mechanisms of Defects in Insulin Action in Genetic Syndromes Associated with Insulin Resistance

SIMEON I. TAYLOR, ALESSANDRO CAMA, DOMENICO ACCILI, EIICHI IMANO, RACHEL LEVY-TOLEDANO, CATHERINE FRAPIER, HIROKO KADOWAKI & TAKASHI KADOWAKI

In young women, insulin resistance is frequently associated with hyperandrogenism and acanthosis nigricans. This association has been observed in patients with a wide variety of causes of insulin resistance. Hyperandrogenism is a common feature in women in whom the primary cause of disease is a mutation in the insulin receptor gene [1,2]. Some obese patients present a similar clinical syndrome although the cause of insulin resistance has not been elucidated [3,4]. In addition, hyperandrogenism has been described in premenopausal women who develop extreme insulin resistance as a consequence of autoantibodies directed against the insulin receptor [5]. This close association, irrespective of the biochemical cause of insulin resistance, has led to the hypothesis that hyperandrogenism and acanthosis nigricans are consequences of the insulin-resistant state. In particular, it has been proposed that hyperinsulinemia has "toxic" effects upon the ovary and skin that cause hyperandrogenism and acanthosis nigricans, respectively [5–7]. This chapter will focus upon genetic causes of extreme insulin resistance, with special emphasis on mutations in the insulin receptor gene identified in young women with the syndrome of type A extreme insulin resistance (i.e. insulin resistance in association with acanthosis nigricans and hyperandrogenism, in the absence of obesity or lipoatrophy) (Fig. 20.1) [1,6].

Insulin receptors

Human insulin receptor gene

The gene encoding the human insulin receptor is composed of 22 exons and spans more than 120 kb on chromosome 19 [8,9]. There are

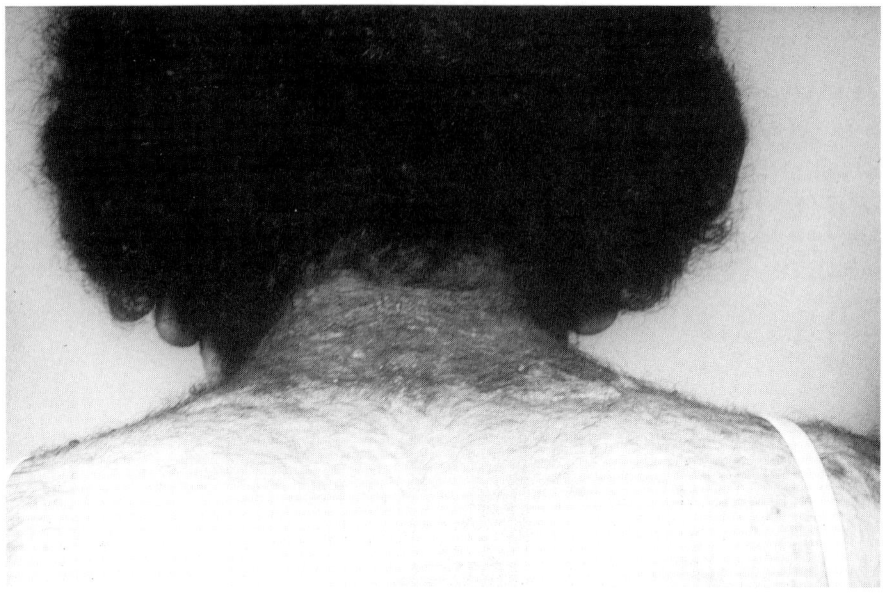

Fig. 20.1 Photograph of patient with type A extreme resistance to insulin. This photograph of patient A-5 illustrates acanthosis nigricans on the back of her neck. The hirsutism noted on her back reflects hyperandrogenism due to increased ovarian production of testosterone [1,2,40].

multiple sites for the initiation of transcription in the region 300–600 base pairs (bp) upstream from the initiator methionine codon [10–12]. Five species of mRNA ranging in size from 5 to 11 kb have been identified [11,13]. The major variation in size is due to variable lengths of 3'-untranslated RNA, resulting from the use of alternate polyadenylation signals [11]. At least one example of alternate splicing has been identified. Exon 11, encoding amino acids 720–731, can either be included or excluded from the mature mRNA [14,15]. In some tissues, such as liver, the majority of mRNA molecules that encode the receptor contain the nucleotide sequence that corresponds to exon 11. Other cell types (e.g. cultured lymphoblasts transformed with Epstein–Barr virus (EBV)) contain exclusively the mRNA without the exon 11 sequence. However, many tissues (e.g. muscle and adipose tissue) contain both splicing variants of mRNA for the insulin receptor. It has been reported that deletion of the 12 amino acids encoded by exon 11 increases the affinity of the receptor for insulin [16].

Structure of the insulin receptor

The insulin receptor gene encodes a single polypeptide that undergoes *N*-linked glycosylation to yield a 190-kDa precursor of the insulin receptor [13,17–20]. This precursor undergoes additional post-translational processing to yield the mature receptor. First, the precursor undergoes proteolytic cleavage into two separate subunits [17,18]. Second, the high-mannose form of *N*-linked carbohydrate undergoes maturation with removal of mannose and glucose residues and the addition of other sugars, which include sialic acid [17,18]. Other post-translational modifications occur, including fatty acylation [21] and *O*-linked glycosylation [22,23].

The basic structural unit of the mature insulin receptor is a heterodimer formed by the α- and β-subunits. The α,β dimers further dimerize to produce a heterotetrameric $\alpha_2\beta_2$ species (Fig. 20.2).

THE α-SUBUNIT

The α-subunit *in situ* is entirely extracellular and provides the binding site for insulin [13,24]. Although the binding site has not been definitively mapped, several lines of evidence suggest that the binding site may be located in the N-terminal portion of the α-subunit [25,26]. Nevertheless, when a cDNA that encoded only the α-subunit was expressed by transfection in 3T3 cells, it was not possible to detect a truncated receptor with high binding activity, possibly because isolated α-subunits are unstable [27]. In contrast, similar transfection studies have demonstrated that a truncated receptor that contains the α-subunit plus the extracellular domain of the β-subunit does retain insulin-binding activity. This observation suggests that the receptor's β-subunit may participate directly or indirectly in formation of the insulin-binding site.

When a bivalent cross-linking reagent such as disuccinimidyl suberate is added to the tetrameric receptor, it is possible covalently to cross-link two α-subunits. Furthermore, in the native receptor, there appear to be disulfide bonds between adjacent α-subunits, which have been tentatively mapped to the cysteine residues at positions 435, 468 and/or 524 [28].

THE β-SUBUNIT

The β-subunit contains the transmembrane domain that anchors the receptor in the plasma membrane, and it possesses enzymatic activity as a tyrosine-specific protein kinase [29,30]. When insulin binds to the extracellular domain of the receptor, the tyrosine kinase activity of the receptor is activated. A growing body of evidence supports the hypothesis that activation of the tyrosine kinase plays a necessary role in mediating insulin action upon the target cell. Mutational analysis of the insulin receptor provides some of the most convincing evidence, as shown below.

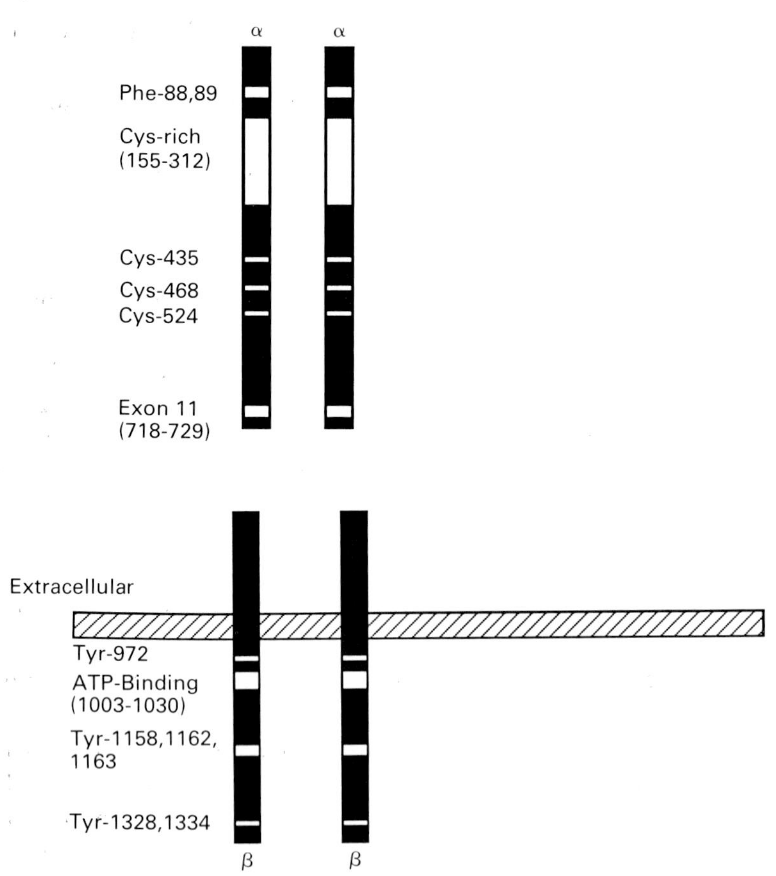

Fig. 20.2 Structural map of the insulin receptor. Key structural landmarks are identified at the left of the drawing of the receptor. Phe^{88}, Phe^{89} [26], and the cysteine-rich domain [13,25] have all been implicated as playing a role in the insulin-binding domain. Cys^{435}, Cys^{468}, and Cys^{524} are candidates for contributors to sulfhydryl groups involved in the formation of the disulfide bonds between adjacent α-subunits [28]. Exon 11 is an exon that has been described as undergoing variable splicing [14,15]. As described in the text, the five [37,38] or six [36] tyrosine residues that are sites of autophosphorylation are indicated. The consenus sequence for an ATP-binding domain is located between amino acid residues 1003 and 1030 [31–35].

Adenosine triphosphate (ATP)-binding site

The site for binding of the substrate ATP is highly conserved in all protein kinases. The conserved ATP-binding motif in the insulin receptor consists of the $\mathbf{Gly}^{1003}$-X-$\mathbf{Gly}^{1005}$-X-X-$\mathbf{Gly}^{1008}$ . . . $\mathbf{Lys}^{1030}$ sequence, with the conserved amino acids indicated in bold (Fig. 20.2) [31]. When Lys^{1030} is mutated, the tyrosine kinase activity of the receptor is abolished and the ability of the receptor to mediate the various biologic actions of insulin [32–34] disappears. In addition, another mutation in the ATP-binding site, substitution of valine for Gly^{1008}, impairs tyrosine kinase activity and also causes insulin resistance *in vivo* [35].

Sites of tyrosine phosphorylation

The binding of insulin to the receptor causes autophosphorylation of tyrosine residues in the receptor [29,30]. The autophosphorylation of the receptor stimulates the activity of the tyrosine kinase to phosphorylate other protein substrates. There are at least two clusters of tyrosine residues that are autophosphorylated in response to insulin (Fig. 20.2): (i) tyrosine residues 1158, 1162, and 1163; and (ii) tyrosine residues 1328 and 1334 [36–38]. When Tyr^{1162} and Tyr^{1163} are replaced with phenylalanine, tryosine kinase activity is impaired, as is the ability of the receptor to mediate the action of insulin [39]. In addition, another potential phosphorylation site is located at Tyr^{972}, adjacent to an acidic amino acid (Glu^{971}) in a consensus sequence for a tyrosine-phosphorylation site. However, there is disagreement in the literature with respect to the question of whether or not Tyr^{972} is phosphorylated [36–38]. In any case, when Tyr^{972} is mutated to phenylalanine, the ability of the receptor to mediate insulin action is impaired, possibly as a result of an impairment of the phosphorylation of substrates by the tyrosine kinase [38].

Mutations in the insulin receptor gene

Type A extreme insulin resistance appears to be a genetic disease. Mutations have been identified in the insulin receptor gene in the small number of patients who have been investigated in detail (Table 20.1) [35,40–48]. Nevertheless, there may be genetic heterogeneity in the syndrome. The mechanism of insulin action is complex, and normal insulin action requires the participation of the products of many genes. Thus, it is possible that, in some patients, insulin resistance may be caused by mutations at other genetic loci.

Table 20.1 Patients with mutations in the insulin receptor gene*

Patient	Genotype	References
Type A extreme insulin resistance		
A-1	Amber^{133}/Ser^{462}	41
A-5 and A-8	Val^{382} (homozygous)	40
BI-1	Thr^{1134}/WT	46
BI-2	Ser^{1200}/WT	44, 45
Chiba-1	$\Delta^{\text{Exon 17(3')}-22}$/?	47
Chiba-2	$\Delta^{\text{Exon 14}}$/?	48
Kyushu-1 and -2	Ser^{735} (homozygous)	42, 43
Sapporo-1	Val^{1008}/?	35
Rabson–Mendenhall syndrome		
RM-1	Lys^{15}/Opal^{1000}	41
Leprechaunism		
Ark-1	Glu^{460}/Amber^{672}	50
Geldermalsen	Pro^{233} (homozygous)	62
Minn-1	Opal^{897}/Unidentified mutation	49
Winnipeg	Arg^{209} (homozygous)	41

* Listed are the mutations in the insulin receptor gene that have been identified in patients with genetic forms of insulin resistance. Missense mutations are identified by the amino acid substitution encoded by the mutation. WT refers to a wild-type allele that encodes a receptor with a normal amino acid sequence. A question mark refers to an allele that is thought to be normal, in cases where the nucleotide sequence has been reported for only a portion of the protein-coding domain. Amber and Opal refer to nonsense mutations corresponding to codons UAG and UGA, respectively. Deletion mutations are abbreviated as $\Delta^{\text{Exon 17(3')}-22}$ (a deletion beginning after codon 1012 in the 3′ part of exon 17 and extending downstream through exons 18–22) and $\Delta^{\text{Exon 14}}$ (a deletion of exon 14).

The degree of insulin resistance is extremely variable in this syndrome. For example, some patients are so severely insulin resistant that they have fasting hyperglycemia and overt diabetes despite having fasting plasma levels of insulin of more than 100 μU/ml (normal ≤20 μU/ml [1,40,41]). This type of patient may require several thousand units of insulin per day to achieve acceptable control of the level of glucose in the plasma. There are relatively few patients with such severe insulin resistance. We have investigated several patients in this category, all of whom have had two mutant alleles of the insulin receptor gene (Table 20.1). For example, two sisters (patients A-5 and A-8) were members of a consanguineous kindred and were homozygous for a missense mutation in the insulin receptor gene [40]. Another patient (patient A-1) was a compound heterozygote, having inherited two different mutations, one from her father and one from her mother [1,41]. However, it is more common for patients to have less severe insulin resistance. In fact, in most patients with this syndrome, the fasting levels of insulin are elevated in the range 20–100 μU/ml. Such levels are sufficient to prevent fasting hyperglycemia although most of these patients have impaired glucose tolerance [1,2,6]. Several patients in this category have been investigated. They appear to be heterozygous for a single mutation that causes insulin resistance in a dominant (or codominant) fashion (Table 20.1) [35,44–47].

Patients with two mutant alleles: homozygotes and compound heterozygotes

PATIENT A-1

Patient A-1 is a compound heterozygote who inherited two mutant alleles of the insulin receptor gene (Table 20.1) [1,41].

Nonsense mutation

In one allele, there is a nonsense mutation in which the normal TGG codon that encodes tryptophan at position 133 in the α-subunit of the insulin receptor is replaced by a TAG chain-termination codon [41]. This nonsense mutation has two effects. First, like most premature chain-termination mutations [49], it has a *cis*-dominant effect such that the level of the mRNA transcribed from the allele with the nonsense mutation is decreased by 80–90% [41]. Second, the mutant allele encodes a truncated receptor that consists of only the 132 amino acids at the amino terminus of the α-subunit. The truncated receptor lacks the transmembrane domain to anchor it to the plasma membrane, and it lacks the tyrosine kinase domain required to mediate insulin action. Thus, from a physiologic point of view, the allele with the nonsense mutation at codon 133 is essentially nonfunctional. The level of the mRNA with the nonsense mutation is decreased by 80–90% so that very little of the truncated receptor is synthesized. Moreover, such a truncated receptor would not be expected to be expressed on the cell surface, and it would not be predicted to have any biologic activity.

Nonsense mutations have also been identified at codons 672, 897, and 1000 in the insulin receptor gene in patients with leprechaunism [49,50] and the Rabson–Mendenhall syndrome [41], two other syndromes associated with insulin resistance.

Missense mutation

In the patient's second allele of the insulin receptor gene, there is a missense mutation: the wild-type AAT codon encoding asparagine at position 462 in the α-subunit of the insulin receptor is replaced by an AGT codon that encodes serine [41]. This mutation has the effect of rendering the binding of insulin relatively insensitive to changes in pH. A mutation causing a similar phenotype was identified previously in a patient with leprechaunism [50,51]. It is noteworthy that the other mutation mapped to a position in the receptor just two amino acids away: substitution of glutamate for lysine at position 460 in the α-subunit [50]. Both the normal human insulin receptor and the Glu^{460}-mutant receptor bind insulin with maximal affinity at a pH of about 8. With the wild-type receptor, a decrease of the pH to 6.8 causes an 85% decrease in the binding affinity. In contrast, with the Glu^{460}-mutant receptor, the binding affinity is decreased by only 55% at pH 6.8 [51]. This abnormal behavior at low pH not only provides a biochemical marker for the mutation but, in addition, it has important physiologic implications. Ordinarily, after the binding of insulin, the complex of insulin with its receptor is internalized into endosomes. The endosomes contain proton pumps that acidify the lumens of these vesicles. In fact, the interior of the endosome is estimated to have a pH of about 5.5. The acidic conditions within the endosome are thought to play a key role in dissociating ligands from their receptors. Thus, the Glu^{460}-mutant receptor binds insulin more tightly within the endosome, such that the process of dissociation is retarded. Furthermore, in addition to the retardation of dissociation to the complex, the Glu^{460}-mutant receptor is degraded more rapidly [52,53]. Thus, it seems likely that the cause of insulin resistance is a decreased number of insulin receptors on the cell surface, which is the result of an accelerated rate of receptor degradation [52–54].

PATIENT CHIBA-2

An *Alu-Alu* recombination, resulting in the deletion of exon 14, was identified in one allele of the insulin receptor gene of an obese adolescent girl with insulin resistance, hyperandrogenism, and acanthosis nigricans (Table 20.1) [48]. The deletion of exon 14 leads to a frameshift such that there is premature chain termination of the polypeptide after amino acid 867 in the fusion protein encoded by the mutant allele. Data were not presented to indicate whether it is possible to detect either the mRNA transcribed from the mutant allele or the fusion protein that it would encode [48]. In fact, as described above for nonsense mutations, any type of mutation (including deletion mutations) that causes premature chain termination can be associated with a *cis*-acting effect that would decrease the levels of mRNA derived from that allele.

In addition to acanthosis nigricans, hyperandrogenism, and hyperinsulinemia, this patient has fasting hyperglycemia and overt diabetes mellitus. Because her mother, who also was heterozygous for the allele with the nonsense mutation, was neither diabetic nor hyperinsulinemic, it was hypothesized that the daughter was most likely a compound heterozygote who had inherited a second mutant allele from her father. Consistent with this hypothesis, it is noteworthy that the father had borderline impaired glucose tolerance. In addition, it was stated that the tyrosine kinase activity of the father's insulin receptors was impaired [48]. Although it is a plausible hypothesis that the patient inherited a second mutation from the father, the hypothesis must be regarded as speculative, pending the availability of direct data.

PATIENTS A-5 AND A-8

Patients A-5 and A-8 are two sisters who are members of a consanguineous kindred in which the parents are first cousins [40]. Both parents are heterozygous carriers of a mutant allele that was inherited from one of the great-grandparents. In addition, the patients have four unaffected siblings, all of whom are heterozygous carriers of the mutation. However, the two sisters with type A extreme insulin resistance are both homozygous for a mutation in which the TTC codon that encodes phenylalanine at position 382 in the α-subunit of the wild-type insulin receptor is replaced by a GTC codon that encodes valine (Table 20.1) [40]. To evaluate the significance of the substitution of valine for phenylalanine at position 382, the cDNA of the mutant form of the receptor was expressed by transfection in cultured cells. These studies demonstrated that the Val^{382} mutation impairs transport of the receptor through the endoplasmic reticulum and Golgi apparatus [40]. As a consequence of the defect in intracellular transport of the receptor, there is a decrease in the number of receptors transported to the plasma membrane, and there is a decrease in the number of receptors expressed on the cell surface [40]. Furthermore, the Val^{382} mutation causes a second defect. Although it does not decrease the affinity with which the receptor binds insulin, the Val^{382} mutation inhibits the ability of insulin to activate the tyrosine kinase activity of the receptor. Thus, the patient's insulin resistance results from two functional defects, both of which are caused by the Val^{382} mutation: a decrease in the number of receptors on the cell surface, as a result of impaired transport of receptors to the cell surface [40]; and a defect in the ability of insulin to activate the receptor's tyrosine kinase activity [55].

We have identified two additional mutations that impair intracellular transport of receptors through the endoplasmic reticulum and Golgi apparatus to the cell surface (Table 20.1). Leprechaun/Winnipeg was homozygous for a mutation in which arginine was substituted for His^{209} [41]. Patient RM-1 (a patient with the Rabson–Mendenhall syndrome) was a compound heterozygote for a nonsense mutation at codon 1000 and a missense mutation that substituted lysine for Asn^{15} [41]. Neither of these two mutations prevented insulin from activating the receptor's tyrosine kinase activity. However, the Lys^{15} mutation caused a fivefold reduction in the affinity of the receptor for insulin [41,56].

PATIENTS KYUSHU-1 AND KYUSHU-2

Two sisters with type A extreme insulin resistance have been described who are homozygous for a mutation in which serine is substituted for arginine at position 735, the last amino acid in the tetrabasic amino acid sequence (Arg-Lys-Arg-Arg) at the site of proteolytic processing (Table 20.1). These sisters also belong to a consanguineous pedigree. The Ser^{735} mutation prevents proteolytic processing of the precursor to the receptor into two subunits. As shown in studies of the patients' cultured cells, the uncleaved receptor has a decreased affinity for insulin [57,58]. Presumably, it is the failure of cleavage into subunits that causes the reduction in the binding affinity. However, the possibility has not been entirely ruled out that the point mutation *per se* causes a decrease in the receptor's affinity for insulin below that which would be observed with the uncleaved precursor with the wild-type sequence.

Patients heterozygous for a single mutant allele

Several patients have been described who are heterozygous for a mutation in one allele of the insulin receptor gene, with the second allele appearing to be normal (Table 20.1). In several cases, only a portion of the coding sequence of the second allele has been determined [35,46–48,59]. Furthermore, even if the entire coding sequence has been analyzed [41,45], it is impossible to rule out entirely the possibility that there may be a mutation elsewhere in this very large gene. For example, there might be a mutation in a regulatory domain located either in an intron or in DNA located either upstream from the first exon or downstream from the last exon. Nevertheless, a sufficient number of these "heterozygotes" have been identified to render it likely that some mutations can cause insulin resistance in a dominant (or codominant) fashion. The evidence to support this conclusion is especially convincing in those kindreds in which there are multiple

Table 20.2 Classification of mutations in the insulin receptor gene*

Class 1: decreased biosynthesis of receptors
Nonsense mutations (codons 133, 672, 897, and 1000 [41, 49, 50])
Unidentified *cis*-acting mutations that decrease levels of mRNA [49]
Class 2: impaired transport of receptors to plasma membrane
Lys^{15}, Arg^{209}, and Val^{382} [40, 41]
Class 3: decreased affinity for insulin
Lys^{15} and Ser^{735} [41, 56–58]
Class 4: defect in insulin-stimulated tyrosine kinase activity
Val^{382}, Thr^{1134}, Val^{1008}, and Ser^{1200} [35, 40, 44–46]
Class 5: impaired ability of acid pH to dissociate insulin from its receptor
Glu^{460} and Ser^{462} [41, 50, 51, 53, 54]
Unclassified
Pro^{233} [62]
Deletions: exon 14 [48] or exons 17(3')–22 [47]

* Mutations in the insulin receptor gene are classified according to the mechanism whereby they cause insulin resistance. The classification is based upon a modification of the classification proposed by Brown and Goldstein for mutations in the gene for the receptor for low-density lipoprotein [63]. Some mutations (Lys^{15} and Val^{382}) are included in two classes because they impair the function of the insulin receptor by more than one mechanism. Several mutations are listed as unclassified because sufficient data are not available to allow their classification. References are shown in brackets.

affected individuals who share only one allele in common (i.e. the allele in which the mutation was originally identified) [46,59].

Defects in the receptor's tyrosine kinase activity

Missense mutations in the intracellular domain of the β-subunit of the insulin receptor have been identified in three kindreds (Tables 20.1 and 20.2) In two cases, the mutation was identified in young women with type A extreme insulin resistance: a mutation in which threonine was substituted for Ala^{1134} in patient BI-1 [46] and a mutation in which serine was substituted for Trp^{1200} in patient BI-2 [44,45]. A third mutation, substitution of valine for Gly^{1008}, was identified in a young man with insulin resistance and acanthosis nigricans [35]. Of course, because the definition of type A insulin resistance requires the presence of hyperandrogenism, the diagnosis is not ordinarily applied to male patients. Nevertheless, with respect to the mechanism of insulin resistance and the etiology of the acanthosis nigricans, it seems likely that this young man has the masculine equivalent of type A insulin resistance.

Gly^{1008} is the third glycine residue in the highly conserved Gly^{1003}-X-Gly^{1005}-X-X-Gly^{1008} ... Lys^{1030} motif [31,35] that provides part of the binding site for ATP, the donor of phosphate in the tyrosine kinase reaction. The fact that this mutation distorts the ATP-binding site of the tyrosine kinase domain is entirely consistent with the observation that the mutant receptor is deficient in tyrosine kinase activity [35]. Ala^{1134} and Trp^{1200} are both highly conserved amino acid residues in the amino acid sequences of tyrosine kinases but their precise roles in the structure and function of the enzyme are not understood [31].

What is the mechanism whereby these mutations cause the phenotype of insulin resistance to be dominant? Although this question has not been answered with certainty, the leading hypothesis relates to the oligomeric structure of the receptor. If mutant heterodimers ($\alpha\beta_m$) of the insulin receptor and wild-type heterodimers ($\alpha\beta_{wt}$) associate with one another randomly and with equal affinity, then three different heterotetramers would form in a ratio of 1:2:1, namely, $\alpha_2(\beta_{wt})_2$, $\alpha_2\beta_m\beta_{wt}$, and $\alpha_2(\beta_m)_2$. If the hybrid heterotetramer ($\alpha_2\beta_m\beta_{wt}$) were impaired with respect to its tyrosine kinase activity, then a mutation in a single allele might lead to a 75% reduction in the tyrosine kinase activity of insulin receptors.

Gene deletions

Although most of the reported mutations in the insulin receptor gene are point mutations, two deletion mutations have also been described (Table 20.1). The first such deletion mutation to be investigated was identified in a girl with type A insulin resistance (patient Chiba-1) and in her mother. There was a deletion of the portion of the insulin receptor gene that encoded most of the intracellular domain of the β-subunit of the receptor [47]. The proximal end of the deletion was at codon 1012 in exon 17; the distal end of the deletion was not mapped. Analysis of the nucleotide sequence led to the prediction that the mRNA would have an open reading frame for 65 amino acids after codon 1012. Thus, this mutant allele would encode a receptor with a truncated intracellular domain fused to 65 amino acids of an unrelated amino acid sequence at the carboxyl terminus. Data were not presented to indicate whether it is possible to detect either the mRNA transcribed from the mutant allele or the fusion protein that it would encode [47]. In fact, it is possible that this deletion mutation, through any of several possible mechanisms, might decrease the levels of mRNA derived from this allele.

Nonsense mutations

The father of a patient with leprechaunism (leprechaun/Ark-1) is heterozygous for a mutant allele with a nonsense mutation at codon 672. He is hyperinsulinemic and resistant to insulin, although not as severely resistant as his daughter [50,54]. We have shown that the protein-coding sequence of the father's second allele of the insulin receptor gene is normal [41]. Thus, it seems likely that the phenotype of insulin resistance is caused by heterozygosity for this allele with a nonsense mutation, and that insulin resistance is inherited in a codominant fashion [54]. Consistent with the conclusion, there is a 60–70% decrease in binding of [^{125}I]insulin to the father's circulating moncytes. Furthermore, the data suggest that the level of expression of the normal allele of the insulin receptor gene does not increase to compensate for the nonsense mutation. In fact, because the father is hyperinsulinemic with plasma insulin levels that are five- to tenfold greater than those in the normal range [54], it is likely that his receptors become down-regulated *in vivo*. Rather than compensating for the resistance to insulin, this down-regulation would exacerbate the decrease in the number of insulin receptors on the surface of his cells. In fact, when the contribution due to down-regulation is eliminated by cultivating EBV-transformed lymphoblasts in long-term tissue culture, the number of insulin receptors on the cell surface is normal, albeit in the lower half of the normal range.

Mutations that map outside the 22 exons of the protein-coding sequence of the insulin receptor gene

We investigated a patient with leprechaunism (leprechaun/Minn-1) who was a compound heterozygote for two different mutations, both of which had *cis*-acting effects whereby they decreased the level of mRNA for the insulin receptor [49]. One allele had a nonsense mutation at codon 897. The second allele had normal nucleotide sequence in all 22 exons, as well as in the DNA immediately flanking each of the exons. This second allele, with the unidentified mutation, was inherited from the patient's mother. In the mother, the allele with the unidentified mutation was paired with a presumably normal allele. Because of the existence of silent polymorphisms that differentiated the two alleles in the mother, it was possible to quantitate the levels of mRNA transcribed from each allele [49]. Despite their coexistence in the same cell, the two alleles were expressed at very different levels in the mother's cells.

Approximately 90% of the mRNA for insulin receptors in the mother's cells was transcribed from the normal allele, while only 10% was derived from the allele with the unidentified mutation. These data strongly support the conclusion that the "unidentified mutation" maps to the locus of the insulin receptor, but is outside the protein-coding sequence of the gene.

Classification of mutations in the insulin receptor gene

Based upon the particular mechanism whereby each mutation impairs insulin receptor function, five classes of mutations in the insulin receptor gene can be proposed (Table 20.2). Some mutations decrease the number of insulin receptors on the cell surface: by decreasing the rate of biosynthesis of the receptor (Class 1), by inhibiting the intracellular transport of receptors to the cell surface (Class 2), or by accelerating the rate of degradation of the receptor (Class 5). When insulin binds to the extracellular domain of the receptor, the binding activates a tyrosine-specific protein kinase activity associated with the intracellular domain of the receptor [16]. Activation of the tyrosine kinase activity plays a necessary role in mediating some or all of the biologic actions of insulin. Some mutations impede the action of insulin, either by decreasing the affinity with which the receptor binds insulin (Class 3), or by inhibiting tyrosine kinase activity, thereby impairing the ability of the receptor to transmit a signal across the plasma membrane (Class 4).

With some mutations, insulin resistance is inherited in a codominant pattern. Thus, individuals who are heterozygous for the mutation may have a moderate degree of insulin resistance [41,48,50,59], comparable to that which is observed in patients with the common form of noninsulin-dependent diabetes mellitus (NIDDM). This situation raises the possibility that heterozygosity for mutations in the insulin receptor gene may contribute to the development of insulin resistance in some patients with NIDDM. Alternatively, it is possible that some patients with NIDDM might be homozygous for mutations that cause mild impairment of the functions of the insulin receptor. Thus far, there are relatively few data that directly address this question. Nevertheless, the protein-coding sequence of the insulin receptor gene has been determined for three Pima Indians with NIDDM and/or insulin resistance. In all three cases, the sequence was found to be normal [60,61]. Recent advances in technology have enormously facilitated the task of identifying mutations, and it should now be possible to determine the prevalence of mutations in the insulin receptor gene in the general population. In addition, it will be possible to determine whether mutations in the insulin receptor gene contribute to the pathogenesis of insulin resistance in common syndromes, such as NIDDM and polycystic ovary syndrome.

References

1 Kahn CR, Flier JS, Bar RS, Archer JA, Gorden P, Martin MM, Roth J. The syndromes of insulin resistance and acanthosis nigricans. Insulin-receptor disorders in man. N Engl J Med 1976; 294:739–45.

2 Taylor SI, Kadowaki T, Kadowaki H, Accili D, Cama A, McKeon C. Mutations in insulin-receptor gene in insulin-resistant patients. Diabetes Care 1990; 13:257–79.

3 Flier JS, Eastman RC, Minaker KL, Matteson D, Rowe JW. Acanthosis nigricans in obese women with hyperandrogenism. Characterization of an insulin-resistant state distinct from the type A and B syndromes. Diabetes 1985; 34:101–7.

4 Barbieri RL, Ryan KJ. Hyperandrogenism, insulin resistance, and acanthosis nigricans syndrome: a common endocrinopathy with distinct pathophysiologic features. Am J Obstet Gynecol 1983; 147:90–101.

5 Taylor SI, Dons RF, Hernandez E, Roth J, Gorden P. Insulin resistance associated with androgen excess in women with autoantibodies to the insulin receptor. Ann Intern Med 1982; 97:851–5.

6 Taylor SI. Receptor defects in patients with extreme insulin resistance. Diabetes Metab Rev 1985; 1:171–202.

7 Fradkin JE, Eastman RC, Lesniak MA, Roth J. Specificity spillover at the hormone receptor—exploring its role in human disease. N Engl J Med 1989; 320:640–5.

8 Yang-Feng TL, Francke U, Ullrich A. Gene for human insulin receptor: localization to site on chromosome 19 involved in pre-B-cell leukemia. Science 1985; 228:728–31.

9 Seino S, Seino M, Nishi S, Bell GI. Structure of the human insulin receptor gene and characterization of its promoter. Proc Natl Acad Sci USA 1989; 86:114–18.

10 Mamula PW, Wong KY, Maddux BA, McDonald AR, Goldfine ID. Sequence and analysis of promoter region of human insulin-receptor gene. Diabetes 1988; 37:1241–6.

11 Tewari DS, Cook DM, Taub R. Characterization of the promoter region and 3′-end of the human insulin receptor gene. J Biol Chem 1989; 264:16238–45.

12 McKeon C, Moncada V, Pham T, Salvatore P, Kadowaki T, Accili D, Taylor SI. Structural and functional analysis of the insulin receptor promoter. Mol Endocrinol 1990; 4:647–56.

13 Ullrich A, Bell JR, Chen EY, Herrera R, Petruzelli LM, Dull TJ, Gray A, Coussens L, Liao YC, Tsubokawa M, Mason A, Seeburg PH, Grunfeld C, Rosen OM, Ramachandran J. Human insulin receptor and its relationship to the tyrosine kinase family of oncogenes. Nature 1985; 313:756–61.

14 Seino S, Bell GI. Alternative splicing of human insulin receptor messenger RNA. Biochem Biophys Res Commun 1989; 159:312–16.

15 Moller DE, Yokota A, Caro JF, Flier JS. Tissue-specific expression of two alternatively spliced insulin receptor mRNAs in man. Mol Endocrinol 1989; 3:1263–9.

16 McClain D, Mosthaf L, Ullrich A. Properties of the two naturally occurring alternate forms of the insulin receptor. Diabetes 1989; 38(suppl. 2):1A.

17 Hedo JA, Kasuga M, Van Obberghen E, Roth J, Kahn CR. Direct demonstration of glycosylation of insulin receptor subunits by biosynthetic and external labeling: evidence for heterogeneity. Proc Natl Acad Sci USA 1981; 78:4791–5.

18 Hedo JA, Kahn CR, Hayashi M, Yamada Km, Kasuga M. Biosynthesis and glycosylation of the insulin receptor. Evidence for a single polypeptide presursor of the two major subunits. J Biol Chem 1983; 258:10020–6.

19 Deutsch PJ, Wan CF, Rosen OM, Rubin CS. Latent insulin receptors and possible receptor precursors in 3T3-L1 adipocytes. Proc Natl Acad Sci USA 1983; 80:133–6.
20 Jacobs SJ, Kull FCJ, Cuatrecasas P. Monensin blocks the maturation of receptors for insulin and somatomedin C: identification of receptor precursors. Proc Natl Acad Sci USA 1983; 80:1228–31.
21 Hedo JA, Collier E, Watkinson A. Myristyl and palmityl acylation of the insulin receptor. J Biol Chem 1987; 262:954–7.
22 Herzberg VL, Grigorescu F, Edge AS, Spiro RG, Kahn CR. Characterization of insulin receptor carbohydrate by comparison of chemical and enzymatic deglycosylation. Biochem Biophys Res Commun 1985; 129:789–96.
23 Collier E, Gorden P. The insulin receptor contains *O*-linked oligosaccharide. Diabetes 1989; 38(suppl. 2):178A.
24 Pilch PF, Czech MP. Interaction of cross-linking agents with the insulin effector system of isolated fat cells. Covalent linkage of ^{125}I-insulin to a plasma membrane receptor protein of 140 000 daltons. J Biol Chem 1979; 254:3375–81.
25 Waugh SM, DiBella EE, Pilch PF. Isolation of a proteolytically derived domain of the insulin receptor containing the major site of cross-linking/binding. Biochemistry 1989; 28:3448–55.
26 DeMeyts P, Gu J-L, Shymko RM, Kaplan BE, Bell GI, Whittaker J. Identification of a ligand-binding region of the human insulin receptor encoded by the second exon of the gene. Mol Endocrinol 1990; 4:409–16.
27 Whittaker J, Okamoto A. Secretion of soluble functional insulin receptors by transfected NIH3T3 cells. J Biol Chem 1988; 263:3063–6.
28 Frias I, Waugh SM. Probing the $\alpha-\alpha$ subunit interface region in the insulin receptor, location of interhalf disulfide(s). Diabetes 1989; 38(suppl. 2):60A.
29 Kasuga M, Karlsson FA, Kahn CR. Insulin stimulates the phosphorylation of the 95 000-dalton subunit of its own receptor. Science 1982; 215:185–7.
30 Kasuga M, Zick Y, Blithe DL, Crettaz M, Kahn CR. Insulin stimulates tyrosine phosphorylation of the insulin receptor in a cell-free system. Nature 1982; 298:667–9.
31 Hanks SK, Quinn AM, Hunter T. The protein kinase family: conserved features and deduced phylogeny of the catalytic domains. Science 1988; 241:42–52.
32 Chou CK, Dull TJ, Russell DS, Gherzi R, Lebwohl D, Ullrich A. Human insulin receptors mutated at the ATP-binding site lack protein tyrosine kinase activity and fail to mediate postreceptor effects of insulin. J Biol Chem 1987; 262:1842–47.
33 Ebina Y, Araki E, Taira M, Shimada F, Mori M, Craik CS, Siddle K, Pierce SB, Roth RA, Rutter WJ. Replacement of lysine residue 1030 in the putative ATP-binding region of the insulin receptor abolishes insulin- and antibody-stimulated glucose uptake and receptor kinase activity. Proc Natl Acad Sci USA 1987; 84:704–8.
34 McClain DA, Maegawa H, Lee J, Dull TJ, Ullrich A, Olefsky JM. A mutant insulin receptor with defective tyrosine kinase displays no biologic activity and does not undergo endocytosis. J Biol Chem 1987; 262:14663–71.
35 Odawara M, Kadowaki T, Yamamoto R, Shibasaki Y, Tobe K, Accili D, Bevins C, Mikami Y, Matsuura N, Akanuma Y, Takaku F, Taylor SI, Kasuga M. Human diabetes associated with a mutation in the tyrosine kinase domain of the insulin receptor. Science 1989; 245:66–8.
36 Tornqvist HE, Gunsalus JR, Nemenoff RA, Frackelton HR, Pierce MW, Avruch J. Identification of the insulin receptor tyrosine residues undergoing insulin-stimulated phosphorylation in intact rat hepatoma cells. J Biol Chem 1989; 263:350–9.
37 White MF, Shoelson SE, Keutmann H, Kahn CR. A cascade of tyrosine autophosphorylation in the beta-subunit activates the phosphotransferase of the insulin receptor. J Biol Chem 1988; 263:2969–80.
38 White MF, Livingston JN, Backer JM, Lauris V, Dull TJ, Ullrich A, Kahn CR. Mutation of the insulin receptor at tyrosine 960 inhibits signal transmission but does not affect its tyrosine kinase activity. Cell 1988; 54:641–9.

39 Ellis L, Clauser E, Morgan DO, Edery M, Roth RA, Rutter WJ. Replacement of insulin receptor tyrosine residues 1162 and 1163 compromises insulin-stimulated kinase activity and uptake of 2-deoxyglucose. Cell 1986; 45:721–32.
40 Accili D, Frapier C, Mosthaf L, McKeon C, Elbein S, Permutt MA, Ramos E, Lander E, Ullrich A, Taylor SI. A mutation in the insulin receptor gene that impairs transport of the receptor to the plasma membrane and causes insulin-resistant diabetes. EMBO J 1989; 8:2509–17.
41 Kadowaki T, Kadowaki H, Rechler MM, Serrano-Rios M, Roth J, Gorden P, Taylor SI. Five mutant alleles of the insulin receptor gene in patients with genetic forms of insulin resistance. J Clin Invest 1990; 86:254–64.
42 Yoshimasa Y, Seino S, Whittaker J, Kakehi T, Kosaki A, Kuzuya H, Imura I, Bell GI, Steiner DF. Insulin-resistant diabetes due to a point mutation that prevents insulin proreceptor processing. Science 1988; 240:784–7.
43 Kobayashi M, Sasaoka T, Takata Y, Ishibashi O, Sugibayashi M, Shigeta Y, Hisatomi A, Nakamura E, Tamaki M, Teraoka H. Insulin resistance by unprocessed insulin proreceptors: point mutation at the cleavage site. Biochem Biophys Res Commun 1988; 153:657–63.
44 Moller DE, Flier JS. Detection of an alteration in the insulin-receptor gene in a patient with insulin resistance, acanthosis nigricans, and the polycystic ovary syndrome (type A insulin resistance). N Engl J Med 1988; 319:1526–9.
45 Moller DE, Yokota A, Ginsberg-Fellner F, Flier JS. Funtional properties of a naturally occurring $Trp^{1200} \rightarrow Ser^{1200}$ mutation of the insulin receptor. Mol Endocrinol 1990 (in press).
46 Moller DE, Yokota A, White MF, Pazianos AG, Flier JS. A naturally occurring mutation of insulin receptor Ala^{1134} impairs tyrosine kinase function and is associated with dominantly inherited insulin resistance. J Biol Chem 1990 (in press).
47 Taira M, Taira M, Hashimoto N, Shimada F, Suzuki Y, Kanatsuka A, Nakamura F, Ebina Y, Tatibana M, Makino H, Yoshida S. Human diabetes associated with a deletion of the tyrosine kinase domain of the insulin receptor. Science 1989; 245:63–6.
48 Shimada F, Taira M, Suzuki Y, Hashimoto N, Nozaki O, Taira M, Tatibana M, Ebina Y, Tawata M, Onaya T, Makino H, Yoshida S. Insulin-resistant diabetes associated with partial deletion of insulin-receptor gene. Lancet 1990; 335:1179–81.
49 Kadowaki T, Kadowaki H, Taylor SI. A nonsense mutation causing decreased levels of insulin receptor mRNA: detection by a simplified technique for direct sequencing of genomic DNA amplified by polymerase chain reaction. Proc Natl Acad Sci USA 1990; 87:658–62.
50 Kadowaki T, Bevins CL, Cama A, Ojamaa K, Marcus-Samuels B, Kadowaki H, Beitz L, McKeon C, Taylor SI. Two mutant alleles of the insulin receptor gene in a patient with extreme insulin resistance. Science 1988; 240:787–90.
51 Taylor SI, Roth J, Blizzard RM, Elders MJ. Qualitative abnormalities in insulin binding in a patient with extreme insulin resistance: decreased sensitivity to alterations in temperature and pH. Proc Natl Acad Sci USA 1981; 78:7157–61.
52 McElduff A, Hedo JA, Taylor SI, Roth J, Gorden P. Insulin receptor degradation is accelerated in cultured lymphocytes from patients with genetic syndromes of extreme insulin resistance. J Clin Invest 1984; 74:1366–74.
53 Kadowaki H, Kadowaki T, Cama A, Marcus-Samuels B, Rovira A, Bevins CL, Taylor SI. Mutagenesis of lysine-460 in the human insulin receptor: effects upon receptor recycling and cooperative interactions among binding sites. J Biol Chem 1990 (in press).
54 Taylor SI, Marcus-Samuels B, Ryan-Young J, Leventhal S, Elders MJ. Genetics of the insulin receptor defect in a patient with extreme insulin resistance. J Clin Endocrinol Metab 1986; 62:1130–5.
55 Accili D, Mosthaf L, Ullrich A, Taylor SI. A mutation in the extracellular domain of the insulin receptor impairs the ability of insulin to stimulate receptor autophosphorylation. J Biol Chem 1990 (in press).

56 Kadowaki T, Kadowaki H, Taylor SI. Mutational analysis of insulin receptor. Diabetes 1990; 39(suppl. 1):114A.
57 Kakehi T, Hisatomi A, Kuzuya H, Yoshimasa Y, Okamoto M, Yamada K, Nishimura H, Kosaki A, Nawata H, Umeda F, Ibayashi H, Imura H. Defective processing of insulin receptor precursor in cultured lymphocytes from a patient with extreme insulin resistance. J Clin Invest 1988; 81:2020–2.
58 Kobayashi M, Sasaoka T, Takata Y, Hisatomi A, Shigeta Y. Insulin resistance by uncleaved insulin propreceptor. Emergence of binding site by trypsin. Diabetes 1988; 37:653.
59 Lekanne Deprez RH, Potter van Loon BJ, van der Zon GC, Moller W, Lindhout D, Klinkhamer MP, Krans HM, Maassen JA. Individuals with only one allele for a functional insulin receptor have a tendency to hyperinsulinaemia but not to hyperglycaemia. Diabetologia 1989; 32:740–4.
60 Moller DE, Yokota A, Flier JS. Normal insulin-receptor cDNA sequence in Pima Indians with NIDDM. Diabetes 1989; 38:1496–500.
61 Cama A, Patterson A, Kadowaki T, Siegel G, D'Ambrosio D, Lillioja S, Roth J, Taylor SI. Cloning of insulin receptor cDNA from an insulin-resistant Pima Indian. J Clin Endocrinol Metab 1990; 70:1155–61.
62 Klinkhamer M, Groen NA, van der Zon GCM, Lindhout D, Sandkuyl LA, Krans HM, Moller W, Maassen JA. A leucine-to-proline mutation in the insulin receptor in a family with insulin resistance. EMBO J 1989; 8:2503–7.
63 Brown MS, Goldstein JL. A receptor-mediated pathway for cholesterol homeostasis. Science 1986; 232:34–47.

Chapter 21
Effects of Insulin on Ovarian Steroidogenesis

ROBERT L. BARBIERI

Hyperandrogenism is one of the most common endocrinopathies that affect women of reproductive age. In a small minority of hyperandrogenic women, a "specific" cause of the hyperandrogenism can be identified. For example, specific etiologic causes of hyperandrogenism include tumors of the adrenal or ovary, congenital or acquired adrenal hyperplasia, Cushing's disease, acromegaly, hyperprolactinemia, and various drugs. However, for most hyperandrogenic women, no specific etiologic cause of the hyperandrogenism can be identified. These cases are often diagnosed as examples of polycystic ovary syndrome (PCO). Proposed pathogenetic mechanisms for PCO include primary abnormalities of the hypothalamic–pituitary unit, the ovary, and the adrenal [1,2]. It is likely that PCO is an "end-stage" endocrinopathy that can be caused by many different mechanisms. Major advances in our understanding of PCO will require the identification of specific causes of PCO at the molecular level. A unique opportunity to identify a specific molecular cause of PCO is provided by recent clinical observations that demonstrate that there is a strong association between hyperinsulinemia and hyperandrogenism in women of reproductive age [3,5]. Our basic hypothesis is that chronic hyperinsulinemia stimulates the biosynthesis of ovarian thecal and stromal androgens and perturbs the normal growth and differentiation of granulosa cells. Before reviewing the effects of hyperinsulinemia on ovarian steroidogenesis, we shall summarize the clinical evidence that supports a casual relationship between hyperinsulinemia and hyperandrogenism.

The association between hyperinsulinemia and hyperandrogenism

Many clinical observations have suggested that there is a strong relationship between hyperinsulinemia and hyperandrogenism. For example, in 1921, Achard and Thiers [5] described a syndrome of hyperandrogenism in obese, noninsulin-dependent diabetic women. An association between hyperinsulinemia and hyperandrogenism has also been reported in isolated cases of women with Kahn type A and type B diabetes [4], lipoatropic diabetes, and leprechaunism [6]. However, these case reports did not include detailed quantitative biochemical evidence of an association between hyperinsulinemia and hyperandrogenism. In addition, none of the investigators explicitly stated that the observed clinical association between severe hyperinsulinemia and hyperandrogenism might represent a causal relationship.

Burghen and coworkers [7] were the first investigators to report a strong statistical relationship between hyperinsulinemia and hyperandrogenism. These investigators used immunoassays to measure circulating levels of insulin, testosterone, and androstenedione in eight obese women with PCO and six obese women without PCO [7]. It is noteworthy that they actually "overcontrolled" for obesity. The obese women without PCO were significantly more obese than the obese women with PCO (percent ideal body weight: 210 vs. 166, $P < 0.05$). These investigators reported statistically significant ($P < 0.01$) positive correlations between fasting levels of insulin and androstenedione ($r = 0.65$) and fasting levels of insulin and testosterone ($r = 0.72$). In addition, they observed a strong correlation between glucose-stimulated plasma insulin and testosterone ($r = 0.85$, $P < 0.001$). These observations in obese women with PCO have been confirmed by many other investigators [3,6,8–10]. A common criticism of these data is that the obesity "caused" the findings. This criticism is untenable because a correlation between hyperinsulinemia and hyperandrogenism has been demonstrated in women with normal body mass and PCO [8]. In addition, insulin resistance and hyperinsulinemia have been reported to be present in women with PCO, irrespective of obesity.

Three hypotheses could account for the strong association between hyperinsulinemia and hyperandrogenism: (i) hyperandrogenism causes hyperinsulinemia; (ii) hyperinsulinemia causes hyperandrogenism; and (iii) an unidentified "third factor" causes both hyperinsulinemia and hyperandrogenism. Each of these hypotheses is discussed below.

Most of the available evidence suggests that, in women, hyperandrogenism alone cannot account for the associated hyperinsulinemia.

In men, circulating concentrations of total testosterone are in the range of 5 ng/ml. This concentration of testosterone is not associated with significant hyperinsulinemia. In hyperandrogenic women with PCO, circulating concentrations of total testosterone are in the range of 1 ng/ml. If this concentration of testosterone causes hyperinsulinemia, a major difference in the insulin response to testosterone must exist between men and women. There is no evidence to support such a contention. Numerous dynamic studies suggest that, in women with hyperinsulinemia and hyperandrogenism, the hyperandrogenism does not cause the insulin resistance. For example, Nagamani and colleagues [11] have demonstrated that, in women with ovarian hyperandrogenism and hyperinsulinemia, bilateral oophorectomy eliminated the hyperandrogenism but was not associated with a reduction in the severity of the hyperinsulinemia. Geffner and Chang [12] treated hyperandrogenic, hyperinsulinemic women with a long-acting gonadotropin-releasing hormone agonist (GnRH agonist). The GnRH agonist therapy produced complete resolution of the hyperandrogenism, but it did not alter the hyperinsulinemia. Finally, Pasquali and associates [13] reported that, in women with PCO and hyperinsulinemia, drug therapy with the "progestational anti-androgen" cyproterone acetate caused a decrease in circulating androgens but did not improve the hyperinsulinemia. In all three studies, decreases in concentrations of circulating androgens were not associated with decreases in the severity of hyperinsulinemia. The results of these studies do not support the hypothesis that hyperandrogenism causes severe insulin resistance and hyperinsulinemia in women of reproductive age.

The association between hyperinsulinemia and hyperandrogenism observed in women with PCO may be caused by an unidentified "third factor" that produces both the hyperinsulinemia and the hyperandrogenism. It is difficult to reject the "third factor hypothesis" definitively because a large number of possible "third factors" exists. However, the evidence that severe hyperinsulinemia causes hyperandrogenism is so strong that it is unlikely a "third factor" plays a critical causative role. It is possible that one or more "third factor(s)" modulates the causative relationship between hyperinsulinemia and hyperandrogenism. The hypothesis that hyperinsulinemia causes hyperandrogenism is supported by multiple, separate lines of investigation. The data that support this hypothesis include: (i) diverse disease states that result in severe hyperinsulinemia (Kahn type A and type B diabetes, leprechaunism [4,6,10] and lipoatrophic diabetes) are uniformly associated with hyperandrogenism; (ii) the acute administration of insulin to women with PCO causes an increase in circulating androstenedione [14]; (iii) the administration of glucose to hyperinsulinemic hyperandrogenic women results in an increase in circulating levels of insulin and androgens [9]; (iv) in women, weight loss, fasting, or a hypocaloric diet is associated with a decrease in circulating levels of androgens [15]; and (v) *in vitro*, insulin stimulates production of human ovarian stromal androgens, possibly by interacting via an ovarian insulin-like growth factor I (IGF-I) receptor [16].

The genetic evidence that links hyperinsulinemia and hyperandrogenism is reviewed below.

The HAIR-AN syndrome

The syndrome of hyperandrogenism (HA), insulin resistance (IR), and acanthosis nigricans (AN) is an "experiment of nature" that provides a unique opportunity to identify a specific cause of functional ovarian hyperandrogenism [3]. As noted above, hyperandrogenism is the state of increased production and action of androgens. In most cases of the HAIR-AN syndrome, the ovary is the primary site of the overproduction of androgens. Insulin resistance is a condition in which a "normal" concentration of insulin produces an abnormally attenuated biologic effect, e.g. glucose clearance. In all cases where pancreatic function is intact, insulin resistance results in a compensatory hyperinsulinemia.

Acanthosis nigricans (see Chapter 30) is a dermatologic disorder that presents as the development of velvety, mossy, verrucous, hyperpigmented skin, usually over the nape of the neck, in the axillae, beneath the breasts and occasionally in other body folds. The pathologic changes in acanthosis nigricans are usually limited to the epidermis. The most salient pathologic features are papillomatosis, hyperkeratosis, and hyperpigmentation. Skin tags are often found in or near areas of acanthosis nigricans. Acanthosis can be caused by "benign" or malignant disease processes. When acanthosis nigricans is caused by a malignancy, an adenocarcinoma is usually present (in the stomach, pancreas, or colon). When acanthosis nigricans is caused by a benign process, severe insulin resistance can usually be demonstrated to be present. A good clinical rule is that, in young women who do not have an adenocarcinoma, the presence of acanthosis nigricans strongly suggests the presence of insulin resistance (see Chapter 32).

In 1921, Achard and Thiers [5] described the association of hyperandrogenism and noninsulin-dependent (adult onset) diabetes mellitus. Since that time, numerous clinical reports have been published describing the association of insulin resistance and acanthosis nigricans or of hyperandrogenism and acanthosis nigricans. However, the first clear realization that hyperandrogenism, insulin resistance, and acanthosis nigricans might be causally related was not reported until recently. In 1976, Kahn and associates [4] described three cases of hyperandrogenism, insulin resistance, and acanthosis nigricans. In these three cases, the insulin resistance was due to a functional defect in the insulin-receptor system (type A), which resulted in severe compensatory hyperinsulinemia. These investigators hypothesized that the acanthosis nigricans was a dermatologic manifestation of the chronic hyperinsulinemia. Kahn and colleagues [4] did not comment on any possible causal relationship between the hyperinsulinemia and hyperandrogenism. In 1982, Taylor and associates [17] reported that some women with type B insulin resistance (with antibodies to the insulin-receptor system) had an associated hyperandrogenism. Taylor *et al.* [17] postulated that the hyperinsulinemia might cause the hyperandrogenism.

Type A and type B insulin resistance are due to dramatically different causes. Type A insulin resistance is often due to a genetic defect that results in impaired function of insulin receptors. In many individuals with type A insulin resistance, the defect can be demonstrated in childhood. In contrast, type B insulin resistance arises most often in women with autoimmune diseases, such as systemic lupus erythematosus, rheumatoid arthritis, and Sjogren's syndrome. Type B insulin resistance is usually due to a disease acquired in adulthood. Although type A and type B insulin resistance are due to different molecular mechanisms, both result in hyperinsulinemia and hyperandrogenism. The observation that two genetically different causes of insulin resistance both resulted in hyperandrogenism suggests that hyperinsulinemia causes hyperandrogenism. Our basic hypothesis is that both insulin and luteinizing hormone (LH) regulate ovarian stromal and thecal production of androgens.

A few salient points pertinent to the HAIR-AN syndrome should be emphasized.

1 In all cases studied to date, the overproduction of androgens occurs predominantly in the ovary. In the HAIR-AN syndrome, ovarian stromal hyperthecosis is a common pathologic finding.

2 The severity of the insulin resistance is highly correlated with the severity of the hyperandrogenism.

3 Low-normal profiles of gonadotropins are common in the HAIR-AN syndrome and suggest that a hormone or hormones, other than the gonadotropins, contributes to the stimulation of the ovarian production of androgens.

4 Gonadotropins play an essential role in the development of the

HAIR-AN syndrome. Administration of combined estrogen–progesterone pills, or GnRH agonists, to women with the HAIR-AN syndrome results in a decrease in serum levels of testosterone. In addition, girls with Kahn type A diabetes do not usually develop severe virilization until the hypothalamic generator of pulses of GnRH becomes activated during pubertal development. Since many cases of Kahn type A diabetes are due to a genetic defect, this observation suggests that luteinizing hormone (LH) and follicle-stimulating hormone (FSH) are required for the full expression of the phenotype.

5 Reduction in ovarian overproduction of androgens by medical or surgical means does not markedly improve the insulin resistance.

6 The acanthosis nigricans is an epiphenomenon and does not play a central role in the development of the disease process. The acanthosis nigricans is probably due to chronic hyperinsulinemia (and possibly to hyperandrogenism). Acanthosis nigricans is a good clinical marker of severe insulin resistance.

Recent advances in molecular biology have made it possible to sequence the entire insulin receptor gene in women with ovarian hyperandrogenism and to identify the precise change(s) in the DNA that are associated with the HAIR-AN phenotype (see Chapter 20). For example, Moller and Flier [18] studied the insulin receptor gene in a woman with the HAIR-AN syndrome. cDNA prepared from fibroblast cell lines and lymphocyte cell lines was amplified by the polymerase chain reaction (PCR). Specific amplified segments of DNA were cloned into M13 phage and sequenced. The insulin receptor is a heterotetrameric glycoprotein containing two alpha subunits and two beta subunits. A single precursor protein of 1346 amino acids, containing one alpha subunit and one beta subunit, is synthesized from the 4-kb coding region of the mRNA sequence [19]. Amplified DNA from this patient revealed one important base change (from TGG to TCG) at codon 1200 in only one allele, which resulted in the replacement of a tryptophan residue by a serine residue. Codon 1200 is in a region of the beta subunit of the insulin receptor that is involved in expression of the tyrosine kinase activity of the receptor. It is likely that the base change at codon 1200 results in an insulin receptor that has lost its ability to act as a tyrosine kinase and is nonfunctional. The loss of function by the insulin receptor results in severe insulin resistance and a compensatory hyperinsulinemia. In turn, it is our contention that the severe, chronic hyperinsulinemia synergizes with LH to stimulate the ovarian production of androgens seen in this patient. The observation that a point mutation in only one allele for the insulin receptor produces the HAIR-

AN phenotype suggests that certain mutations in the tyrosine kinase domain of the beta subunit may be "dominant."

Yoshimasa *et al.* [20] reported another example of a point mutation in the insulin receptor gene that produced the phenotype of the HAIR-AN syndrome. In the woman studied by this group, hyperandrogenism, insulin resistance and acanthosis nigricans were present (HAIR-AN syndrome). The woman was the product of a consanguineous marriage. Genomic DNA was prepared from lymphocytes transformed with Epstein–Barr virus and digested with Eco RI. Specific sequences were cloned with lambda-EMBL-4. Clones encoding amino acids 655–993 of the insulin receptor were identified and the DNA of one clone was sequenced. The sequence revealed a point mutation at codon 735 (AGG to AGT), which resulted in the substitution of a serine residue for an arginine residue, in the four-base processing site of the proreceptor molecule. As a result of the mutation at the processing site, the propeptide could not be cleaved to the mature alpha and beta subunits, and a functional insulin receptor could not be generated. Both alleles of the insulin receptor gene contained the same point mutation. This observation suggests that a mutation at codon 735 in "recessive." This loss of function of the insulin receptor then resulted in severe insulin resistance and, in our view, hyperandrogenism.

In addition to the adult forms of the HAIR-AN syndrome, such as Kahn type A insulin resistance, pediatric patients with leprechaunism can also be afflicted with the HAIR-AN syndrome. Leprechaunism is a rare genetic syndrome characterized by intrauterine and neonatal retardation of growth, reduced subcutaneous fat, unusual facies, severe insulin resistance with compensatory hyperinsulinemia, and early death. Girls with leprechaunism frequently have polycystic ovaries, hyperandrogenism and acanthosis nigricans [21,22]. Kadawaki *et al.* [23] recently demonstrated that in one patient with leprechaunism, point mutations in the DNA that encoded for the alpha subunit of the insulin receptor resulted in a nonfunctional insulin receptor, and this defect probably produced the HAIR-AN syndrome. The patient described by Kadawaki *et al.* was a compound heterozygote. One allele of the insulin receptor gene had a mutation at nucleotide 1507 (codon 460), which resulted in the substitution of a glutamic acid residue for a lysine residue. This mutation in the alpha subunit probably resulted in decreased affinity of the receptor for insulin. The other allele had a mutation at nucleotide 2143 (C to T, codon 671) which resulted in a stop signal. As a result, both the transmembrane and tyrosine kinase domains of the receptor were missing.

An important genetic principle is that a phenotypic trait (such as the HAIR-AN syndrome) that segregates in a family linked to a single gene marker indicates that the trait is caused by the gene. Accili and colleagues [24] have recently reported a linkage analysis of one pedigree with the HAIR-AN syndrome. In this family, a marriage between first cousins produced two daughters having the HAIR-AN syndrome (Kahn type A diabetes), three unaffected daughters and one unaffected son. cDNA for the insulin receptor has been cloned from one affected sister and demonstrated a single missense mutation in both alleles of the insulin receptor gene, with a resultant substitution of a valine residue for a phenylalanine residue at position 382 of the alpha subunit. Analysis of restriction fragment length polymorphisms (RFLPs) demonstrated that the two affected sisters are homozygous for this mutation while the two parents and the unaffected siblings are heterozygous carriers. By use of the homozygosity mapping method, a logarithm of the odds (LOD) score of 2.25 was calculated for this pedigree (see Chapter 6). This LOD score supports the hypothesis that the mutation in the insulin receptor gene causes the HAIR-AN phenotype. It is of interest that transfection of cDNA for the mutant receptor into NIH-3T3 cells demonstrated that the substitution of valine for phenylalanine at position 382 impairs post-translational processing and retards the transport of the insulin receptor to the plasma membrane. The mutation causes insulin resistance by decreasing the number of insulin receptors on the cell surface.

The importance of the observation that point mutations in the insulin receptor gene can result in the HAIR-AN syndrome cannot be underestimated. This is the first example of a specific genetic analysis of ovarian hyperandrogenism ("polycystic ovary syndrome"), and it should encourage detailed genetic analysis of large pedigrees with familial PCO. In addition, these observations suggest that any cause of severe hyperinsulinemia, such as obesity, may result in ovarian hyperandrogenism. This hypothesis is strengthened by the observation that acquired causes of insulin-receptor dysfunction are also associated with ovarian hyperandrogenism.

Effects of insulin on ovarian function

Classical concepts of ovarian steroidogenesis focus on LH and FSH as the major regulators of the functions of ovarian granulosa and theca cells. Recently, many growth factors (transforming growth factor (TGF), epidermal growth factor (EGF), fibroblast growth factor (FGF), etc.) have been implicated as important determinants of ovarian function. Significant attention has been focused on insulin and IGF-I as important modulators of the ovarian response to gonadotropins. A review of the relevant literature is complicated by the fact that different species (e.g. human, rat, swine), different cell types (granulosa cells, luteinized granulosa cells, theca cells, stroma) and different hormones (insulin, IGF-I, IGF-II) have been utilized in experimental model systems. In this review, we will focus on the response of human theca and stroma to insulin and IGF-I. To provide historical perspective, the development of the concept of ovarian response to insulin and IGF-I will be reviewed.

Channing *et al.* [25] were the first investigators to examine in detail the effects of insulin on the functions of swine granulosa cells *in vitro*. Swine granulosa cells from small (1–2mm), medium (3–5 mm) and large (6–12 mm) follicles were grown in serum-free medium. Addition of 1000 μU/ml of insulin to the culture medium resulted in morphologic changes that included an increase in numbers of lipid-filled vacuoles and an increase in cell volume. Insulin also produced a marked increase in the number of viable cells per culture. In granulosa cells from small and medium follicles, insulin had minimal effects on secretion of progestin. In granulosa cells from large follicles, insulin (1000 μU/ml) alone produced an 800% increase in secretion of progestin. Insulin plus LH or FSH resulted in more secretion of progestin than that observed with LH or FSH alone. The investigators concluded that insulin produced a generalized increased responsiveness of granulosa cells.

In support of these observations, Veldhuis and colleagues [26] reported that insulin stimulated the biosynthesis of progesterone in porcine granulosa cells obtained from small (1–3 mm) follicles. At a concentration of serum in the culture medium of 4%, 1 μg/ml insulin produced a 7-fold and 12-fold increase in the production of progesterone on days 2 and 4 of culture, respectively. Insulin (1 μg/ml) also augmented the secretion of progesterone in response to 8-bromo-cyclic AMP. In their report, Veldhuis and colleagues [26] did not examine the interaction between insulin and gonadotropins in the regulation of steroidogenesis. Davoren and Hsueh [27] reported that insulin (100 ng/ml) increased the sensitivity of rat granulosa cells to FSH by two- to threefold. Insulin augmented FSH-induced biosynthesis of progestin and estrogen. Of particular interest is the result that insulin stimulated 3β-hydroxysteroid dehydrogenase activity, but it did not stimulate 20α-hydroxysteroid dehydrogenase activity. Human granulosa cells also appear to respond to insulin. For example, in human granulosa cells obtained from follicles of 0.4–2.0 cm in diameter in the follicular phase of the menstrual cycle, insulin (500 ng/ml) caused a threefold increase in FSH-stimulated aromatase activity. In general, in the case of granulosa cells, the concentration of insulin required to stimulate steroidogenesis significantly is in the range of 50 ng/ml to 1 μg/ml. In severely insulin-resistant women, circulating levels of insulin seldom exceed 50 ng/ml.

As noted above, many women with the HAIR-AN syndrome have a genetic defect that prevents normal functioning of the insulin receptor and results in a compensatory, chronic hyperinsulinemia. If the insulin receptor is defective, how can hyperinsulinemia cause the ovarian abnormalities? One possibility is that insulin at high concentrations stimulates ovarian IGF-I receptors. IGF-I receptors are present in ovarian tissue, and they appear to modulate steroidogenic responses to stimulation by gonadotropins. For example, Veldhuis and colleagues [29] demonstrated that IGF-I alone could produce a 50-fold increase in the production of progesterone in swine granulosa cells over a 48–96-hour period. Platelet-derived growth factor (PDGF), EGF, FGF, desoctapeptide insulin and porcine relaxin did not stimulate the biosynthesis of progesterone. High-affinity, low-capacity IGF-I binding sites were demonstrated on the swine granulosa cells (K_d, 0.69 nM; 0.57 pmol IGF-I bound per mg DNA). In addition, Adashi and colleagues [30] demonstrated that, in rat granulosa cells, IGF-I (50 ng/ml) enhanced the FSH-mediated (10 ng/ml) accumulation of progesterone approximately tenfold.

Insulin and IGF-I also regulate theca and stromal responsiveness to gonadotropins. Unlike cultures of granulosa cells, thecal cultures present complex methodologic problems. One experimental model that has been extensively tested involves preparation of "thecal" cultures from cells harvested by dispersion with collagenase of ovaries of immature hypophysectomized rats. The major steroid produced by these "theca-interstitial" cell cultures is androsterone. These cultures are not "pure" and contain multiple types of cell, including granulosa cells. Erickson and Case [31] were the first to report that, using this system, insulin enhanced HCG-stimulated production of androsterone 3.6-fold. This observation has been replicated by Hernandez and colleagues [32] and Cara and Rosenfield [33]. Hernandez and colleagues [32] reported that insulin (1 μg/ml) and HCG (1 ng/ml) stimulated the secretion of androsterone by immature rat theca-interstitial cells 1.5- and 2.6-fold, respectively. Combined treatment with both agents resulted in a 5.7-fold amplification of HCG-stimulated production of androsterone. The insulin effect was time and dose dependent with a minimal time requirement of 72 hours. High-affinity, low-capacity binding sites for insulin were demonstrated (K_d, 0.17 nM; 5000 sites/cell).

Cara and Rosenfield [33] have reported similar findings. Luteinizing hormone alone, but not insulin or IGF-I alone, stimulated the accumulation of androsterone in ovarian thecal-interstitial cells obtained from immature rats. Insulin (100 ng/ml) plus LH (10 ng/ml) caused significantly greater accumulation of androsterone than that observed with LH alone (240 ng/ml vs. 17 ng/ml). Similarly, IGF-I (100 ng/ml) plus LH (10 ng/ml) resulted in significantly greater accumulation of androsterone than that seen with LH alone (302 ng/ml vs. 17 ng/ml). The combination of IGF-I plus insulin did not increase the accumulation of androsterone above that observed with each hormone alone. High-affinity, low-capacity IGF-I receptors were demonstrated in the theca-interstitial cells (K_d, 1.3 nM). Half-maximal inhibition of binding of ^{125}I-labeled IGF-I occurred at a concentration of insulin of 300 nM.

In addition to stimulating accumulation of androgen in rat ovarian theca-interstitial cells, insulin also stimulated the accumulation of androgen in porcine thecal cells [34]. Porcine thecae were microdissected from follicles 1–8 mm in diameter. The thecae were dispersed by treatment with hyaluronidase and collagenase and placed in primary culture. The thecal cultures produced significant quantities of progesterone (P) and androstenedione. Testosterone, dihydrotestosterone, estrone and estradiol could not be detected in the culture media. Alone LH (50 ng/ml) significantly stimulated the accumulation of P and androstenedione. Insulin alone (500 ng/ml and 20 μg/ml) significantly stimulated the accumulation of P, but not that of androstenedione. Insulin plus LH caused a significantly greater accumulation of P and androstenedione than that observed with LH alone.

The "insulin hypothesis" states that chronic hyperinsulinemia causes the human ovary to secrete excessive quantities of androgens. Data to support this hypothesis have been derived from experiments designed to examine the effects of insulin on human ovarian thecal and stromal production of androgen. Barbieri and colleagues [16,35] reported data on the effects of LH and insulin on the thecal and stromal production of androgens. In incubations of theca obtained from a woman with the HAIR-AN syndrome, LH alone (25 ng/ml) stimulated the accumulation of androstenedione, testosterone, progesterone and estradiol. Insulin alone (500 ng/ml) stimulated accumulation of androstenedione and testosterone but not that of progesterone or estradiol. In incubations of stroma obtained from four women with the HAIR-AN syndrome, insulin along (500 ng/ml) stimulated the accumulation of androstenedione in incubations of stroma from three of the four women and the accumulation of testosterone in incubations of stroma from one of the four women. In stromal incubations from three of the four hyperandrogenic women, insulin alone (500 ng/ml) caused greater accumulation of androstenedione and testosterone than did LH alone (25 ng/ml). Insulin-like growth factor I (50 ng/ml) also stimulated the accumulation of androstenedione and testosterone. Relaxin and IGF-II did not stimulate the synthesis of androgens. Incubations of ovarian stroma from three nonhyperandrogenic, normally cycling women demonstrated low levels of accumulation of androgens. Insulin alone (500 ng/ml) and LH alone (25 ng/ml) produced no significant increases in the accumulation of androgens. Insulin (500 ng/ml) plus LH (25 ng/ml) produced a small but significant increase in the accumulation of androgens.

These studies suggest that the ovarian tissue from women with the HAIR-AN syndrome is responsive to insulin *in vitro*, at the same time that the women appear to be insulin resistant with respect to carbohydrate metabolism. The mechanisms responsible for this heterogeneity of response is unclear. One possibility is that certain genetic abnormalities in the insulin receptor can result in insulin resistance with respect to carbohydrate metabolism, while other functions of the receptor (e.g. stimulation of cell growth) may be preserved. This hypothesis is supported by the observation that women with the HAIR-AN syndrome are relatively resistant to becoming ketotic. Alternatively, as noted above, insulin may exert its effects on ovarian theca and stroma by interacting with IGF-I receptors. This possibility is a critical issue that requires further investigation.

Hyperinsulinemia and PCO

The role of hyperinsulinemia in the pathogenesis of ovarian hyperandrogenism in certain rare genetic forms of PCO (e.g. the HAIR-AN syndrome) is clear. The role of hyperinsulinemia in the pathogenesis of the common forms of PCO is less clear. At least two pathways exist by which insulin may interact with LH to produce the PCO phenotype [1]. Insulin has been demonstrated to augment the induction by FSH of receptors for LH in granulosa cells and to augment the effects of LH on the granulosa cells via postreceptor mechanisms [36]. Through a variety of molecular mechanisms elevated concentrations of LH plus elevated concentrations of insulin (both common in PCO) may synergize to produce premature luteinization of granulosa cells in small follicles. Early exposure of granulosa cells in small follicles to high concentrations of LH and insulin may prevent the full expression of the potential of these cells for mitotic growth. Instead of growing, the granulosa cells exposed to high concentrations of LH and insulin may differentiate (luteinize) prematurely. As a result, no large follicles would develop, and ovulation would not occur. This hypothesis could explain the accumulation of large numbers of small follicles associated with PCO [2].

Simultaneously, the high concentrations of LH and insulin will stimulate thecal and stromal growth and the secretion of androgens. Excessive ovarian production of androgens will result in the androgenic phenotype seen in PCO. Further investigation is required to fully delineate, through genetic-linkage studies, the role of mutations in the insulin receptor in the development of PCO. In addition, until the intracellular signaling mechanisms utilized by the ovarian receptors for insulin and IGF-I are fully characterized, the puzzle will remain incompletely solved. It is likely that data generated in the next decade will convince all investigators that insulin plays as central a role in the development of PCO as does LH.

Acknowledgments

Supported in part by HD 24563-01.

References

1 Goldzieher JW. Polycystic ovary disease. Fertil Steril 1981; 35:371–9.
2 Yen SSC. The polycystic ovary syndrome. Clin Endocrinol 1980; 12:77–98.
3 Barbieri RL, Ryan KJ. Hyperandrogenism, insulin resistance and acanthosis nigricans syndrome: a common endocrinopathy with distinct pathophysiological features. Am J Obstet Gynecol 1983; 147:90–101.
4 Kahn CR, Flier JS, Bar RS, Archer JA, Gorden P, Martin MM, Roth J. The syndromes of insulin resistance and acanthosis nigricans. N Engl J Med 1976; 294:739–42.
5 Achard C, Thiers J. Le virilisme pilaire et son association a l'insuffisanse glycolytique (diabete a femme de barbe). Bull Acad Natl Med (Paris) 1921; 86:51–83.
6 Barbieri RL, Hornstein MD. Hyperinsulinemia and hyperandrogenism: cause and effect. Endocrinol Metab Clin North Am 1988; 17:685–703.
7 Burghen GA, Givens JR, Kitabchi AE. Correlation of hyperandrogenism with hyperinsulinemia in polycystic ovarian disease. J Clin Endocrinol Metab 1980; 50:113–15.
8 Chang RJ, Nakamura RM, Judd HL. Insulin resistance in nonobese patients with polycystic ovarian disease. J Clin Endocrinol Metab 1983; 57:356–60.
9 Smith S, Ravnikar VA, Barbieri RL. Androgen and insulin response to an oral glucose challenge in hyperandrogenic women. Fertil Steril 1987; 48:72–7.
10 Barbieri RL, Smith S, Ryan KJ. The role of hyperinsulinemia in the pathogenesis of ovarian hyperandrogenism. Fertil Steril 1988; 50:197–212.
11 Nagamani M, Dinh TV, Kelver ME. Hyperinsulinemia in hyperthecosis of the ovaries. Am J Obstet Gynecol 1986; 154:384–9.
12 Geffner ME, Kaplan SA, Bersch N, Chang JR. Persistence of insulin resistance in polycystic ovarian disease after inhibition of ovarian steroid secretion. Fertil Steril 1986; 45:327–33.
13 Pasquali R, Casimirri F, Venturoli S. Insulin resistance in patients with polycystic ovaries: its relationship to body weight and androgen levels. Acta Endocrinol 1983; 104:110–15.
14 Dunaif AM, Graf M. Insulin administration alters gonadal steroid metabolism

independent of changes in gonadotropin secretion in insulin-resistant women with the polycystic ovary syndrome. J Clin Invest 1989; 83:23–9.

15 Barbieri RL. The role of adipose tissue and hyperinsulinemia in the development of hyperandrogenism in women. In: Frisch RE, ed. Adipose Tissue and Reproduction. Basel: Karger, 1990.

16 Barbieri RL, Makris A, Randall RW, Daniels G, Kistner RW, Ryan KJ. Insulin stimulates androgen accumulation in incubations of ovarian stroma from women with hyperandrogenism. J Clin Endocrinol Metab 1986; 62:904–10.

17 Taylor SI, Dons RF, Hernandez E, Roth J, Gorden P. Insulin resistance associated with androgen excess in women with autoantibodies to the insulin receptor. Ann Intern Med 1982; 97:851–4.

18 Moller DE, Flier JS. Detection of an alteration in the insulin-receptor gene in a patient with insulin resistance, acanthosis nigricans and the polycystic ovary syndrome (type A insulin resistance). N Engl J Med 1988; 319:1526–9.

19 Kahn CR, White MF. The insulin receptor and the molecular mechanism of insulin action. J Clin Invest 1988; 82:1151–6.

20 Yoshimasa Y, Seino S, Whittaker J. Insulin-resistant diabetes due to a point mutation that prevents insulin receptor processing. Science 1988; 240:784–7.

21 Geffner ME, Kaplan SA, Bersch N. Leprechaunism *in vitro*: insulin action despite genetic insulin resistance. Pediat Res 1987; 22:286–91.

22 D'Ercole AJ, Underwood LE, Grokle J. Leprechaunism: studies on the relationship among hyperinsulinemia, insulin resistance and growth retardation. J Clin Endocrinol Metab 1979; 48:495–8.

23 Kadawaki T, Berins C, Cama A. Two mutant alleles of the insulin receptor gene in a patient with extreme insulin resistance. Science 1988; 240:787–90.

24 Accili D, Frapier C, Mosthat L, McKeon C, Elbein SC, Permutt MA. A mutation in the insulin receptor gene that impairs transport of the receptor to the plasma membrane and causes insulin-resistant diabetes. EMBO J 1989; 8:2509–17.

25 Channing C, Tsai V, Sachs D. Role of insulin, thyroxine and cortisol in luteinization of porcine granulosa cells grown in chemically defined media. Biol Reprod 1976; 15:235–41.

26 Veldhuis JD, Kolp LA, Toaff ME, Strauss JF, Demers LM. Mechanisms subserving the tropic actions of insulin on ovarian cells: *in vitro* studies using swine granulosa cells. J Clin Invest 1983; 72:1046–51.

27 Davoren JB, Hsueh AJW. Insulin enhances FSH-stimulated steroidogenesis by cultured rat granulosa cells. Mol Cell Endocrinol 1984; 35:97–102.

28 Garzo VG, Dorrington JH. Aromatase activity in human granulosa cells during follicular development and the modulation by FSH and insulin. Am J Obstet Gynecol 1984; 148:657–60.

29 Veldhuis JD, Furlanetto RW. Tropic actions of human somatomedin C–insulin-like growth factor 1 on ovarian cells: *in vitro* studies with swine granulosa cells. Endocrinology 1985; 116:1235–42.

30 Adashi EY, Resnick CE, Svoboda ME, Van Wyk JJ. Somatomedin C synergizes with FSH in the acquisition of progestin biosynthetic capacity by cultured rat granulosa cells. Endocrinology 1985; 116:2135–42.

31 Erickson GF, Case E. Epidermal growth factor antagonizes ovarian theca-interstitial cytodifferentiation. Mol Cell Endocrinol 1933; 31:71–6.

32 Hernandez ER, Resnick CE, Holtzclaw WD, Payne DW, Adashi EY. Insulin as a regulator of androgen biosynthesis by cultured rat ovarian cells: cellular mechanisms underlying physiological and pharmocological actions. Endocrinology 1988; 122:2034–43.

33 Cara JF, Rosenfield RL. Insulin-like growth factor-I and insulin potentiate LH-induced androgen synthesis by rat ovarian thecal-interstial cells. Endocrinology 1988; 123:733–9.

34 Barbieri RL, Makris A, Ryan KJ. Effects of insulin on steroidogenesis in cultured porcine ovarian theca. Fertil Steril 1983; 40:237–41.
35 Barbieri RL, Makris A, Ryan KJ. Insulin stimulates androgen accumulation in incubations of human ovarian stroma and theca. Obstet Gynecol 1984; 64:73s–80s.
36 May JV, Schomberg DW. Granulosa cell differentiation *in vitro*: effect of insulin on growth and functional integrity. Biol Reprod 1981; 25:421–31.

Chapter 22
Effects of Insulin on Steroidogenesis *In Vivo*

JOHN E. NESTLER, JOHN N. CLORE &
WILLIAM G. BLACKARD

An increasing body of evidence suggests that insulin plays an important role in the regulation of steroidogenesis and that hyperinsulinemia causes the hyperandrogenism experienced by some women with polycystic ovary syndrome (PCO) [1–3]. The concept that insulin may play a role in PCO emerged from the observation that young women who are insulin resistant and hyperinsulinemic due to a lack of insulin receptors are often virilized [4]. It was subsequently demonstrated that women with PCO are also insulin resistant and hyperinsulinemic, and that a positive correlation exists between fasting serum insulin levels and serum androgens (androstenedione and testosterone) in these women [5–13]. What remained uncertain was whether this correlation represented a cause-and-effect relationship or merely an epiphenomenon, and, if a cause-and-effect relationship existed, whether the hyperinsulinemia was a cause or consequence of the hyperandrogenism.

Taylor and colleagues were the first to propose that overproduction of testosterone in women with insulin resistance may result from a direct effect of hyperinsulinemia on the ovaries [14], and several other investigators have since provided evidence to support this hypothesis [1,3,15,16]. These investigators noted that it is unlikely that the hyperinsulinemia of PCO occurs as a result of hyperandrogenism for the following reasons. In women with PCO who have undergone either subtotal [17] or total [13] removal of the ovaries, or in whom androgens have been suppressed by the use of a long-acting agonist of gonadotropin-releasing hormone (GnRH) [18,19], insulin resistance persists. Prepubertal women with acanthosis nigricans are hyperinsulinemic, yet elevated serum androgen levels do not appear until several years after the diagnosis of insulin resistance [20]. Men have androgen levels 10- to 30-fold higher than those in women, yet they do not demonstrate insulin resistance. These observations suggest that, if a cause-and-effect relationship exists, it is more likely that it is the hyperinsulinemia of PCO that causes the accompanying hyperandrogenism.

In support of the above-mentioned hypothesis, there is abundant evidence from experiments *in vitro*, both with animal and human tissues, demonstrating regulation of the biosynthesis of steroid hormones by insulin [1]. In addition, human ovaries possess insulin receptors [21–23], suggesting a role for this peptide in ovarian function. What has remained to be demonstrated is an effect *in vivo* of insulin on serum androgens in women with PCO. Until recently, attempts to document such an effect in either normal women or in women with PCO have yielded conflicting results. Such earlier studies utilized either the hyperinsulinemic-euglycemic clamp technique [24–27] or an oral glucose-tolerance test [12] to raise insulin levels. In these studies serum androstenedione levels increased variably [12,25,27], while serum testosterone was reported to increase [12,26], to decrease [27], or to remain unchanged [24,25] (Table 22.1).

The inability to demonstrate convincingly an increase in serum androgens in these studies may have been due to the relatively brief periods of insulin elevation (3–16 hours). In addition, evidence suggests that steroidogenic pathways of normal women may be less responsive to stimulation by insulin than those of women with PCO. Ovarian tissues removed from women with hyperandrogenism exhibit enhanced release of androstenedione and testosterone in response to insulin, whereas

Table 22.1 Effects of acute experimentally induced hyperinsulinemia on serum concentrations of testosterone (T) and androstenedione (A) in women.

Investigators	Subjects	Degree of hyperinsulinemia	T	A
Insulin–glucose clamp studies				
Nestler *et al.* [24]	Normal (5)	High	NC	
	PCO (1)		NC	
Stuart *et al.* [25]	Normal (11)	Low to high	NC	↑
	PCO (3)		NC	↑
Micic *et al.* [26]	PCO (6)	Low to moderate	↑	
Dunaif *et al.* [27]	Normal (5)	High	NC	NC
	PCO (10)		↓	↑
Oral glucose challenge study				
Smith *et al.* [12]	Normal (7)	Low	NC	NC
	PCO (5)		↑	↑

NC, no change; ↑, increased; ↓, decreased.

ovarian tissues removed from normal women remain unaffected by insulin treatment [28]. Moreover, this disparity has also been noted in studies *in vivo* where experimentally induced hyperinsulinemia appears to alter serum concentrations of sex steroids in women with PCO, but not those in normal women [12,27]. Thus, the failure to demonstrate an effect of hyperinsulinemia on serum androgens of normal women [24] may merely reflect the lack of a predisposition to hypersecretion of androgens by the steroidogenic tissues of these subjects.

To avoid the limitations of short-term, insulin–glucose clamps and examine the role of chronic physiologic hyperinsulinemia on androgen levels in PCO, we employed diazoxide to lower serum insulin levels in five obese women with this disorder [29]. Administration of diazoxide uniformly suppressed fasting and glucose-stimulated release of insulin and resulted in a 17% decrease in serum total testosterone from 2.5 ± 0.4 nmol/l to 2.1 ± 0.3 nmol/l ($P < 0.007$; Fig. 22.1). Serum sex hormone-binding globulin levels rose in all five subjects during diazoxide administration from a mean value of 13.2 ± 1.0 nmol/l to 21.7 ± 4.1 nmol/l, but this elevation was not statistically significant ($P = 0.09$) (Fig. 22.1). Because of the concurrent decrease in serum concentrations of testosterone and the increase in those of sex hormone-binding globulin, the amount of serum testosterone that was not bound to sex hormone-binding globulin fell by 28% from 190 ± 30 pmol/l to 140 ± 20 pmol/l ($P < 0.01$).

Administration of diazoxide did not affect the frequency of pulses of luteinizing hormone (LH), the amplitude of LH pulses, the mean LH level, the mean level of follicle-stimulating hormone (FSH), the molar ratio of LH to FSH, or the integrated response of LH levels to stimulation by GnRH. These data suggest that hyperinsulinemia mediates the hyperandrogenism of obese women with PCO through direct actions on the metabolism of testosterone.

The next questions to be answered were (i) do physiologic insulin levels play a regulatory role in the androgen status of nonobese women with normal menses, and (ii) does diazoxide itself directly alter androgen homeostasis. To address these issues, we recently assessed the effect of insulin suppression with diazoxide on the androgen status of five nonobese, healthy women by studying them in a similar fashion. In marked contrast to our results in obese women with PCO, we found that treatment with diazoxide altered neither serum concentrations of androgens nor those of sex hormone-binding globulin in these healthy women with normal levels of circulating insulin (JE Nestler, R Singh, DW Matt, JN Clore, WG Blackard, submitted for publication). This result suggests that either (i) normal women are not as sensitive to

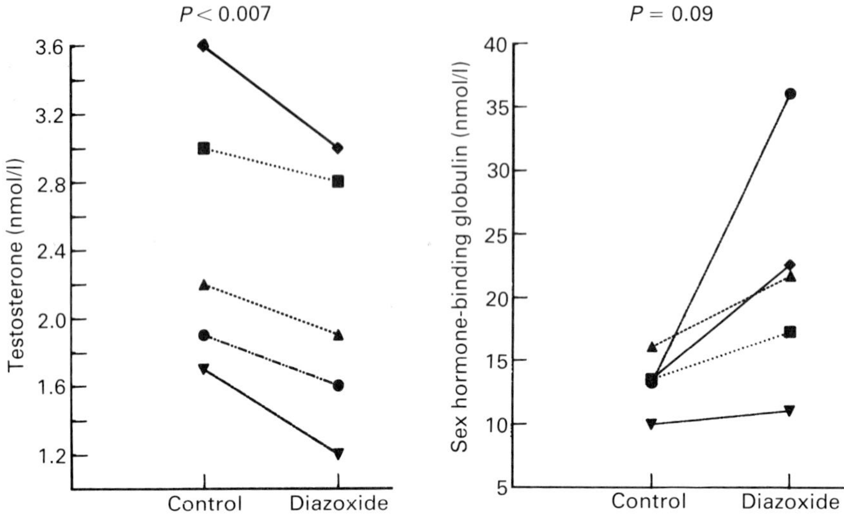

Fig. 22.1 Serum levels of testosterone and sex hormone-binding globulin in five obese women with PCO during a control period and after 10 days of insulin suppression with diazoxide. (Adapted from Nestler *et al* [29].)

insulin's actions on androgen homeostasis as are women with PCO or (ii) insulin concentrations in the physiologic range do not play an important role in regulating serum levels of testosterone. As noted before, evidence exists suggesting that androgenic pathways of normal women may be less responsive to stimulation by insulin than those of women with PCO [12,27,28]. Alternatively, it has been postulated that in PCO elevated serum insulin levels affect androgenic pathways via cross-reactions with the insulin-like growth factor I (IGF-I) receptor [30]. Concentrations of insulin in the physiologic range may be too low to permit significant association with receptors for IGF-I. Thus, insulin may not regulate serum androgen levels under physiologic conditions.

The various above-mentioned observations also indicate that diazoxide does not directly affect serum levels of testosterone or sex hormone-binding globulin *in vivo*. Thus, the reduction in serum levels of testosterone observed when diazoxide is administered to obese women with PCO [29] is indeed due to suppression of insulin release and not to independent properties of diazoxide. These results lend further support to the hypothesis that the hyperinsulinemia of PCO is responsible in part for the hyperandrogenism, and they also suggest that women with PCO may possess an inherent (perhaps genetically transmitted) susceptibility to the hyperandrogenic effects of insulin.

An additional mechanism whereby hyperinsulinemia could result in hyperandrogenism would be the direct and independent reduction in levels of sex hormone-binding globulin in serum. Since testosterone is highly bound to sex hormone-binding globulin, a decrease in serum levels of sex hormone-binding globulin would increase the availability of unbound testosterone to tissues. Several lines of evidence suggest that hyperinsulinemia does indeed reduce serum levels of sex hormone-binding globulin. Studies *in vitro* indicate that insulin suppresses production of sex hormone-binding globulin by cultured hepatoma cells [31]. Furthermore, epidemiologic studies have demonstrated an inverse correlation between serum levels of insulin and serum levels of sex hormone-binding globulin in obese Mexican-American women [32] and obese healthy women [33]. These inverse correlations are independent of serum levels of androgens or the degree of adiposity.

To examine this issue specifically, we recently studied the effects of insulin suppression with diazoxide on serum levels of sex hormone-binding globulin under conditions where serum levels of androgens and estrogen remained unchanged [34]. After the suppression of gonadotropin release and of ovarian steroidogenesis with a long-acting agonist of GnRH, six obese women with PCO were given diazoxide to inhibit insulin release. Since ovarian steroidogenesis had been suppressed in these women, diazoxide did not alter serum levels of androgens or estrogen, but it did cause a significant increase in serum concentrations of sex hormone-binding globulin. Since diazoxide does not affect the production of sex hormone-binding globulin by cultured HepG2 cells (SR Plymate, unpublished observations), and since it does not alter serum levels of sex hormone-binding globulin in nonobese healthy women with normal levels of circulating insulin (see above), these observations suggest that the increase in serum levels of sex hormone-binding globulin after the administration of diazoxide is directly due to suppression of insulin release, and that hyperinsulinemia can reduce serum levels of sex hormone-binding globulin in obese women with PCO independently of any effect on serum sex steroids.

It should be noted that raising [27] or lowering [29] serum insulin levels alters serum levels of androgens without affecting serum concentrations or the release of gonadotropins. However, when gonadotropin release is suppressed in women with PCO by the administration of a long-acting agonist of GnRH, ovarian androgen levels fall markedly [19,34], and inhibition of insulin release with diazoxide does not further lower serum androgen levels [34]. Taken together, these observations suggest that (i) hyperinsulinemia can *directly* stimulate ovarian production of androgens without affecting the release of gonadotropin, and

(ii) gonadotropins exert a permissive effect that allows insulin-stimulated production of androgens to occur. Thus, the presence of gonadotropin-stimulated ovarian steroidogenesis appears to be required if hyper-insulinemia is to exert its stimulatory actions.

It is not yet known whether hyperinsulinemia produces hyperandrogenism by increasing androgen production or decreasing androgen catabolism, or by a combination of these processes. At the cellular level, hyperinsulinemia could theoretically affect androgen metabolism either via the classical insulin receptor [21–23], perhaps through processes distinct from those responsible for glucose transport (e.g. by the generation of second messengers [35]), or by cross-reacting with receptors for IGF-I [23]. Insulin-like growth factor I is a potent stimulator of LH-induced synthesis of androgens by interstitial cells [36]. The activity of IGF-I is modulated by a low-molecular-weight binding protein termed the 34-kDa insulin-like growth factor-binding protein (34k IGFBP), which has been detected in human follicular fluid [37], is growth hormone independent [38] and insulin dependent [39]. Since insulin can inhibit the synthesis of some insulin-like growth factor-binding proteins [40], an intriguing indirect mechanism whereby insulin might produce hyperandrogenism would be via reduction of intrafollicular levels of 34k IGFBP, which would increase the concentration of unbound IGF-I available for the stimulation of androgen production. Indeed, serum levels of 34k IGFBP have been found to be low in women with PCO, and they are inversely correlated with serum levels of insulin [41,42].

Given the above observations, we have formulated the scheme illustrated in Fig. 22.2 to explain how hyperinsulinemia might result in hyperandrogenism in a susceptible woman. According to this hypothesis, hyperinsulinemia increases the ovarian production of androgens. Although multiple studies *in vivo* support the validity of this concept in women with PCO, the absence of any effect of hyperinsulinemia on serum levels of androgens of normal women, and the fact that many obese (and consequently hyperinsulinemic) women are not hyperandrogenemic, remain to be explained. One possible explanation for this inconsistency is that women with PCO are genetically predisposed to stimulation by insulin of ovarian androgen production, i.e. there is a "PCO gene" that needs to be present if hyperinsulinemia is to exert an effect. We call this hypothesis the "iceberg hypothesis," as illustrated in Fig. 22.3. The often familial nature of PCO [43] suggests that this hypothesis may indeed be valid. Additional studies contrasting the effects of hyperinsulinemia in normal

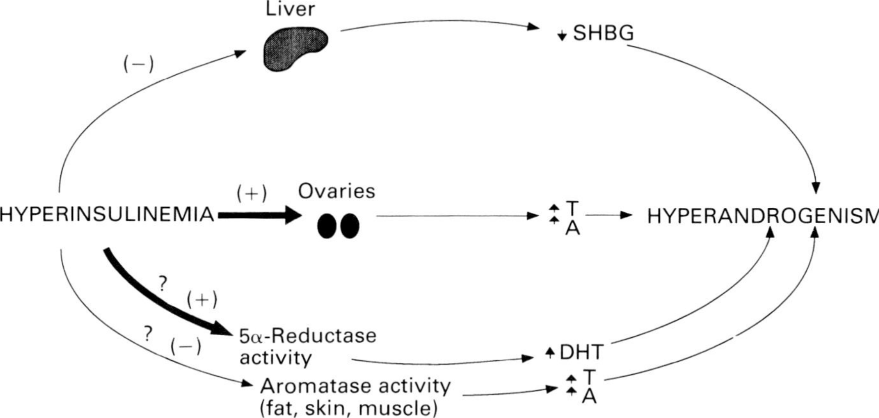

Fig. 22.2 Theoretical scheme illustrating the mechanisms whereby hyperinsulinemia could produce hyperandrogenism in women with PCO. T = testosterone; A = androstenedione; DHT = dihydrotestosterone; SHBG = sex hormone-binding globulin.

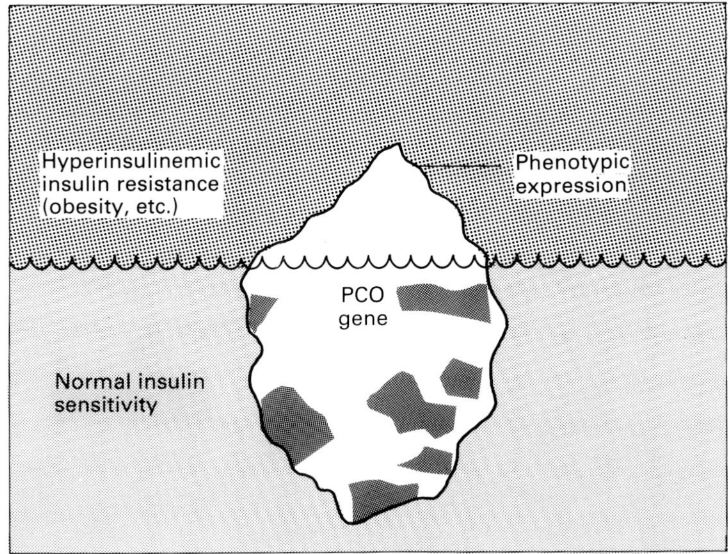

Fig. 22.3 The "iceberg hypothesis," which postulates that both hyperinsulinemia and a genetic predisposition to the androgenic actions of insulin are required for phenotypic expression of PCO.

women with those in women with PCO are needed to examine this possibility in greater detail.

An alternate explanation for the discrepancy observed in studies where experimentally induced hyperinsulinemia resulted in a rise in serum levels of androstenedione in women with PCO, but not in normal women, takes into account the relatively greater contribution of the ovaries to circulating levels of androstenedione in women with PCO (compared to normal women) and postulates opposing effects of hyperinsulinemia on ovarian vs. adrenal androstenedione production. Indirect support for this construct is provided by the following observations. We have shown that in normal men serum levels of androstenedione decrease markedly during experimentally induced hyperinsulinemia [44]. In contrast, serum levels of androstenedione either do not change [45] or they increase [25,27] in normal women studied under similar conditions. In men, the adrenals are the primary source of circulating androstenedione [46], whereas in women during the follicular phase of the menstrual cycle the ovaries and adrenals contribute equally to peripheral levels of androstenedione [47]. Evidence from studies *in vitro* suggests that insulin may affect different human steroidogenic tissues in dissimilar ways, e.g. insulin stimulates ovarian aromatase activity [48] but inhibits cytotrophoblastic aromatase activity [49]. As illustrated in Table 22.2, the seemingly divergent data obtained *in vivo* from men and women could potentially be explained by inhibition of adrenal production of androgens by insulin (which would result in a decrease in serum levels of androstenedione in men), coupled with stimulation of ovarian production of androstenedione by insulin (which, in women, would compensate for the inhibition of adrenal production and result in no net change in serum levels of androstenedione). Since the contribution of the ovaries to serum levels of androstenedione is increased to 80% in women with PCO [46], this contribution would explain how hyperinsulinemia could result in elevated serum levels of androstenedione in these women while seemingly exerting no effect in normal women. Studies examining the specific and separate actions of hyperinsulinemia on ovarian vs. adrenal production of androgens are needed to evaluate this possibility.

An additional mechanism whereby hyperinsulinemia could contribute to hyperandrogenism is via suppression of overall aromatase activity, which would decrease the rate of catabolism of androgens. This mechanism is unlikely to constitute the *sole* mechanism that is responsible for hyperandrogenism, but it may represent a contributory factor. The overall effect of insulin on aromatase activity in women is unknown. Garzo and Dorrington demonstrated a stimulatory effect of insulin on the aromatase activity of human granulosa cells from normal women [48], but a recent study suggests that insulin treatment is relatively ineffective in altering the aromatase activity of granulosa cells from women with PCO [50]. Furthermore, Veldhuis and colleagues

Table 22.2 Theoretical scheme of the way in which hyperinsulinemia would alter serum levels of androstenedione if it exerted opposing effects on ovarian vs. adrenal production of androstenedione.

	Relative contribution to circulating androstenedione		Predicted change in serum androstenedione if insulin stimulates ovarian and inhibits adrenal production of androstenedione
	Ovaries	Adrenals	
Men	—	>90%	↓↓
Normal women	50%	50%	No change
Women with PCO	80%	20%	↑

found that insulin suppressed aromatase activity in swine granulosa cells [51], and we ourselves have demonstrated an inhibitory effect of insulin on placental aromatase activity [49]. A study designed to assess the effect of insulin on net whole-body aromatase activity *in vivo* (i.e. inclusive of fat, muscle, ovaries, etc.) seems warranted.

It remains to be determined whether or not hyperinsulinemia affects the activity of tissue 5α-reductase, the enzyme that converts testosterone to its active metabolite, dihydrotestosterone, in various tissues. It is of interest, however, that insulin may augment 5α-reductase activity in isolated rat hepatocytes [52], and Pasupuleti and Horton have recently shown *in vitro* that IGF-I increases 5α-reductase activity in rat skin fibroblasts [53]. Hyperinsulinemia-stimulated 5α-reductase activity, mediated via either the insulin receptor or IGF-I receptor, may represent yet another mechanism whereby hyperinsulinemia could amplify the actions of testosterone at the tissue level, with resultant clinical hyperandrogenism.

Some women with PCO manifest elevated serum levels of dehydroepiandrosterone sulfate (DHEAS) with normal or minimally elevated serum levels of testosterone, suggestive predominantly of excess adrenal production of androgens. We have examined the effects of acute hyperinsulinemia on adrenal androgens in a study employing the hyperinsulinemic-euglycemic clamp technique [24]. Five normal women received an infusion of insulin for 12–16 hours, such that a mean concentration of insulin of $1832 \pm 292\,\mu$U/ml was achieved, while the serum concentration of glucose was clamped at 116 ± 5 mg/dl. During this study, serum concentrations of DHEAS decreased progressively, declining by 39% at 12 hours (144 ± 29 vs. $234 \pm 35\,\mu$g/dl at zero time; $P < 0.01$). This steady decline in serum levels of DHEAS in response to hyperinsulinemia was shown not to be due to diurnal variation, suppression of adrenocorticotropic hormone (ACTH) release, or alterations in serum levels of prolactin. More recently, other investigators have demonstrated an inverse correlation between fasting serum levels of insulin and DHEAS in hyperandrogenic women [12], as well as a decrease in serum levels of DHEAS when serum levels of insulin were raised to within the physiologic range (150–200 μU/ml) in normal women [45].

We have shown that this insulin-mediated suppression of serum levels of DHEAS is not mediated by increased clearance due to enhanced (i) hydrolysis of DHEAS to DHEA, (ii) conversion of DHEAS/DHEA to androstenedione, and/or (iii) urinary excretion of these steroids [44]. Recent evidence suggests that hyperinsulinemia reduces serum levels of DHEA by inhibiting production, and that this mechanism may be especially relevant in women with PCO [54]. A possible mechanism whereby hyperinsulinemia might specifically decrease adrenal production of androgens, without affecting adrenal production of glucocorticoids or mineralocorticoids, involves inhibition of 17,20-lyase activity. This possibility warrants further investigation (see Chapter 23).

The decline in serum levels of DHEAS under conditions of both physiologic [45] and supraphysiologic [24,44] elevations of serum levels of insulin is of particular interest, since many women with PCO have abnormal patterns of adrenal steroidogenesis and the adrenal androgen whose level in serum is most commonly elevated in these women is DHEAS. If insulin plays a role in the metabolism of DHEA/DHEAS, it may be that abnormalities in tissue sensitivity to insulin or secretion/action of insulin result in adrenal hyperandrogenism.

In summary, it is becoming increasingly apparent that hyperinsulinemia is an almost universal feature of women with PCO and that hyperinsulinemia may play an important role in the pathogenesis of this syndrome by affecting multiple facets of androgen homeostasis. Nonetheless, many questions remain unanswered and warrant further investigation. Such unresolved issues include, but are not limited to, the following.

1 Are women with PCO more susceptible to insulin-induced hyperandrogenism than healthy women? Does a genetic factor, inherited by women with PCO, predispose these women to the hyperandrogenic effects of hyperinsulinemia?

2 Can women predisposed to developing PCO be prospectively identified by monitoring serum androgen levels while insulin levels are either increased or decreased?

3 What are the effects of hyperinsulinemia on adrenal vs. ovarian secretion of androgens? Can opposing effects of insulin on these two glands account for the apparent discrepancy between the effects of hyperinsulinemia on healthy women (no change in serum levels of androstenedione) vs. women with PCO (increase in serum levels of androstenedione)?

4 Does hyperinsulinemia alter serum levels of ovarian or adrenal androgens by affecting the rate of production, the rate of clearance, or both the rates of production and clearance for these steroids?

5 Does hyperinsulinemia affect androgenic processes by activating the classical insulin receptor or by cross-reacting with the receptor for IGF-I?

6 Can the hyperandrogenism of women with PCO be ameliorated by dietary changes that reduce the prevailing level of hyperinsulinemia?

7 Does hyperinsulinemia alter 5α-reductase or net whole-body aromatase activity?

8 Does insulin resistance play a pathogenic role in PCO in women who manifest primarily adrenal hyperandrogenism?

The relationship between hyperinsulinemia and hyperandrogenism in PCO clearly remains a fertile and exciting area of investigation; one which should yield novel information about the pathogenesis, as well as new treatment modalities, for this common disorder.

Acknowledgments

We would like to thank Drs Cornelius Barlascini, Keith Usiskin, Linda Powers, Stephen Plymate, Dennis Matt, Kenneth Steingold, Roshnara Singh, Jerome Strauss III, the staff of the General Clinical Research Center of the Medical College of Virginia, and Bettie Duke (CLINFO Systems Analyst) who helped conduct the studies emanating from our laboratory. The research from our laboratory was supported in part by NIH grants RR-00065 and DK-18904, and by grants from the Virginia Affiliate of the American Diabetes Association and the Thomas F. and Kate Miller Jeffress Memorial Trust.

References

1 Poretsky L, Kalin MF. The gonadotropic function of insulin. Endocr Rev 1987; 8:132–41.

2 Barbieri RL, Smith S, Ryan KJ. The role of hyperinsulinemia in the pathogenesis of ovarian hyperandrogenism. Fertil Steril 1988; 50:197–212.

3 Nestler JE, Clore JN, Blackard WG. The central role of obesity (hyperinsulinemia) in the pathogenesis of the polycystic ovary syndrome. Am J Obstet Gynecol 1989; 161:1095–7.

4 Kahn CR, Flier JS, Bar RS, Archer JA, Gorden P, Martin MM, Roth J. The syndrome of insulin resistance and acanthosis nigricans. N Engl J Med 1976; 294:739–45.

5 Burghen GA, Givens JR, Kitabchi AE. Correlation of hyperandrogenism with hyperinsulinism in polycystic ovarian disease. J Clin Endocrinol Metab 1980; 50:113–16.
6 Chang RJ, Nakaruma RM, Judd HL, Kaplan SA. Insulin resistance in nonobese patients with polycystic ovarian disease. J Clin Endocrinol Metab 1983; 57:356–9.
7 Pasquali R, Casimirri F, Venturoli S, Paradisi R, Mattioli L, Capelli M, Melchionda N, Labo G. Insulin resistance in patients with polycystic ovaries: its relationship to body weight and androgen levels. Acta Endocrinol 1983; 104:110–16.
8 Pasquali R, Fabbri R, Venturoli S, Paradisi R, Antenucci D, Melchionda N. Effect of weight loss and antiandrogenic therapy on sex hormone blood levels and insulin resistance in obese patients with polycystic ovaries. Am J Obstet Gynecol 1986; 154:139–44.
9 Shoupe D, Kumar DD, Lobo RA. Insulin resistance in polycystic ovary syndrome. Am J Obstet Gynecol 1983; 147:588–92.
10 Shoupe D, Lobo RA. The influence of androgens on insulin resistance. Fertil Steril 1984; 41:385–8.
11 Stuart CA, Peters EJ, Prince MJ, Richards G, Cavallo A, Meyer WJ. Insulin resistance with acanthosis nigricans: the roles of obesity and androgen excess. Metabolism 1986; 35:197–205.
12 Smith S, Ravnikar VA, Barbieri RL. Androgen and insulin response to an oral glucose challenge in hyperandrogenic women. Fertil Steril 1987; 48:72–7.
13 Nagamani M, Minh TV, Kelver ME. Hyperinsulinemia in hyperthecosis of the ovaries. Am J Obstet Gynecol 1986; 154:384–9.
14 Taylor SI, Dons RF, Hernandez E, Roth J, Gorden P. Insulin resistance associated with androgen excess in women with autoantibodies to the insulin receptor. Ann Intern Med 1982; 97:851–5.
15 Flier JS, Eastman RC, Minaker KL, Matteson D, Rowe JW. Acanthosis nigricans in obese women with hyperandrogenism. Characterization of an insulin-resistant state distinct from the type A and B syndromes. Diabetes 1985; 34:101–7.
16 Barbieri RL, Ryan KJ. Hyperandrogenism, insulin resistance, and acanthosis nigricans syndrome: a common endocrinopathy with distinct pathophysiologic features. Am J Obstet Gynecol 1983; 147:90–101.
17 Imperato-McGinley J, Peterson RE, Sturla E, Dawood Y, Bar RS. Primary amenorrhea associated with hirsutism, acanthosis nigricans, dermoid cysts of the ovaries and a new type of insulin resistance. Am J Med 1978; 65:389–95.
18 Geffner ME, Kaplan SA, Bersch N, Golde DW, Landaw EM, Chang RZ. Persistence of insulin resistance in polycystic ovarian disease after inhibition of ovarian steroid secretion. Fertil Steril 1986; 45:327–33.
19 Dunaif A, Green G, Futterweit W, Dobrjansky A. Suppression of hyperandrogenism does not improve peripheral or hepatic insulin resistance in the polycystic ovary syndrome. J Clin Endocrinol Metab 1990; 70:699–704.
20 Richards GE, Cavallo A, Meyer III WJ, Prince MJ, Peters EJ, Stuart CA, Smith ER. Obesity, acanthosis nigricans, insulin resistance, and hyperandrogenemia: pediatric perspective and natural history. J Pediatr 1985; 107:893–7.
21 Poretsky L, Smith D, Seibel M, Pazianos A, Moses AC, Flier JS. Specific insulin binding sites in human ovary. J Clin Endocrinol Metab 1984; 59:809–11.
22 Jarrett II JC, Ballejo G, Tsibris JCM, Spellacy WN. Insulin binding to human ovaries. J Clin Endocrinol Metab 1985; 60:460–3.
23 Poretsky L, Grigorescu F, Seibel M, Moses AC, Flier JS. Distribution and characterization of insulin and insulin-like growth factor I receptors in normal human ovary. J Clin Endocrinol Metab 1985; 61:728–34.
24 Nestler JE, Clore JN, Strauss III JF, Blackard WG. The effects of hyperinsulinemia on serum testosterone, progesterone, dehydroepiandrosterone sulfate, and cortisol levels in normal women and in a woman with hyperandrogenism, insulin resistance, and acanthosis nigricans. J Clin Endocrinol Metab 1987; 64:180–4.

25 Stuart CA, Prince NJ, Peters EJ, Meyer WJ. Hyperinsulinemia and hyperandrogenemia: *in vivo* response to insulin infusion. Obstet Gynecol 1987; 69:921–5.
26 Micic D, Popovic V, Nesovic M, Sumarac M, Dragasevic M, Kendereski A, Markovic D, Djordjevic P, Manojlovic D, Micic J. Androgen levels during sequential insulin euglycemic clamp studies in patients with polycystic ovary disease. J Steroid Biochem 1988; 31:995–9.
27 Dunaif A, Graf M. Insulin administration alters gonadal steroid metabolism independent of changes in gonadotropin secretion in insulin-resistant women with the polycystic ovary syndrome. J Clin Invest 1989; 83:23–9.
28 Barbieri RL, Makris A, Randall RW, Daniels G, Kistner RW, Ryan KJ. Insulin stimulates androgen accumulation in incubations of ovarian stroma obtained from women with hyperandrogenism. J Clin Endocrinol Metab 1986; 62:904–10.
29 Nestler JE, Barlascini CO, Matt DW, Steingold KA, Plymate SR, Clore JN, Blackard WG. Suppression of serum insulin by diazoxide reduces serum testosterone levels in obese women with polycystic ovary syndrome. J Clin Endocrinol Metab 1989; 68:1027–32.
30 Nissley SP, Rechler MM. Somatomedin/insulin-like growth factor tissue receptors. Clin Endocrinol Metab 1984; 13:43–67.
31 Plymate SR, Matej LA, Jones RE, Friedl KE. Inhibition of sex hormone-binding globulin production in the human hepatoma (Hep G2) cell line by insulin and prolactin. J Clin Endocrinol Metab 1988; 67:460–4.
32 Haffner SM, Katz MS, Stern MP, Dunn JF. The relationship of sex hormones to hyperinsulinemia and hyperglycemia. Metabolism 1988; 37:683–8.
33 Peiris AN, Sothmann MS, Aiman EJ, Kissebah AH. The relationship of insulin to sex hormone-binding globulin: role of adiposity. Fertil Steril 1989; 52:69–72.
34 Nestler JE, Powers LP, Matt DW, Steingold KA, Plymate SR, Rittmaster RS, Clore JN, Blackard WG. A direct effect of hyperinsulinemia on serum sex hormone-binding globulin levels in obese women with polycystic ovary syndrome. J Clin Endocrinol Metab 1991; 72:83–9.
35 Gulati P. Skett P. The effect of the insulin mediator on the metabolism of androst-4-ene-3,17-dione in isolated rat hepatocytes. Biochem Pharmacol 1989; 38:4415–18.
36 Cara JF, Rosenfield RL. Insulin-like growth factor I and insulin potentiate luteinizing hormone-induced androgen synthesis by rat ovarian thecal-interstitial cells. Endocrinology 1988; 123:733–9.
37 Seppala M, Wahlstrom T, Kosimies AI, Tenhunen A, Rutanen E-M, Koistinen R, Huhtaniemi I, Bohn H, Stenman U-H. Human preovulatory follicular fluid, luteinized cells of hyperstimulated preovulatory follicles, and corpus luteum contain placental protein 12. J Clin Endocrinol Metab 1984; 58:505–10.
38 Baxter RC, Cowell CT. Diurnal rhythm of growth hormone-independent binding protein for insulin-like growth factors in human plasma. J Clin Endocrinol Metab 1987; 62:432–40.
39 Suikkari A-M, Koivisto VA, Rutanen E-M, Yki-Jarvinen H, Karonen S-L, Seppala M. Insulin regulates the serum levels of low molecular weight insulin-like growth factor-binding protein. J Clin Endocrinol Metab 1988; 66:266.
40 Conover CA, Lee PDK. Insulin regulation of insulin-like growth factor-binding protein production in cultured HepG2 cells. J Clin Endocrinol Metab 1990; 70:1062–7.
41 Pekonen F, Laatikainen T, Buyalos R, Rutanen E-M. Decreased 34K insulin-like growth factor binding protein in polycystic ovarian disease. Fertil Steril 1989; 51:972–5.
42 Suikkari A-M, Ruutiainen K, Erkkola R, Seppala M. Low levels of low molecular weight insulin-like growth factor-binding protein in patients with polycystic ovarian disease. Hum Reprod 1989; 4:136–9.
43 Givens JR. Familial polycystic ovarian disease. Endocrinol Metab Clin North Am 1988; 17:771–84.

44 Nestler JE, Usiskin KS, Barlascini CO, Welty DF, Clore JN, Blackard WG. Suppression of serum dehydroepiandrosterone sulfate levels by insulin: an evaluation of possible mechanisms. J Clin Endocrinol Metab 1989; 69:1040–6.
45 Diamond MP, Grainger D, Gill AL, Zych K, Knab G, DeFronzo RA. Exogenous and endogenous elevation of circulating insulin levels are associated with acute reduction in levels of dehydroepiandrosterone sulfate (DHEAS), but not androstenedione (A), testosterone (T), or free testosterone (FT). Scientific program and abstracts for the 36th annual meeting of the Society for Gynecologic Investigation, 1989, p. 293 (Abstract 424).
46 Brooks RV. Androgens: physiology and pathology. In: Makin HLJ, ed. Biochemistry of Steroid Hormones, 2nd edn. Boston: Blackwell Scientific Publications, 1984, pp. 565–94.
47 Abraham GE. Ovarian and adrenal contribution to peripheral androgens during the menstrual cycle. J Clin Endocrinol Metab 1974; 39:340–6.
48 Garzo VG, Dorrington JH. Aromatase activity in human granulosa cells during follicular development and the modulation of follicle-stimulating hormone and insulin. Am J Obstet Gynecol 1984; 148:657–62.
49 Nestler JE. Modulation of aromatase and P450 cholesterol side-chain cleavage enzyme activities of human placental cytotrophoblasts by insulin and insulin-like growth factor I. Endocrinology 1987; 121:1845–52.
50 Erickson GF, Magoffin DA, Cragun JR, Chang RJ. The effects of insulin and insulin-like growth factors-I and -II on estradiol production by granulosa cells of polycystic ovaries. J Clin Endocrinol Metab 1990; 70:894–902.
51 Veldhuis JD, Kolp LA, Toaff ME, Strauss III JF, Demers LM. Mechanisms subserving the trophic actions of insulin on ovarian cells. J Clin Invest 1983; 72:1046–57.
52 Hussin AH, Skett P. The effect of insulin on steroid metabolism in isolated rat hepatocytes. Biochem Pharmacol 1987; 36:3155–9.
53 Pasupuleti V, Horton R. Insulin-like growth factor can alter steroid 5α-reductase activity and formation of dihydrotestosterone in skin. Clin Res 1990; 38:99A (Abstract).
54 Farah MJ, Givens JR, Kitabchi AE. Bimodal correlation between the circulating insulin level and the production rate of dehydroepiandrosterone: positive correlation in controls and negative correlation in the polycystic ovary syndrome with acanthosis nigricans. J Clin Endocrinol Metab 1990; 70:1075–81.

Chapter 23
Acute Augmentation of Plasma Androstenedione and Dehydroepiandrosterone by Euglycemic Insulin Infusion: Evidence for a Direct Effect of Insulin on Ovarian Steroidogenesis

CHARLES A. STUART & MANUBAI NAGAMANI

The association of hyperinsulinemia and hyperandrogenemia in women has been documented by several investigators [1–6]. There is no evidence that excess androgen secretion results in insulin resistance [7,8] but both *in vivo* [9–11] and *in vitro* studies [12–14] have shown that either direct or indirect stimulation of androgen production can be caused by increased insulin concentrations. Studies in normal women and in women with polycystic ovary syndrome (PCO) have demonstrated that euglycemic hyperinsulinemia acutely increased plasma androstenedione [9,11] concentrations without any increase in plasma testosterone [9–11] or dehydroepiandrosterone sulfate (DHEAS) [10,11]. The studies described below evaluate the acute effects of hyperinsulinemia on plasma androgen concentrations in normal women and insulin-resistant women.

Materials and methods

Euglycemic insulin clamp studies

After giving informed written consent, subjects were admitted to the General Clinical Research Center of the University of Texas Medical Branch at Galveston on a protocol approved by the Institutional Review Board. All subjects were maintained on a balanced diet, isocaloric with their customary dietary intake as determined by the research dietitian of the Clinical Research Center. For some of these studies, five-step multidose euglycemic insulin clamp studies were performed using previously described modifications [1,15] of the method of Rizza and coworkers [16]. After a 2-hour baseline period, four sequential, increasing dose, 2-hour insulin infusions were administered at 15, 40, 120, and 240 mU/m^2/min to achieve plasma insulin concentrations of approximately 5, 25, 75, 250 and 750 μU/ml respectively. For other studies, a single primed insulin infusion of 3 hours' duration at 40 or 120 mU/m^2/min was performed after a 2-hour baseline period. The rate of infusion of 15% dextrose was adjusted continuously based on the Biostator Monitor (Ames Instruments, Miles, Indianapolis, IN) glucose readout to maintain the blood glucose at 85 mg/dl during the entire insulin infusion. In the three patients with noninsulin-dependent diabetes mellitus (NIDDM), the insulin infusion was given until euglycemia 85 mg/dl was achieved (20–45 min) and then continued for another 3 hours maintaining euglycemia. Blood was drawn every 10 min from an intermittent sampling line, and glucose was measured with a YSI Glucose analyzer (Yellow Springs Instrument Company, Yellow Springs, OH) as an independent check on the Biostator glucose monitor. Blood was drawn every 10 min during the last 30 min of the baseline and the insulin infusion periods. These four samples from each period were pooled for determination of plasma concentrations of the hormones of interest.

Hormone assays

Plasma androgens were measured by radioimmunoassay of plasma extracts after fractionation by column chromatography as previously described [1]. Luteinizing hormone (LH) and follicle-stimulating hormone (FSH) were measured by radioimmunoassay [17]. Adrenocorticotropic hormone (ACTH) was measured in unextracted plasma as previously described [18]. Cortisol was measured in unextracted plasma by double-antibody radioimmunoassay [19].

Statistics

Comparison of baseline and insulin infusion-related plasma concentrations of hormones were made using the analysis of variance (ANOVA) with repeated measures within groups with Sheffee post hoc test and using Student's t test for comparison between the two groups. All group data are presented as mean ± standard error of the mean, unless otherwise specifically stated.

Results

Effect on androstenedione production in normal women of euglycemic insulin infusions at physiologic and supraphysiologic plasma insulin concentrations

Six normal women were studied after an overnight fast. Table 23.1 contains the plasma concentrations of glucose, insulin, androstenedione, testosterone and cortisol during the five periods of the sequential multi-dose euglycemic clamps. If physiologic plasma insulin concentrations are defined as 5–150 μU/ml based on the insulin concentrations seen in normal subjects in response to a standard meal [20], only plasma androstenedione was significantly augmented at physiologic insulin concentrations (28 and 73 μU/ml). At higher insulin concentrations, the androstenedione concentrations were not different from the baseline value. Plasma cortisol did not change and plasma testosterone tended to decrease (not statistically significant). Whether the decline in plasma androstenedione in periods 4 and 5 are because of a biphasic insulin dose response or a desensitization to insulin related to the duration of the insulin infusion cannot be determined from these data.

The effect of supraphysiologic insulin concentrations on plasma androstenedione and dehydroepiandrosterone (DHEA) in insulin-resistant women

Six women underwent single-dose euglycemic clamp studies with a 2-hour baseline period and a 3-hour insulin infusion at 120 mU/m^2/min. Three of these subjects had NIDDM and three had hirsutism, hyper-

Table 23.1 Androstenedione response to euglycemic hyperinsulinemia in six normal females*.

	Glycemic clamp period				
	1	2	3	4	5
Plasma glucose (mg/ml)	8 ± 1	85 ± 1	86 ± 1	85 ± 1	86 ± 1
Plasma insulin (μU/ml)	9 ± 1	28 ± 2	73 ± 5	246 ± 15	718 ± 5
Plasma androstenedione (ng/ml)	89 ± 10	117 ± 18**	120 ± 22**	101 ± 19	88 ± 13
Plasma testosterone (ng/dl)	37 ± 4	39 ± 5	36 ± 3	32 ± 5	31 ± 4
Plasma cortisol (μg/dl)	7 ± 1	7 ± 2	9 ± 2	9 ± 1	8 ± 1

* All data are mean ± SEM.
** Significantly different from baseline period ($P < 0.05$) by ANOVA paired measures.

androgenemia, and oligomenorrhea. The mean plasma insulin concentration achieved during the infusion was 301 ± 23 μU/ml. Figure 23.1 displays the effect of the insulin infusion on plasma testosterone, androstenedione, and DHEA in these subjects. Plasma testosterone was not altered but androstenedione concentration was augmented to 220% of baseline and DHEA went to 163% of baseline. Plasma cortisol did not change (6 ± 1 μg/dl baseline vs. 8 ± 2 μg/dl during insulin infusion).

The roles of gonadotropins and ACTH in insulin-related augmentation of plasma concentrations of androstenedione and DHEA

During the euglycemic insulin infusions performed in the insulin-resistant subjects described above, potential associated changes in LH, FSH, and ACTH were evaluated. Table 23.2 shows the results of those determinations. The insulin infusion that resulted in acute increases in androstenedione and DHEA had no effect on serum gonadotropins or plasma ACTH, indicating that these pituitary hormones were not mediating the insulin-related augmentation of weak androgen production.

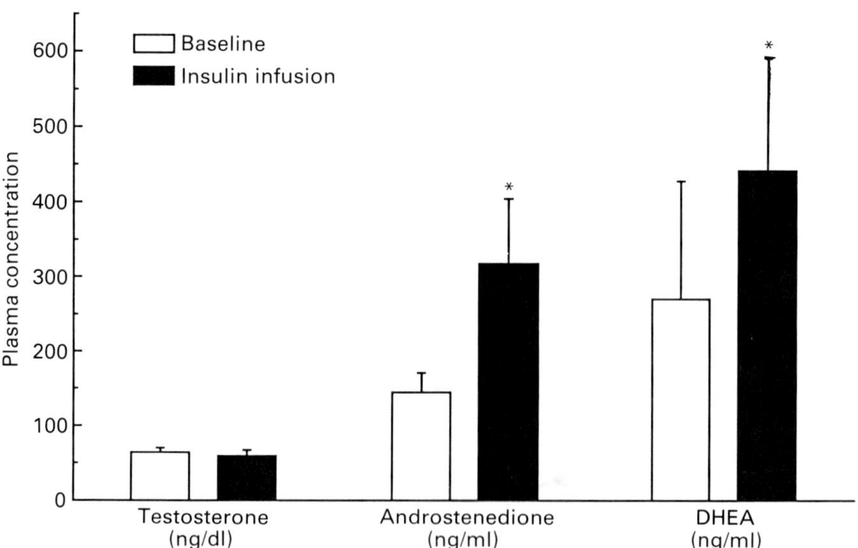

Fig. 23.1 Androgen response to sustained euglycemic hyperinsulinemia in six women with glucose metabolism insulin resistance and hyperinsulinemia. Three women with NIDDM and three with PCO had plasma androgen concentrations quantitated before and during a 3-hour insulin infusion, which achieved an insulin concentration in plasma of 301 μU/ml. The asterisk denotes significant difference from the baseline value ($P < 0.05$, ANOVA, repeated measures).

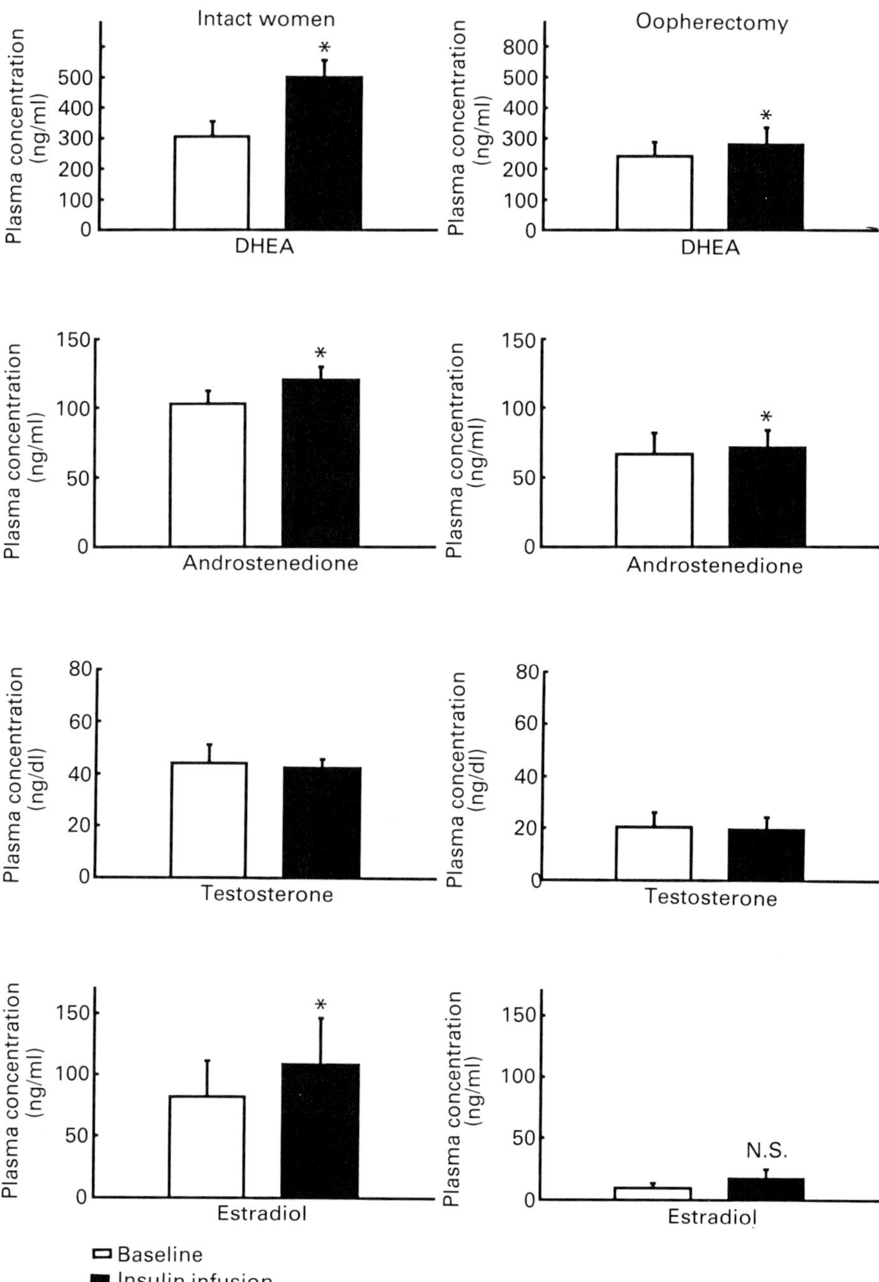

Fig. 23.2 Changes in plasma sex steroids during euglycemic insulin infusion. Five women with surgically removed ovaries and five normal women in the follicular phase of their menstrual cycles were studied with a euglycemic clamp, achieving plasma insulin concentration of 60 μU/ml during the infusion. The asterisk denotes significant difference from the baseline value ($P < 0.05$, ANOVA, repeated measures).

Table 23.2 The effect of insulin infusion on serum concentrations of gonadotropins and plasma ACTH in insulin-resistant females.

	Baseline	Insulin infusion
Serum LH (mIU/ml)	22.8 ± 4.8	23.2 ± 5.6 NS
Serum FSH (mIU/ml)	33.6 ± 14.3	30.1 ± 13.8 NS
Plasma ACTH (pg/ml)	9.8 ± 2.3	11.2 ± 2.6 NS

NS, not significantly different from baseline ($P > 0.05$).

The effect of physiologic increased plasma insulin concentrations on sex steroid production in oophorectomized women

We performed single-dose euglycemic clamp studies on five normal women in the follicular phase of their menstrual cycle and in five women who had undergone bilateral oophorectomy at least 6 weeks previously. None of these women had taken estrogen or progestin-containing medication for at least 3 months prior to study. Insulin concentration was 7 ± 1 μU/ml in the baseline period and achieved 60 ± 5 μU/ml in the insulin infusion period. Figure 23.2 displays the data for the baseline and insulin infusion period for plasma concentrations of DHEA, androstenedione, testosterone, and estradiol. The DHEA and androstenedione concentrations increased in both groups of women. Serum DHEAS was quantitated only in the oophorectomy group and its concentration did not change with insulin infusion (1477 ± 345 pg/ml baseline vs. 1286 ± 242 pg/ml, $P = 0.57$). The baseline concentrations of androstenedione, testosterone, and estradiol, but not that of DHEA, were significantly lower in the oophorectomy group. Estradiol concentration increased with insulin infusion in the intact women but not in the oophorectomy group. The changes above baseline in plasma androstenedione and DHEA due to insulin infusion are shown in Fig. 23.3. In women possessing ovaries, the mean increase in DHEA concentration was five-fold that seen in women without ovaries and the change in androstenedione concentration was nearly four-fold that found in oopherectomy subjects.

Discussion

Hyperinsulinemia is associated with hyperandrogenemia in women with PCO [21,22]. Insulin sensitivity is not altered by either androgen administration [7,8] or androgen suppression [23], suggesting that the

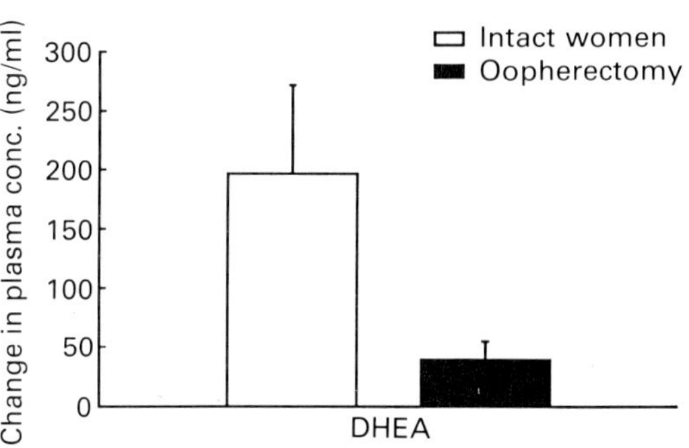

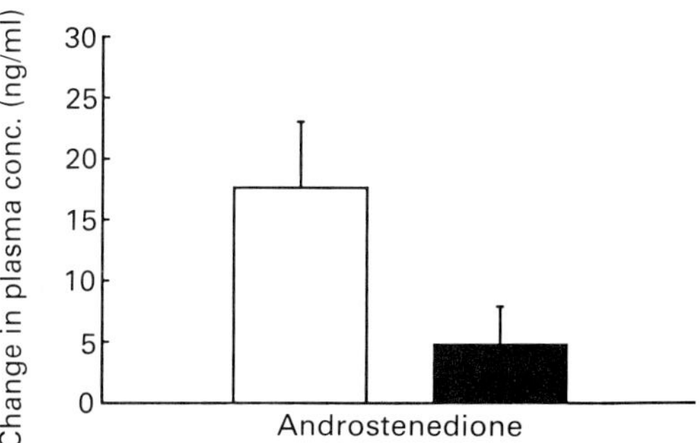

Fig. 23.3 Changes in plasma androstenedione and DHEA during insulin infusion in normal women and women with surgically removed ovaries. The bars represent the calculated change in DHEA or androstenedione occurring during the insulin infusion. The women with adrenal only responded significantly less than those with both adrenals and ovaries intact ($P < 0.01$, independent t test).

hyperandrogenemia of PCO is not the cause of the insulin resistance seen in this condition. On the other hand, administration of insulin acutely results in increased plasma concentrations of androstenedione and DHEA in normal women [1,9,24] and in women with PCO [9,24]. The augmented secretion of weak androgens occurs in the absence of acute changes in either plasma testosterone or serum DHEAS concentrations [9–11].

In vitro studies have demonstrated insulin effects directly on ovarian tissue and on pituitary gonadotropin release. Adashi and coworkers showed insulin in culture media increases cultured pituitary cell release of LH [12]. Augmentation of ovarian stromal tissue production of androgens by insulin was documented by Barbieri *et al.* [14]. Thus, it is possible that the *in vivo* effects of insulin infusion could be due to stimulation of pituitary release of gonadotropins or direct stimulation of androgen production in the peripheral target gland. These current studies and those of Dunaif and Graf [11] have shown that the augmented androgen production occurs in the absence of any increase in gonadotropins. We also demonstrated that insulin augmentation of plasma androgens was not associated with increased pituitary ACTH release, excluding an indirect adrenal effect mediated via pituitary ACTH.

The specific biochemical steps in steroidogenesis modulated by insulin that are responsible for these *in vivo* observations are not known. Cholesterol uptake in bovine adrenal cells *in vitro* is stimulated by insulin in the culture medium [25]. Enhanced cholesterol uptake could increase steroid production solely by increased intracellular substrate availability. Insulin may modulate the activity of production of key steroidogenic enzymes (see Chapters 7 and 9) such as 3β-hydroxysteroid dehydrogenase, 17α-hydroxylase, or 17,20-lyase, and thus result in increased production of the enzyme products. Stimulation of early synthetic enzymes but not later steps is consistent with insulin's acute increase in DHEA and androstenedione production without an increase in the subsequent products, DHEAS and testosterone. An insulin effect only on cholesterol availability would be expected to increase the products at each subsequent enzymatic step. The lack of plasma testosterone concentration augmentation by insulin may be related to the majority of testosterone production occurring by peripheral conversion of androstenedione to testosterone outside the ovary and adrenal [26]. Plasma estradiol was acutely augmented by insulin infusion only in women with intact ovaries, consistent with a direct insulin effect on ovarian aromatase activity as previously shown by Garzo and Dorrington *in vitro* [27].

Steroid hormones, unlike peptide hormones, are not stored in substantial quantities in the cell where they are produced. Instead, steroid hormones are rapidly released as soon as they are synthesized. Changes in plasma concentrations of steroid hormones can be due to alteration in either production or plasma clearance. The steroid hormone clearance rates, however, were not directly measured.

The data from oophorectomized women showed a substantial decrease in DHEA response to insulin when compared with the results from intact women with both adrenal and ovaries present. Even though DHEA production is 5–10-fold higher in the adrenal than the ovary and the baseline DHEA concentration was only 20% decreased, insulin-related augmentation of plasma DHEA was fivefold higher in women with ovaries. These data suggest the basal production of DHEA is mostly from the adrenal, but the acute insulin augmentation is predominantly an ovarian effect.

These studies demonstrate that acute increases in plasma concentrations of androstenedione and DHEA occur with sustained physiologic insulin concentrations. In normal women, significant augmentation occurs at 30–75 μU/ml insulin, but not at supraphysiologic concentrations in excess of 300 μU/ml. Patients with resistance to insulin effects on glucose metabolism (PCO and NIDDM patients) have androgen responses to insulin concentration as high as 275 μU/ml but not at 750–10 000 μU/ml [9]. The increases in androstenedione and DHEA during euglycemic insulin infusions are not accompanied by increases in gonadotropins or ACTH, indicating that the effects are not mediated via the pituitary. These data do not exclude a permissive effect of gonadotropins or ACTH on peripheral direct response in the ovaries or adrenals. The comparison of insulin responsiveness of sex steroids in oophorectomized women and normal intact women suggests that both adrenal and ovary respond acutely to hyperinsulinemia, but the ovary is the predominant target tissue. These data demonstrating moderate increases in weak androgen production by physiologically achieved insulin concentrations suggest that hyperinsulinemia caused by glucose metabolism insulin resistance, due to diverse metabolic defects, may commonly play a role in the development or progression of PCO.

References

1 Stuart CA, Peters EJ, Prince MJ, Richards G, Cavalla A, Meyer WJ. Insulin resistance with acanthosis nigricans: the roles of obesity and androgen excess. Metabolism 1986; 35:197–205.

2 Burghen GA, Givens JR, Kitabchi AE. Correlation of hyperandrogenism with hyperinsulinism in polycystic ovarian disease. J Clin Endocrinol Metab 1980; 50:113–16.

3 Chang RJ, Nakamura RM, Judd HL, Kaplan SA. Insulin resistance in nonobese patients with polycystic ovarian disease. J Clin Endocrinol Metab 1983; 57:356–9.

4 Pasquali R, Casimirri F, Venturoli S, Paradisi R, Mattioli L, Capelli M, Melchionda N, Labo G. Insulin resistance in patients with polycystic ovaries: its relationship to body weight and androgen levels. Acta Endocrinol 1983; 104:110–16.

5 Shoupe D, Kumar DD, Lobo RA. Insulin resistance in polycystic ovary syndrome. Am J Obstet Gynecol 1983; 147:588–91.

6 Nagamani M, Dinh TV, Kelver ME. Hyperinsulinemia in hyperthecosis of the ovaries. Am J Obstet Gynecol 1986; 154:384–9.

7 Billiar RB, Richardson D, Schwartz R, Posner B, Little B. Effect of chronically elevated androgen or estrogen on the glucose tolerance test and insulin response in female rhesus monkeys. Am J Obstet Gynecol 1987; 157:1297–302.

8 Dunaif A, Graf M, Mandel J, Laumas V, Dobrjansky A. Characterization of groups of hyperandrogenic women with acanthosis nigricans, impaired glucose tolerance, and/or hyperinsulinemia. J Clin Endocrinol Metab 1987; 65:499–507.

9 Stuart CA, Prince MJ, Peters EJ, Meyer WJ. Hyperinsulinemia and hyperandrogenemia: androgen response to insulin infusion. Obstet Gynecol 1987; 69:921–5.

10 Nestler JE, Clore JN, Strauss JF, Blackard WG. The effects of hyperinsulinemia on serum testosterone, progesterone, dehydroepiandrosterone sulfate, and cortisol levels in normal women and in a woman with hyperandrogenemia, insulin resistance, and acanthosis nigricans. J Clin Endocrinol Metab 1987; 64:180–4.

11 Dunaif A, Graf M. Insulin administration alters gonadal steroid metabolism independent of changes in gonadotropin secretion in insulin-resistant women with the polycystic ovary syndrome. J Clin Invest 1989; 83:23–9.

12 Adashi EY, Hsueh AJW, Yen D. Insulin enhancement of luteinizing hormone and follicle-stimulating hormone release by cultured pituitary cells. Endocrinology 1981; 108:1441–9.
13 Van Houten M, Posner BI, Kopriwa BM, Brawer JR. Insulin binding sites localized to nerve terminals in rat median eminence and arcuate nucleus. Science 1980; 207:1081–3.
14 Barbieri RL, Makris A, Randall RW, Daniels G, Kistner RW, Ryan KJ. Insulin stimulates androgen accumulation in incubations of ovarian stroma obtained from women with hyperandrogenism. J Clin Endocrinol Metab 1986; 62:904–10.
15 Stuart CA, Shangraw RE, Prince MJ, Peters EJ, Wolfe RR. Bedrest-induced insulin resistance occurs primarily in muscle. Metabolism 1988; 37:802–6.
16 Rizza RA, Mandarino LJ, Gerich JE. Dose–response characteristics for effects of insulin on production and utilization of glucose in man. Am J Physiol 1981; 240:E630–E639.
17 Odell WD, Rayford PL, Ross GT. Simplified, partially automated method for radioimmunoassay of human thyroid-stimulating, growth, luteinizing and follicle-stimulating hormones. J Lab Clin Med 1967; 70:973–9.
18 Nicholson WE, Davis DR, Sherell BJ, Orth DN. Rapid radioimmunoassay for corticotropin in unextracted human plasma. Clin Chem 1984; 30:259–65.
19 Murphy BE. Some studies of the protein binding of steroids and their application to the reactive micro and ultramicro measurement of various steroids in body fluids by competitive protein binding radioassay. J Clin Endocrinol Metab 1967; 27:913–29.
20 Genuth SM. Plasma insulin and glucose profiles in normal, obese, and diabetic persons. Ann Intern Med 1973; 79:812–22.
21 Barbieri RL, Smith S, Ryan KJ. The role of hyperinsulinemia in the pathogenesis of ovarian hyperandrogenism. Fertil Steril 1988; 50:197–212.
22 Poretsky L, Kalin MF. The gonadotropic function of insulin. Endocr Rev 1987; 8:132–41.
23 Geffner ME, Kaplan SA, Bersch N, Golde DW, Landow EM, Chang RJH. Persistence of insulin resistance in polycystic ovarian disease after inhibition of ovarian steroid secretion. Fertil Steril 1986; 45:327–33.
24 Prince MJ, Meyer WJ, Smith ER, Stuart CA. Androgen response to insulin infusion is pituitary independent. The Endocrine Society 70th Annual Meeting, 1988, Abstract 749.
25 Ill CR, Lipine J, Gospodarowicz D. Permissive effect of insulin on the adenosine 3′,5′ monophosphate-dependent, up-regulation of low density lipoprotein receptors and the stimulation of steroid release in bovine adrenal cortical cells. Endocrinology 1984; 114:767–75.
26 Judd HL, Yen SAC. Serum androstenedione and testosterone levels during the menstrual cycle. J Clin Endocrinol Metab 1973; 36:475–81.
27 Garzo VG, Dorrington JH. Aromatase activity in human granulosa cells during follicular development and the modulation by follicle-stimulating hormone and insulin. Am J Obstet Gynecol 1984; 148:657–62.

Chapter 24

The Role of Testosterone and Dehydroepiandrosterone on Insulin Resistance and Sensitivity in Hyperandrogenic Females: Use of Activated T-lymphocytes as an *In Vitro* Study Model and its Correlation to *In Vivo* Studies

ABBAS E. KITABCHI, CYNTHIA K. BUFFINGTON, JAMES R. GIVENS & HIROSHI INOUYE

The triad of polycystic ovary syndrome (PCO), acanthosis nigricans, and insulin resistance was first described by Givens *et al.* [1] in a teenage girl with luteoma in 1974 and was further substantiated and classified by Kahn *et al.* [2] in 1976. In 1980, we demonstrated the existence of significant positive correlations between plasma insulin and the two gonadal androgens, testosterone and androstenedione [3]. The direct relationships between hyperinsulinemia and elevated testosterone levels in females has since been shown by others [4–9] and found to hold true with free testosterone as well [10,11]. These studies would suggest that the degree of insulin resistance associated with PCO is dependent upon the severity of each individual's hyperandrogenemic state.

Understanding the etiology of the association between insulin resistance and hyperandrogenemia is of clinical importance for appropriate treatment of the syndrome. Thus, in patients with PCO, insulin may play a role in the pathogenesis of ovarian hyperandrogenism or androgens may lead to hyperinsulinemia. Evidence to suggest that androgens may induce insulin resistance has been provided by studies that have shown that administration of testosterone or its derivatives results in impairment in glucose tolerance and causes hyperinsulinemia in women [12,13], in male athletes [14], in aplastic anemic patients [15] and in laboratory rats [16] (see Chapter 30). Recent evidence, however, suggests that insulin may enhance androgen production. Hyperandrogenemia has been described in hyperinsulinemic, insulin-resistant patients with disorders other than PCO. Furthermore, insulin resistance has been found to persist in PCO patients following surgery or treatment which results in normalization of androgens [17–20]. The manner in which hyperinsulinemia may increase plasma androgen levels in females has not been clearly delineated. However, as is presented elsewhere in this book (see Chapter 18), insulin and insulin-like growth factor I (IGF-I) have been found to enhance ovarian steroidogenesis *in vitro* [21]. Thus, there is evidence that insulin may cause hyperandrogenemia and that androgens may induce insulin resistance. However, it remains unknown if the relationship between androgens and insulin is one of the former stimulating the latter or vice versa. In fact both relationships may exist with different degrees of involvement.

Although the above studies would suggest that insulin resistance is universally associated with hyperandrogenemia, we have recently identified a group of females with an adrenal source of excessive androgens, i.e. elevated dehydroepiandrosterone (DHEA), dehydroepiandrosterone sulfate (DHEAS), who do not have insulin resistance in spite of the fact they are obese and hypertestosteronemic [6]. Furthermore, we found, upon examining basal and glucose-challenged insulin in a large group of women with varying levels of adrenal androgens, that insulin levels were negatively correlated to DHEAS and positively correlated to each individual's erythrocyte insulin binding [6]. Recent studies by Barbieri and associates [8,21] have also demonstrated negative correlations between insulin levels and DHEA in women with PCO. These data would suggest that insulin may regulate DHEA or the reverse.

In support of a role of insulin in modulating plasma concentrations of DHEA (see Chapters 22 and 23), we have recently shown in control and PCO patients a bimodal relationship between basal insulin and DHEA production rates (PR) [22]. We found positive correlations between insulin and DHEA PR in patients with insulin levels $<40\,\mu U/ml$ and negative correlations between DHEA PR and insulin at levels $>40\,\mu U/ml$. Additionally, in our hyperinsulinemic subjects, we found that the metabolic clearance rates (MCR) of DHEA were maximally enhanced. We concluded that the elevated MCR and reduced PR of DHEA of our PCO patients was largely responsible for their low levels of plasma DHEA. *In vitro*, bimodal actions of insulin on androgen production by bovine adrenal cells have likewise been demonstrated [23]. These observations would suggest a functional role of insulin in regulating circulating levels of DHEA.

Negative correlations between DHEA and insulin may suggest that DHEA affects insulin levels. In regard to a role of DHEA in altering insulin, we have found that female patients with high DHEA have low insulin and enhanced insulin binding to their erythrocytes [6]. Other investigators [24–28] using various insulin-resistant animal models have shown that chronic oral administration of DHEA has certain salutary effects on insulin sensitivity, as determined by improved glucose tolerance and reduced insulin levels. Nestler *et al.* [29] have recently found no changes in glucose disposal following DHEA treatment in young, healthy males, and Mortola and Yen [30] found deterioration of insulin sensitivity along with elevated testosterone and dihydrotestosterone levels following oral DHEA administration in postmenopausal females. However, a lack of a positive finding for males as compared to premenopausal females may be gender related and differences between DHEA actions on insulin sensitivity in premenopausal vs. postmenopausal females may involve variations in the metabolic fate of androgens [31,32] or the ratios of DHEA to testosterone and/or dihydrotestosterone. Furthermore, whether DHEA modulation of insulin via improved insulin sensitivity, which is observed in hyperandrogenic females, also occurs in normal subjects remains unclear.

From our studies [3,6] showing negative correlations between DHEA and insulin and positive correlations between testosterone and insulin we have hypothesized that the severity of the insulin-resistant state that is associated with hyperandrogenemia in women is dependent upon the origin of androgen excess, i.e. ovarian vs. adrenal. If this assumption is correct, it follows that levels of DHEA and testosterone and/or the ratios of DHEA/testosterone may be important determinants of insulin sensitivity in women in general, and in patients with hyperandrogenism in particular. To test this hypothesis, we embarked on a rather ambitious plan to examine the relationships between hyperandrogenemia of ovarian and adrenal origin and insulin sensitivity, as assessed by both *in vivo* and *in vitro* parameters. Our study approach has depended not only on selection of specific types of study patients, i.e. those with elevated adrenal androgens vs. those with high testosterone, but also on appropriate selection of insulin-sensitive tissue for both *in vitro* and *in vivo* assessment of insulin sensitivity.

Our search for the selection of an appropriate tissue that would permit simultaneous measurement of both insulin receptor and post-receptor events led us to test the feasibility of using phytohemagglutinin (PHA)-activated T-lymphocytes as a model for studies of insulin resistance and hyperandrogenemia. Circulating T-lymphocytes are a readily available tissue comprising over 85% of the mononuclear population. These cells have both IGF-I and IGF-II receptors [33,34] and, when activated in culture with mitogens or antigens, develop insulin receptors [35–38]. The T-lymphocyte insulin receptor in activated cells, similar to other insulin-sensitive tissue, is subject to down-regulation by insulin

[39] and is highly reflective of both acute (i.e. starvation, insulin infusion) and chronic *in vivo* insulin levels [40–42]. Along with the emergence of the insulin receptor, these cells develop the ability to degrade insulin [38] and to form certain intermediate products of insulin degradation similar to those identified and characterized in other insulin-sensitive tissues [43,44]. Furthermore, along with the development of the insulin receptor, T-lymphocytes become responsive to insulin with regard to glucose and amino acid uptakes [39,45], glucose oxidation [39,45], and pyruvate dehydrogenase (PDH) sensitivity to insulin [38].

In a previous study [46], we examined the appropriateness of using activated T-lymphocytes as a model to identify mechanisms underlying the insulin-resistant state of patients with PCO. Our study population consisted of PCO patients with acanthosis nigricans and basal and glucose-challenged insulin levels 10-fold above those values observed in a group of weight-matched controls. All our PCO patients were hypertestosteronemic and half of these subjects, in addition to being hyperandrogenic, were also diabetic. T-lymphocyte insulin binding in both groups of PCO patients was reduced approximately 45% below weight-matched control values. Similar defects in insulin binding were found with the patients' erythrocytes. From the insulin displacement curves of both types of cell lines, we concluded that the insulin receptor defect found in these patients occurred primarily as a result of a decrease in receptor number rather than a change in binding affinity. Furthermore, we found in our PCO and control subjects that activated T-lymphocyte insulin binding was inversely correlated to each individual's basal insulin ($r = -0.75$) and positively and significantly correlated to erythrocyte insulin binding ($r = +0.85$, $P < 0.001$). Thus, T-lymphocyte insulin binding in these patients' cells was not only reflective of binding activities in other tissue but also recognized each individual's *in vivo* insulin levels.

In the series of studies described above, the activation state of PDH and its responsiveness to insulin were investigated. We found that the activation state of PDH in the absence of insulin was elevated above control values in patients with PCO and normal glucose tolerance, which we hypothesized may be due to their elevated ambient insulin. Maximal enzyme responses to insulin were similar between non-diabetic PCO patients and weight-matched controls. However, PDH responses to submaximal and maximal concentrations of insulin were blunted in our PCO patients with diabetes. When we examined the relationship between oral glucose tolerance test (OGTT) glucose area under the curve and maximal insulin-stimulated PDH responsiveness of all our study subjects, we found a strong negative correlation ($r = -0.87$, $P < 0.001$) showing that the greater the glucose intolerance of an individual, the more severe the impairment in PDH responsiveness. These results would suggest that lesions at the level of the receptor are primarily responsible for the insulin resistance of our particular population of PCO patients but that both receptor and postreceptor defects (i.e. PDH responsiveness to insulin) contribute to the insulin-resistant state of PCO patients with noninsulin-dependent diabetes mellitus (NIDDM). Furthermore, these studies suggest that activated human T-lymphocytes not only recognize ambient insulin levels of the original donor but the individual's glycemic status as well.

Based on the above data, we elected to use T-lymphocytes as one of our *in vitro* tissue models for studies of insulin sensitivity in patients with hyperandrogenemia of ovarian or adrenal origin [47]. Our study population included: (i) eight women with adrenal hyperplasia (AH) and elevated levels of DHEA, DHEAS; (ii) nine patients with PCO, hypertestosteronemia, acanthosis nigricans, and normal luteinizing hormone (LH) and follicle-stimulating hormone (FSH); (iii) eight obese, weight-matched controls (OC); and (iv) six lean normal controls (LC). The PCO group presented with obesity, extreme hyperinsulinemia, acanthosis nigricans, hypertestosteronemia, normal LH and FSH levels, and reduced levels of DHEA, DHEAS. Of these individuals, two were diabetic and two were glucose intolerant as defined by criteria established by the Diabetes Data Group [48] for glucose values following oral glucose challenge. The second group of hyperandrogenic patients presented with obesity, normal basal insulin levels, and elevated adrenal androgens. Of the adrenal hyperandrogenic group, three patients were diagnosed as having adrenal hyperplasia resulting from 21-hydroxylase deficiency and five subjects had elevated DHEA levels due to 3β-hydroxylase-Δ^5-steroid dehydrogenase deficiency. The study population provided us with testosterone levels which ranged from 17 to 239 ng/dl and DHEA values from 113 to 2211 ng/dl. Body mass indices (kg/m^2) were 20.3 ± 1.0, 35.2 ± 2.1, 35.6 ± 5.4, and 39.0 ± 1.7 for the LC, OC, AH, and PCO groups, respectively, and did not significantly differ between the obese groups. *In vivo* insulin sensitivity was assessed by OGTT, insulin/glucose (I/G) ratios, basal insulin, insulin under the OGTT curve (AUC), and hypoglycemic responses to a standard dose of i.v. insulin. *In vitro*, we examined insulin binding to erythrocytes and PHA-activated T-lymphocytes of the study subjects, and additional studies were conducted to examine the direct *in vitro* effects of DHEA and testosterone on T-lymphocyte insulin binding and pyruvate flux.

Figure 24.1 shows the androgen levels of patients in each of the

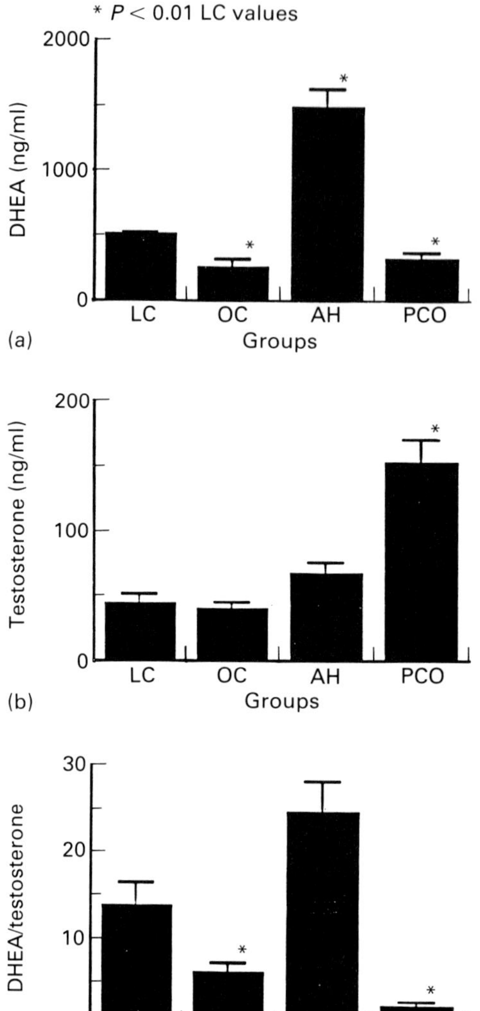

Fig. 24.1 Levels of DHEA (a), testosterone (b), and ratios of DHEA/testosterone (c) of the study population. Values represent the mean ± SEM of 6 LC, 8 OC, 8 AH, and 9 PCO subjects.

study groups. Patients with PCO had testosterone levels (Fig. 24.1a) higher than, and DHEA levels (Fig. 24.1b) lower than, LC values. Due to both their high testosterone and low DHEA levels, DHEA/testosterone ratios (Fig. 24.1c) in the PCO group were less than 20% those of the LC group. The OC females, with low levels of circulating DHEA, also had DHEA/testosterone ratios significantly below LC values. The AH patients had DHEA levels nearly threefold above the average values of the LC group but because of the variability in their testosterone levels, DHEA/

testosterone ratios did not significantly differ from those of the lean controls.

The various *in vivo* indices of insulin sensitivity, i.e. basal insulin, insulin AUC, basal and OGTT I/G ratios, of the study groups are shown in Fig. 24.2a–d. Patients with PCO were clearly insulin resistant with all parameters of insulin sensitivity measuring 7–10-fold above control values. The AH patients had lower basal and glucose-challenged insulin levels and I/G ratios than their weight-matched controls. In fact, the obese AH patients' insulin levels and I/G indices were comparable to LC values. This was also true fot the AH group's hypoglycemic responses to 0.15 U/kg i.v. insulin where glucose levels fell from 87 to 34 mg/dl in contrast to a change of 103 to 75 mg/dl for patients with PCO.

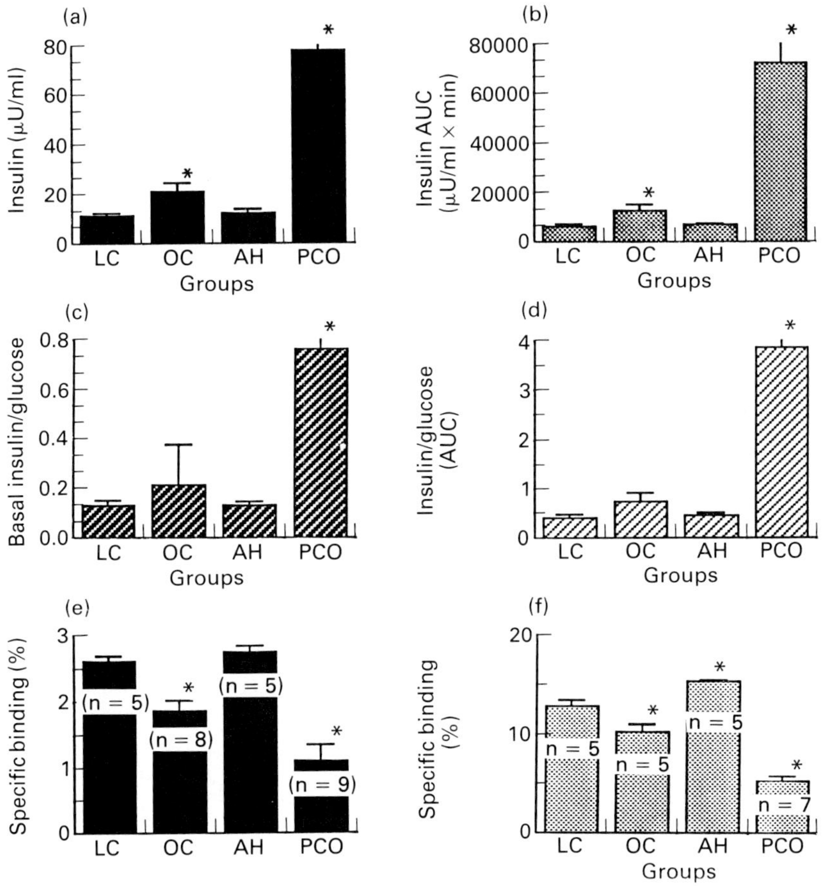

Fig. 24.2 Parameters of insulin sensitivity. Values represent the mean ±SEM of basal insulin levels (a), insulin AUC (b), basal I/G (c), and I/G AUC (d) of 6 LC, 8 OC, 8 AH, and 9 PCO subjects. Average insulin binding activities in T-lymphocytes (e) and erythrocytes (f) are for the number of subjects indicated. $P < 0.05$ LC values.

In vitro, we examined insulin sensitivity at both the receptor and postreceptor levels of insulin action by studying insulin binding and postbinding events in T-lymphocytes and erythrocytes of our study subjects. As seen in Fig. 24.2d, insulin binding to T-lymphocytes of PCO patients was 40% below OC values and 60% below binding activities of the LC group. Insulin binding to T-lymphocytes of the AH patients was comparable to LC values and significantly above binding activities of their weight-matched controls ($P < 0.01$). Insulin binding to erythrocytes was likewise dramatically impaired in patients with PCO (Fig. 24.2e) and significantly above the LC values in cells of the AH patients. From the insulin displacement curves shown in Fig. 24.3a, the higher binding activities in erythrocytes of the AH subjects appeared to occur secondary to an increase in binding affinity. The amount of insulin that produced half-maximal displacement of ^{125}I-labeled insulin from erythrocytes of the AH subjects was 11 ng/ml as compared with 30 and 31 ng/ml for the LC and OC groups, respectively. In contrast, half-maximal radiolabeled insulin displacement in PCO cells occurred with an insulin concentration nearly identical to that of the OC and LC groups, i.e. 31 ng/ml. These observations would suggest that in PCO subjects, impairments in insulin binding are due to a decrease in receptor number rather than to a defect in binding affinity. Furthermore, the data demonstrate that PCO patients have a lesion at the level of the insulin receptor that is not present in patients with hyperandrogenism of adrenal origin.

In addition to defects in insulin binding, insulin resistance may occur if there is an interruption in the transmission of signals responsible for initiation of the cellular responses to insulin. As insulin-mediated activation of receptor tyrosine kinase is believed to represent an important step in generation of the signal(s) responsible for insulin postbinding events [49], impairments in these activities may lead to insulin resistance. With regard to this, reduction in insulin receptor tyrosine kinase activities has been identified in erythrocytes, fibroblasts, monocytes, and Epstein–Barr virus-transformed lymphocytes [50–54] of patients with syndromes of extreme insulin resistance and hyperandrogenism. We have also found impairments in insulin receptor kinase activities in erythrocytes of hypertestosteronemic patients with PCO. As is shown in Fig. 24.3b, basal kinase activities in partially isolated receptors of three PCO subjects was 56% of those values observed in receptors from erythrocytes of three obese controls, i.e. 5.18 ± 0.43 vs. 9.03 ± 0.78, respectively. Kinase responsiveness to insulin in erythrocytes of PCO-1 was similar proportionately to that of the obese controls. However, insulin responsiveness was blunted in PCO-2 and nearly negligible in erythrocytes of PCO-3. Interestingly, PCO-1 had normal glycemic

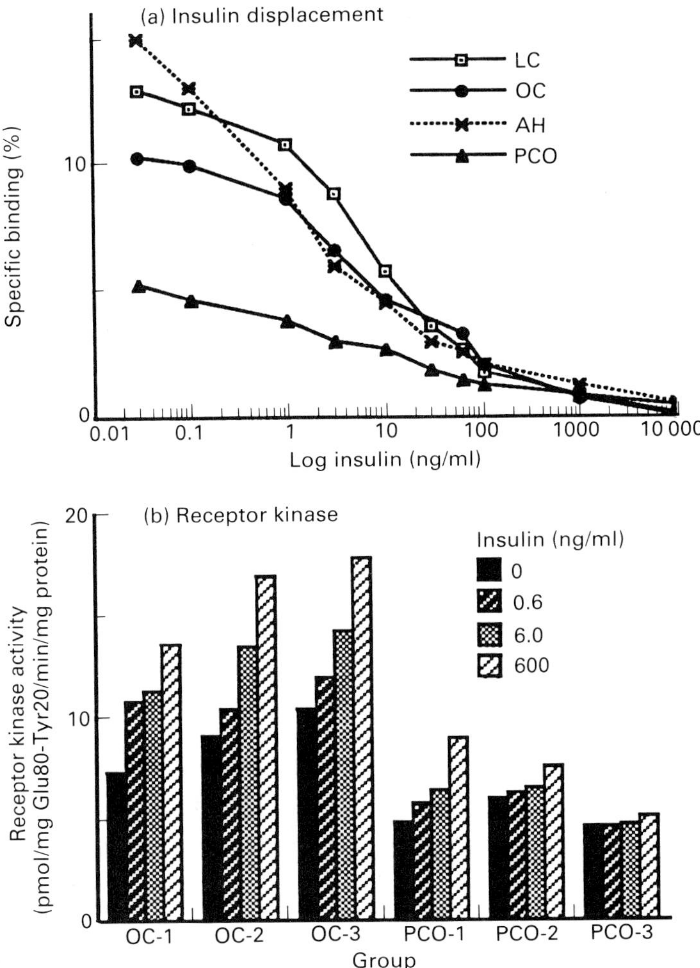

Fig. 24.3 Erythrocyte insulin displacement and receptor kinase activities. (a) shows the displacement of ^{125}I-labeled insulin by unlabeled insulin at concentrations ranging from 0.1 to 10 000 ng/dl. Each point is the average binding activities of 5 LC, 5 OC, 5 AH, and 7 PCO subjects. (b) shows basal and insulin-stimulated receptor kinase activities of partially isolated erythrocyte receptors of 3 OC subjects and 3 patients with PCO.

responses to oral glucose challenge whereas PCO-2 was glucose intolerant and PCO-3 was diabetic.

In previous studies, we [55,56] and others [57] have provided evidence to suggest that certain products of insulin degradation may be important in initiating specific biologic events of insulin action. With regard to insulin degradation, we have measured the percentage of bound insulin degraded in activated T-lymphocytes of our hyperandrogenic patients and their weight-matched and lean controls. We found that the percentage of bound insulin that was degraded over a 30-min period in cells of the LC, OC, PCO, and AH groups were 61%, 45%, 22%, and 62%, respectively. Insulin degradation was significantly below LC values in cells of the OC group ($P < 0.01$) and dramatically impaired in cells of patients with PCO ($P < 0.0001$). In AH patients, insulin degradation was above OC values and comparable to LC degradative activities. Thus, it is possible that one mechanism of increased sensitivity in the AH groups may involve increased production of biologically active insulin degradation products possibly brought about by DHEA-mediated activation of insulin degrading enzyme.

At the postreceptor level of insulin action, insulin resistance may occur secondary to impairments in key regulatory enzymes of glucose metabolism, i.e. glycogen synthase and/or PDH. Podskalny and Kahn [58] have shown in fibroblasts of two type A patients defects in insulin-mediated glycogen synthase and we have found impairments in T-lymphocyte PDH insulin responsiveness in PCO patients with diabetes [46]. When we examined PDH in patients with elevated testosterone vs. those with elevated DHEA, we found that PDH insulin sensitivity was reduced in PCO cells but enhanced above normal control levels in cells of the AH patients [47]. Thus, in obese patients with adrenal hyper-androgenemia both receptor and postreceptor events of insulin action are more sensitive to insulin than in their weight-matched controls. In contrast, PCO patients with high testosterone have defects in both receptor and postreceptor events of insulin action that are more severe than can be explained by their obesity alone.

The *in vivo* and *in vitro* studies described above may suggest that DHEA and testosterone have opposing actions on insulin sensitivity. To test this assumption we have (i) examined the relationships between the various *in vivo* and *in vitro* indices of insulin sensitivity with each individual's level of DHEA and testosterone and (ii) studied the direct *in vitro* effects of DHEA and testosterone on insulin action. Table 24.1 reports the correlation coefficients of these various interrelationships. As can be seen, basal and glucose-challenged insulin levels and I/G indices were positively correlated to testosterone and negatively correlated to DHEA and to the DHEA/testosterone ratios. T-lymphocyte and erythrocyte insulin binding were positively correlated to DHEA and DHEA/testosterone ratios and negatively correlated to testosterone levels. As is schematically illustrated by Fig. 24.4a, the relationship between testosterone and the various indices of insulin sensitivity were exponential such that there was relatively little change in insulin sensitivity with testosterone levels within the normal range, i.e. 20–60 ng/dl.

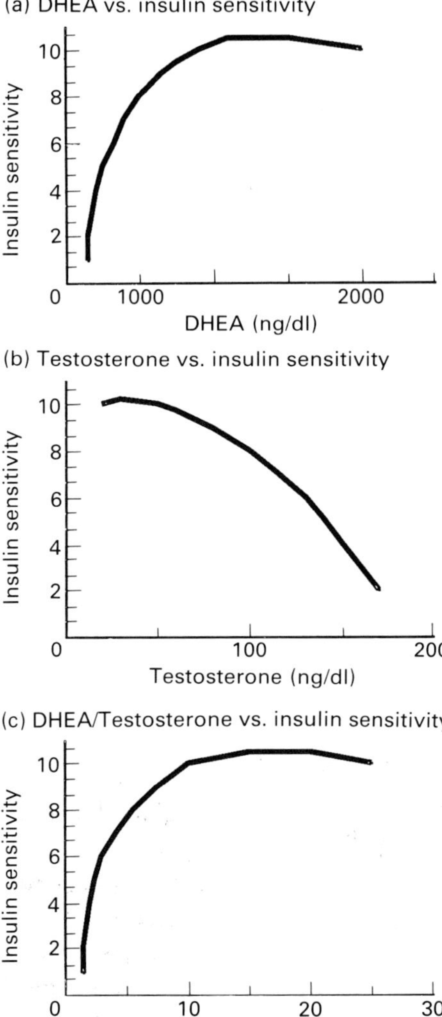

Fig. 24.4 Schematic representation of the relationships between insulin sensitivity and levels of DHEA (a), testosterone (b), and the ratios of DHEA/testosterone (c). The various parameters of insulin sensitivity, i.e. basal insulin, insulin AUC, I/G, I/G AUC, erythrocyte and T-lymphocyte insulin binding, are rated on a scale of 1 to 10 with a score of 1 representing the greatest impairments in these and a score of 10 representing the highest insulin sensitivities.

However, the more severe the individual's hypertestosteronemic state, the more severe their insulin resistance. The relationships between insulin sensitivity and DHEA and/or the ratio of DHEA/testosterone were logarithmic such that in either control or PCO patients small changes in DHEA or DHEA/testosterone were associated with relatively major changes in insulin sensitivity. As reported in Table 24.1, the various parameters of insulin sensitivity were highly correlated to the ratios of DHEA/testosterone with insulin sensitivity at its peak in subjects with ratios of 10 or greater (Fig. 24.4c). These results would suggest

Table 24.1 Insulin sensitivity vs. DHEA (D)/Testosterone (T).

Correlates	r
Basal insulin vs. D/T	−0.76
Basal insulin vs. T	0.73
Basal insulin vs. D	−0.43
Insulin/glucose vs. D/T	−0.75
Insulin/glucose vs. T	0.72
Insulin/glucose vs. D	−0.42
Insulin AUC vs. D/T	−0.81
Insulin AUC vs. T	0.78
Insulin AUC vs. D	−0.45
Insulin/glucose AUC vs. D/T	−0.77
Insulin/glucose AUC vs. T	0.76
Insulin/glucose AUC vs. D	−0.42
T-lymphocyte binding vs. D/T	0.85
T-lymphocyte binding vs. T	−0.63
T-lymphocyte binding vs. D	0.57
Erythrocyte binding vs. D/T	0.91
Erythrocyte binding vs. T	−0.74
Erythrocyte binding vs. D	0.64

that in the female population in general, the ratio of DHEA/testosterone may be an important modulator of insulin sensitivity.

In an attempt to examine the direct effects of androgens on insulin action, we studied changes in T-lymphocyte insulin binding and pyruvate flux in response to DHEA, testosterone, or the combination of the two (Fig. 24.5a). In previous studies, we have found that DHEA enhances T-lymphocyte insulin binding in a time- and dose-dependent fashion [59]. Figure 24.5a shows that DHEA, at a concentration often found in patients with adrenal hyperandrogenemia (1500 ng/dl), significantly stimulates insulin binding in T-lymphocytes of three insulin-resistant PCO patients and three weight-matched controls. Preincubation of cells with testosterone (100 ng/dl) caused little change in binding activities. However, with coincubation of testosterone and DHEA, insulin binding to PHA-activated T-lymphocytes of the control subjects was reduced to values comparable to those found in cells incubated without androgen addition. In PCO subjects, incubation of their cells with DHEA and testosterone reduced binding activities to values 25–40% below those of cells treated with vehicle alone. These observations along with the relatively strong relationships we found between insulin binding and ratios of DHEA/testosterone would suggest that testosterone

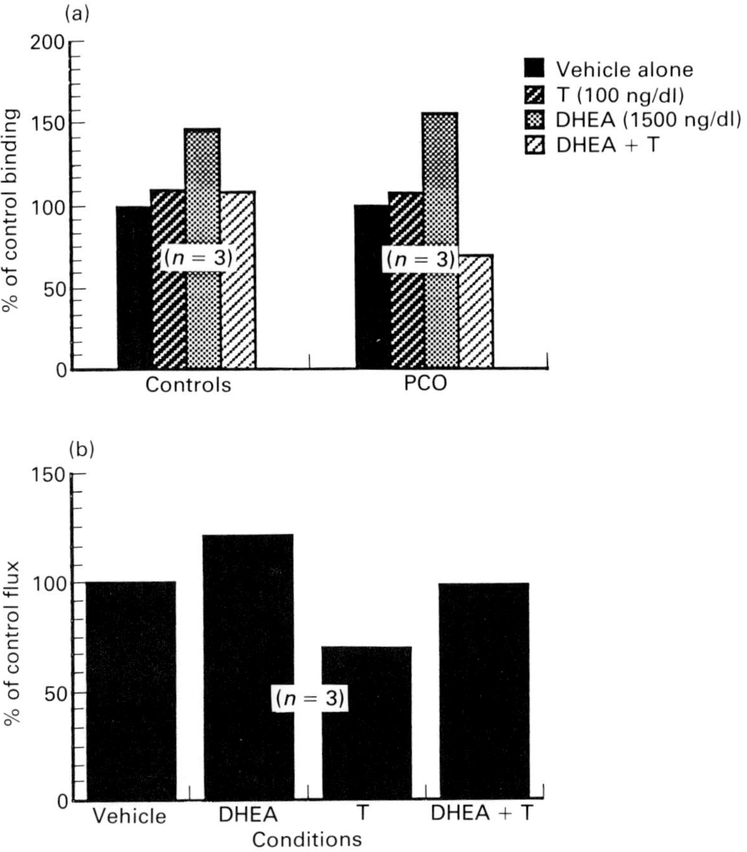

Fig. 24.5 *In vitro* effects of DHEA and testosterone on T-lymphocyte insulin binding (a) [47] and pyruvate flux (b). For measurements of insulin binding and pyruvate flux, T-lymphocytes were preincubated for 18 hours with DHEA (1500 ng/dl) and/or testosterone (100 ng/dl). Insulin binding and pyruvate flux were then determined as described previously [38,46]. Values represent the means of triplicate determinations for cells from each of the study subjects. $P < 0.05$ vehicle alone.

may oppose the actions of DHEA on insulin sensitivity, at least with regard to insulin binding.

In addition to a direct effect of DHEA on insulin binding, we have also found that DHEA, in a dose-dependent fashion, enhances the decarboxylation of 1-^{14}C pyruvate by intact T-lymphocytes [59]. As is shown in Fig. 24.5b, DHEA (1500 ng/dl) stimulated flux by approximately 20% above values observed for cells from control subjects incubated with vehicle alone. Although testosterone had no effect on insulin binding, the androgen inhibited T-lymphocyte pyruvate decarboxylation. Coincubation of cells with both DHEA and testosterone did not restore flux to control values but did increase values above those observed with testosterone alone. Thus, DHEA and testosterone not only have divergent effects on T-lymphocyte insulin binding but also on pyruvate metabolism.

Based on the earlier reports in the literature and our preliminary studies we have proposed that in female subjects not all hyperandrogenemia is associated with insulin resistance. We hypothesize that the extent of insulin resistance is determined by the ambient levels of DHEA and testosterone in general, and the ratio of DHEA/testosterone in particular, regardless of the degree of adiposity or hyperandrogenemia. This means that the lower the ratio of DHEA/testosterone the higher the insulin resistance. Alternatively, the higher the DHEA/testosterone ratio the higher is the insulin sensitivity. Implicit in this hypothesis is that high levels of testosterone are not necessarily associated with insulin resistance if levels of DHEA are elevated. On the other hand, there exist clinical conditions whereby testosterone levels may be low to normal but DHEA is much reduced such that the ratio of DHEA/testosterone is low leading to significant insulin resistance. Therefore, the important modifier is DHEA. These relationships have been studied in specially selected groups of female patients with a wide range of DHEA and testosterone levels. Studies in such a selected population with various ratios of DHEA/testosterone provide evidence to suggest that the greater the ratio of DHEA/testosterone the greater the degree of insulin sensitivity; the critical value above which no further increase in sensitivity is noted is 10. The *in vivo* parameters of insulin resistance studied included basal and glucose-challenged insulin as well as the ratios of I/G and hypoglycemic response to i.v. insulin. The *in vitro* parameters included erythrocyte insulin binding and receptor kinase as well as insulin binding and pyruvate flux in T-lymphocytes where the highest correlation of insulin sensitivity occurred at high ratios of DHEA/testosterone. These observations have also been extended *in vitro* with exogenous use of DHEA and testosterone to study their effects on insulin binding and pyruvate flux.

Although the mechanism of insulin resistance associated with PCO is not well understood, the availability of insulin-sensitive tissue such as activated T-lymphocytes as a model system may provide an opportunity to study hormonal mechanisms of insulin resistance at the molecular level.

Acknowledgments

*This work was supported in part by a grant from the American Diabetes Association (C.K.B.), by a General Clinical Research grant RR 00211,

Division of Research Resources, NIH, and from the Abe Goodman Fund for Diabetes Research.

References

1 Givens JR, Kerber IJ, Wiser WL, Anderson RN, Coleman SA, Fish SA. Remission of acanthosis nigricans associated with polycystic ovarian disease and a stromal luteoma. J Clin Endocrinol Metab 1974; 38:347–55.

2 Kahn CR, Flier JS, Bar RS, Archer JA, Gorden P, Martin MM, Roth J. The syndromes of insulin resistance and acanthosis nigricans: insulin-receptor disorders in man. N Engl J Med 1976; 294:739–45.

3 Burghen GA, Givens JR, Kitabchi AE. Correlation of hyperandrogenism and hyperinsulinism in polycystic ovarian disease. J Clin Endocrinol Metab 1980; 50:112–16.

4 Barbieri RL, Smith S, Ryan KI. The role of hyperinsulinemia in the pathogenesis of ovarian hyperandrogenism. Fertil Steril 1988; 50:197–212.

5 Chang RJ, Nakamura RM, Judd HL, Kaplan SA. Insulin resistance in nonobese patients with polycystic ovarian disease. J Clin Endocrinol Metab 1983; 57:356–9.

6 Schriock ED, Buffington CK, Hubert GD, Kurtz BR, Kitabchi AE, Buster JE, Givens JR. Divergent correlations of circulating dehydroepiandrosterone sulfate and testosterone with insulin levels and insulin receptor binding. J Clin Endocrinol Metab 1988; 66:1329–31.

7 Shoupe D, Kuman DD, Lobo RA. Insulin resistance in polycystic ovary syndrome. Am J Obstet Gynecol 1983; 147:588–92.

8 Smith S, Ravnikar VA, Barbieri RL. Androgen and insulin response to an oral glucose challenge in hyperandrogenic women. Fertil Steril 1987; 48:72–7.

9 Stuart CA, Peters EJ, Prince MJ, Richards G, Cavallo A, Meyer WJ. Insulin resistance and acanthosis nigricans: the roles of obesity and androgen excess. Metabolism 1986; 35:197–205.

10 Dunaif A, Graf M, Mandeli J, Laumas V, Dobrjansky A. Characterization of groups of hyperandrogenic women with acanthosis nigricans, impaired glucose tolerance, and/or hyperinsulinemia. J Clin Endocrinol Metab 1987; 65:499–506.

11 Kiddy DS, Hamilton-Fairley D, Seppala M, Koistinen R, James VHT, Reed MJ, Franks S. Diet-induced changes in sex hormone binding globulin and free testosterone in women with normal or polycystic ovaries: correlation with serum insulin and insulin-like growth factor-I. Clin Endocrinol 1989; 31:757–63.

12 Cole C, Kitabchi AE. Remission of insulin resistance with orthonovum in a patient with polycystic ovarian disease and acanthosis nigricans. Clin Res 1978; 26:412A.

13 Landon J, Wynn V, Samols E. The effect of anabolic steroids on blood sugar and plasma insulin levels in man. Metabolism 1963; 12:924–35.

14 Cohen JC, Hickman R. Insulin resistance and diminished glucose tolerance in powerlifters ingesting anabolic steroids. J Clin Endocrinol Metab 1987; 64:960–3.

15 Woodard RL, Burghen GA, Kitabchi AE. Glucose intolerance and insulin resistance in aplastic anemia treated with oxymetholone. J Clin Endocrinol Metab 1981; 53:905–8.

16 Lewis JJ, Foglia VG, Rodriques RR. The effects of steroids on the incidence of diabetes in rats after subtotal pancreatectomy. Endocrinology 1950; 46:111–21.

17 Dunaif A, Green G, Futterweit W, Dobrjansky A. Suppression of hyperandrogenism does not improve peripheral or hepatic insulin resistance in the polycystic ovary. J Clin Endocrinol Metab 1990; 70:699–704.

18 Geffner ME, Kaplan SA, Bersh N, Golde DW, Landow EM, Chang RJ, Persistence of insulin resistance in polycystic ovarian disease after inhibition of ovarian steroid secretion. Fertil Steril 1986; 43:327–33.

19 Bar RS, Muggeo M, Roth J, Kahn CR, Havrankova J, Imperato-McGinley J. Insulin resistance, acanthosis nigricans, and normal insulin receptors in a young woman: evidence for a postreceptor defect. J Clin Endocrinol Metab 1978; 47:620–5.

20 Nagamani M, Dinh TV, Kelver ME. Hyperinsulinemia in hyperthecosis of the ovaries. Am J Obstet Gynecol 1986; 154:384–9.
21 Barbieri RL, Smith S, Ryan KJ. The role of hyperinsulinemia in the pathogenesis of ovarian hyperandrogenism. Fertil Steril 1988; 50:197–212.
22 Farah MJ, Givens JR, Kitabchi AE. Bimodal correlation between the circulating insulin level and the production rate of dehydroepiandrosterone: positive correlation in controls and negative correlation in the polycystic ovary syndrome with acanthosis nigricans. J Clin Endocrinol Metab 1990; 70:1075–81.
23 Kramer RE, Hubert GD, Buster JE, Andersen RN. Interactions between insulin and ACTH in the control of adrenal cortisol and adrostenedione production in primary cultures of bovine adrenocortical cells. Proceedings of the 71st Annual Meeting of the Endocrine Society, 1989; p. 381.
24 Clearly NJ, Zisk J. Antiobesity effect of two different levels of dehydroepiandrosterone treatment in lean and obese middle-aged female Zucker rats. Int J Obesity 1986; 10:193–204.
25 Coleman DL, Leiter EH, Schwizer RW. Therapeutic effects of dehydroepiandrosterone (DHEA) in diabetic mice. Diabetes 1982; 31:830–3.
26 Gansler RS, Muller S, Cleary MP. Chronic administration of dehydroepiandrosterone (DHEA) reduces pancreatic β-cell hyperplasia and hyperinsulinemia in genetically obese rats. Proc Soc Exp Biol Med 1985; 180:155–62.
27 Mohan PF, Cleary MP. Comparison of dehydroepiandrosterone and clofibric acid treatments on obese Zucker rats. J Nutr 1989; 119:496–501.
28 Shepherd A, Cleary MP. Metabolic alterations after dehydroepiandrosterone treatment in Zucker rats. Am J Physiol 1984; 246:E123–E128.
29 Nestler JE, Barlascini CO, Clore JN, Blackard WG. Dehydroepiandrosterone reduces serum low density lipoprotein levels and body fat but does not alter insulin sensitivity in normal men. J Clin Endocrinol Metab 1988; 66:57–61.
30 Mortola JF, Yen SSC. The impact of oral dehydroepiandrosterone on endocrine–metabolic parameters in postmenopausal women. Abstracts and Papers of the Endocrine Society 72nd Annual Meeting, 1990, p. 237.
31 Leiter EH, Beamer WG, Coleman DL, Longscope C. Androgenic and estrogenic metabolites in serum of mice fed dehydroepiandrosterone—relationship to antihyperglycemic effects. Metabolism 1987; 36:863–9.
32 Schwartz AG, Whitcomb JM, Nyce JW, Lewbart ML, Pashko LL. Dehydroepiandrosterone and structural analogs: a new class of cancer chemopreventive agents. Adv Cancer Res 1988; 51:391–424.
33 Kozak RW, Haskell JF, Greenstein LA, Rehler MM, Waldmann TA, Nissley SP. Type I and II insulin-like growth factor receptors on human phytohemagglutinin-activated T-lymphocytes. Cell Immunol 1987; 109:318–31.
34 Tapson VF, Boni-Schnetzler M, Pilch PF, Center DM, Berman JS. Structural and functional characterization of the human T-lymphocyte receptor for insulin-like growth factor I *in vitro*. J Clin Invest 1988; 82:950–7.
35 Ercolani L, Brown JT, Ginsberg BH. Tunicamycin blocks the emergence and maintenance of insulin receptors on mitogen-activated human T-lymphocytes. Metabolism 1984; 33:309–16.
36 Krug U, Krug F, Cuatrecasas P. Emergence of insulin receptors on human lymphocytes during *in vitro* transformation. Proc Natl Acad Sci USA 1972; 69:2604–8.
37 Helderman JH, Reynolds TC, Strom TB. The insulin receptor as a universal marker of activated lymphocytes. Eur J Immunol 1978; 8:589–95.
38 Buffington CK, El-Sheikh T, Kitabchi AE, Matteri RT. Phytohemagglutinin (PHA)-activated human T-lymphocytes: concomitant appearance of insulin binding, degradation, and insulin mediated activation of pyruvate dehydrogenase. Biochem Biophys Res Commun 1986; 134:412–19.
39 Ercolani L, Lin HL, Ginsberg BH. Insulin-induced desensitization at the receptor and postreceptor level in mitogen-activated human T-lymphocytes. Diabetes 1985;

37:931–7.

40 Helderman JH, Pietri AO, Raskin P. *In vitro* control of T-lymphocyte insulin receptors by *in vivo* modulation of insulin. Diabetes 1983; 32:712–17.

41 Helderman JH. Acute regulation of human lymphocyte insulin receptors: analysis of the glucose clamp. J Clin Invest 1984; 74:1428–35.

42 Helderman JH, Raskin P. The T lymphocyte insulin receptor in diabetes and obesity: an intrinsic binding defect. Diabetes 1980; 29:551–7.

43 Stentz FB, Kitabchi AE, Schilling JW, Schronk LR, Seyer JM. Identification of insulin intermediates and sites of cleavage of native insulin by insulin protease from human fibroblasts. J Biol Chem 1989; 264:20275–81.

44 Stentz FB, Buffington CK, Seyer J, Castle R, Kitabchi AE. Stimulated T-lymphocytes internalize and degrade insulin similar to other insulin requiring cells. Clin Res 1990; 39:34A.

45 Helderman JH. The role of insulin in intermediary metabolism of activated thymic derived lymphocytes. J Clin Invest 1981; 67:1636–42.

46 Buffington CK, Givens JR, Kitabchi AE. Sensitivity of pyruvate dehydrogenase to insulin in activated T-lymphocytes: Lack of responsiveness to insulin in patients with polycystic ovarian disease and diabetes. Diabetes 1990; 39:361–8.

47 Buffington CK, Givens JR, Kitabchi AE. Opposing actions of dehydroepiandrosterone and testosterone on insulin sensitivity: *in vivo* and *in vitro* studies of hyperandrogenic females. Diabetes 1991; 40:693–700.

48 National Diabetes Data Group. Classification and diagnosis of diabetes mellitus and other categories of glucose intolerance. Diabetes 1979; 28:1039–56.

49 Rosen OM. After insulin binding. Science 1987; 237:1452–8.

50 Grigorescu F, Flier JS, Kahn CR. Defect in insulin receptor phosphorylation in erythrocytes and fibroblast associated with severe insulin resistance. J Biol Chem 1984; 259:15003–7.

51 Grunsberger G, Comi RJ, Carpentier JL, Podskalny JM, McElduff A, Taylor SI, Gorden P. Insulin receptor tyrosine kinase activity is abnormal in circulating cells and cultured fibroblasts but normal in transformed lymphocytes from a type A insulin resistant patient. J Lab Clin Med 1988; 112:122–32.

52 Grunsberger G, Comie RJ, Taylor SI, Gorden P. Tyrosine kinase activity of the insulin receptor of patients with type A extreme insulin resistance: studies with circulating mononuclear cells and cultured lymphocytes. J Clin Endocrinol Metab 1984; 59:1152–8.

53 Peters EJ, Stuart CA, Prince MJ. Acanthosis nigricans and obesity: acquired and intrinsic defects in insulin action. Metabolism 1986; 35:807–13.

54 Stuart CA, Pietrzyk RA, Peters EJ, Smith FE, Prince MJ. Autophosphorylation of cultured skin fibroblast insulin receptors from patients with severe insulin resistance and acanthosis nigricans. Diabetes 1989; 38:328–32.

55 Kitabchi AE, Stentz FB, Cole C, Duckworth WC. Accelerated insulin degradation: an alternate mechanism for insulin resistance. Diabetes Care 1979; 2:414–17.

56 Kitabchi AE, Stentz FB, Buffington CK. Insulin degradation products from human fibroblasts stimulate the pyruvate dehydrogenase complex in a cell-free system. Clin Res 1983; 31:882A.

57 Semple JW, Ellis J, Delovitch TL. Processing and presentation of insulin II. Evidence for intracellular plasma membrane associated and extracellular degradation of human insulin by antigen-presenting B-cells. J Immunol 1989; 142:4184–93.

58 Podskalny JM, Kahn RC. Cell culture studies on patients with extreme insulin resistance. II. Abnormal biological responses in cultured fibroblasts. J Clin Endocrinol Metab 1982; 54:269–75.

59 Hidaji F, Buffington C, Kitabchi AE. Dehydroepiandrosterone enhances insulin sensitivity at the receptor and postreceptor levels in human fibroblasts and activated lymphocytes. Clin Res 1990; 39:33A.

Chapter 25
Insulin: an Overview

CHARLES A. STUART

Where does insulin resistance fit into the polycystic ovary syndrome (PCO)? A few important aspects of this question have been established, but several more related issues are not clear.

First, there is an association between hyperinsulinemia and hyperandrogenemia in women. This observation does not by itself provide any clue to differentiate cause and effect. Second, both insulin and insulin-like growth factor I (IGF-I) stimulate steroidogenesis (androgen production) in ovarian tissue *in vitro*. Third, *in vivo* studies have shown that insulin infusion can acutely augment plasma concentrations of weak androgens (androstenedione and dehydroepiandrosterone). Fourth, androgens are not the cause of insulin resistance in PCO. Suppression of androgens and gonadotropins by exogenous estrogen/progesterone treatment in patients with PCO has no effect on insulin resistance. Studies in monkeys have documented no change in insulin sensitivity with administration of androgens. These four observations indicate that insulin may have a primary role in at least some patients with PCO.

What has been pointed out clearly is that there are key questions in PCO and its relationship with insulin still in need of answers. One central issue is the epidemiology of insulin resistance among subsets of PCO. Do all obese patients with polycystic ovaries have moderate-to-severe insulin resistance? Are lean patients with PCO hyperinsulinemic? These are clinical observations that need to be made. Along with the lean and obese subsets, are there major ethnic differences? A second issue under active investigation is the mechanism by which insulin at the concentrations seen in our patients can cause increased androgen production. Glucose transport insulin resistance results in pancreatic compensation by increased insulin secretion. Excess insulin may exert its effects in the ovary through a normal physiologic pathway, which does not exhibit insulin resistance. This pathway could involve a normal insulin receptor and perhaps a signal transduction pathway different from that of glucose transport. Insulin could modulate IGF-I action by suppression of locally produced IGF-binding protein or it may up-regulate cell surface IGF receptors, either of which would amplify IGF-I actions without altering its production rate. Still another option is that excess insulin is crossing over to interact directly with the IGF-I receptor. This last option is not likely since the insulin concentrations in our patients are not high enough to overcome a 200-fold lower affinity of insulin for the IGF-I receptor.

A third unresolved question is whether insulin resistance can explain all the findings of PCO through hyperinsulinemia, i.e. androgen excess *and* gonadotropin dynamic abnormalities.

Finally, a relatively new concept to be considered was put forward by Crowley. Can this hyperinsulinemia seen in many women with PCO be analogous to that in men and be a major risk factor for coronary artery disease? He suggested about the association between PCO and hyperinsulinemia, "Might this be more a public health issue, and maybe less a reproductive issue?"

Section 8
Consequences and Treatment of Polycystic Ovary Syndrome

Chapter 26
Introduction: Consequences and Treatment of Polycystic Ovary Syndrome

ROBERT WILD

In this section we will update and identify the gaps in our knowledge of the long-term implications and therapeutic options for patients with polycystic ovary sydrome (PCO). Historically and currently, we are plagued by problems of definition of the disorder and criteria for inclusion. It should be acknowledged, therefore, that contributors to this section promote a greater understanding of this disorder by bringing their varied disciplines to studies of the problem.

While being extremely sensitive to the cosmetic and psychosexual aspects of the disorder (expanded upon by Anke Erhardt in this section), our group has advanced the thesis that hirsutism is much more than a cosmetic concern. The patient with PCO has significant metabolic derangements that we are only now beginning to recognize and understand. Our first clue in this regard came from our evaluation of familial PCO described in the historical overview in Section 1. Intensive study of one of the multiple families with familial PCO led us to become more aware of the widespread metabolic aberrations. One particular young adult male (Fig. 26.1) has a high ratio of circulating levels of luteinizing hormone (LH) to follicle-stimulating hormone (FSH), as does his sister who was described as having the hyperthecoses variant of classic polycystic ovary. On testicular biopsy of enlarged testicles (probably the result of Leydig cell hyperplasia) we found that this patient has spermatogenic arrest just as his sister's ovaries have multiple atretic follicles. Both he and his sister have acanthosis nigricans and they both exhibit significant insulin resistance. His fasting level of insulin is 100 μU/ml and he has abnormalities in lipoprotein lipids. The family history is dotted with coronary artery disease (Fig. 26.2) [1]. The incidence of carbohydrate abnormalities is high in women with PCO. Dunaif updates our knowledge about diabetes and PCO in Chapter 30.

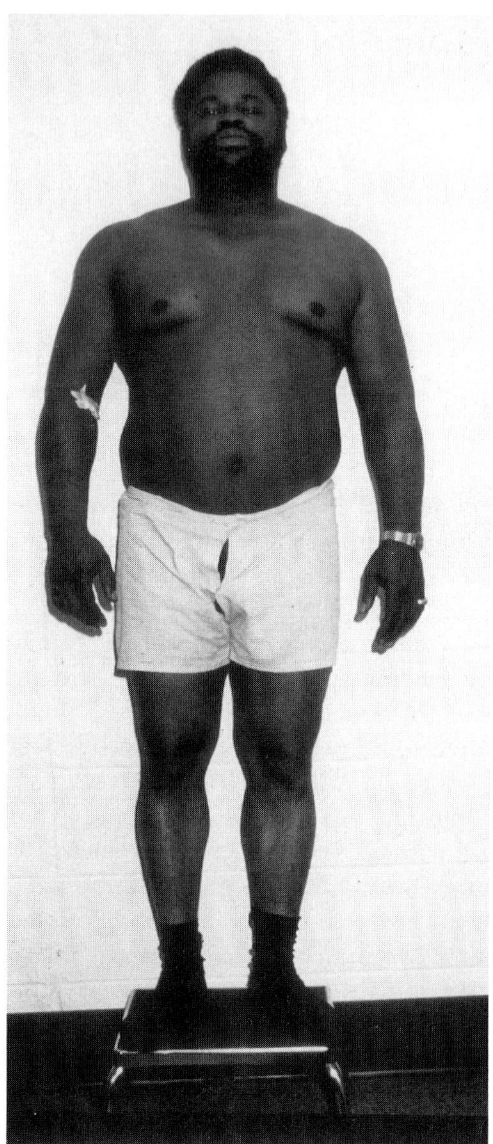

Fig. 26.1 Brother of a patient with familial PCO (hyperthecoses variant) who has a high ratio of levels of LH to FSH, Leydig cell hyperplasia, spermatogenic arrest, acanthosis nigricans and elevated fasting levels of insulin.

One of the first metabolic aberrations and frightening consequences of PCO to be described is the not infrequent occurrence of endometrial cancer. The youngest patient with PCO and endometrial cancer that the author has diagnosed was 19 years old. There are now many well-documented cases of endometrial cancer in teenage patients with PCO. Classically, endometrial cancer is thought to develop in an endocrine

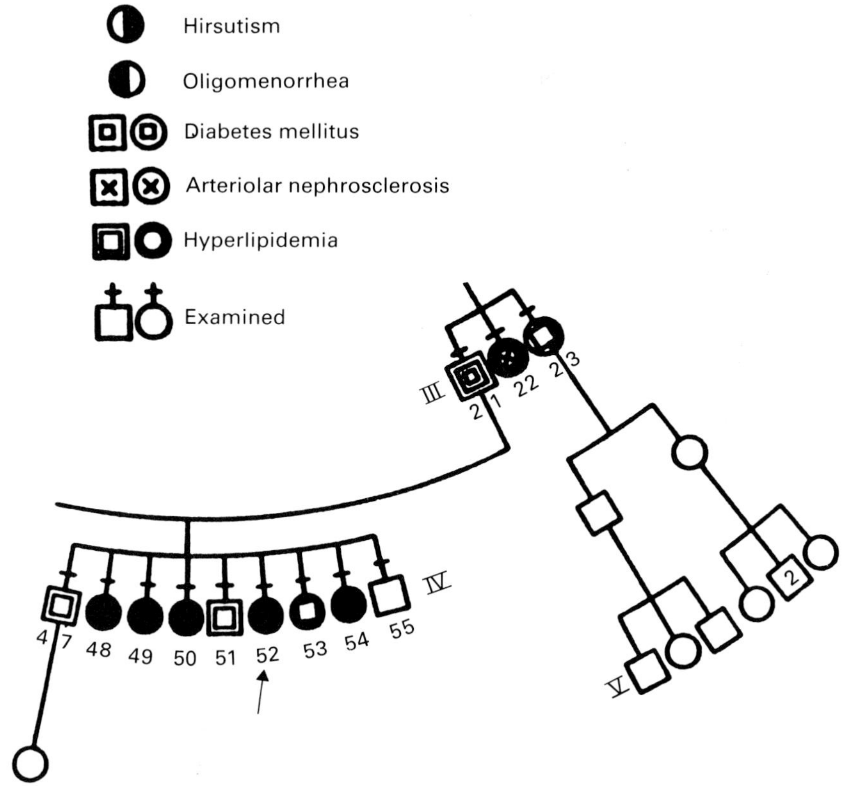

Fig. 26.2 Family tree of familial PCO illustrating prevalence of premature coronary vascular disease and carbohydrate abnormalities. (Reprinted, with permission, from Givens *et al.* [1].)

milieu of unopposed estrogen. The frequent occurrence of insulin resistance in patients with PCO and the recent description of insulin-like growth factor I (IGF-I) receptors in differing histologic grades of endometrial cancer challenge us to determine the exact mechanism whereby patients with PCO are at increased risk for this disease. The frequency of the development of endometrial cancer should, however, alert the clinician to the importance of endometrial sampling in assessing the consequences and treatment of PCO.

One of the dilemmas with PCO has been the well-known dichotomy between clinical manifestations and degree of hyperandrogenism. Historically, this dichotomy has led to much confusion in both the research and the clinical arenas. This problem is compounded by psychosocial implications. Patients not uncommonly can seek help for ovulatory dysfunction and infertility and on the surface they may deny any cosmetic issues. Body-image problems can come between patient and physician. For example, if induction of ovulation is successful, who in our healthcare system looks out for the patient's long-term metabolic issues?

In the past decade or so research has been concentrated on the peripheral target tissue in attempts to explain the common dichotomy between clinical symptoms and degree of hyperandrogenism. The understanding that 5α-reductase activity in the peripheral target tissue acts as an endocrine organ in and of itself (expanded upon by Rogerio Lobo in his discussion of hyperandrogenism in Chapter 27) has shed some light on this apparent paradox.

We became interested in the physiologic consequences associated with PCO as a result of the original studies of Givens and colleagues in the 1970s [2]. Classic treatment with Orthonovum (2 mg) was utilized to suppress LH-dependent hyperandrogenism (Fig. 26.3). This treatment was supplemented by efforts to determine the degree of suppression of adrenal function in PCO [3]. The diurnal rhythmicity of androstenedione was diminished in parallel with decreasing concentrations of dehydroepiandrosterone sulfate (DHEAS), suggesting that this combination preparation of sex steroids inhibits adrenal hyperandrogenism and that DHEAS is a good marker for this effect (Fig. 26.4) [3].

Two landmark observations came from these studies of diurnal changes in levels of hormones. First, two individuals receiving this oral contraceptive had cardiovascular events in their second decade of life. Second, the frequently cited observation was made that basal concentrations of insulin and androgen are related [4]. We now know that hyperinsulinism is an independent risk factor for coronary vascular disease (CVD).

To begin to test the hypothesis that women with PCO are at an increased risk for CVD, we first compared lipoprotein lipid profiles of women with PCO to those in normal women [5]. Women with PCO have higher triglyceride and lower high-density lipoprotein (HDL)-cholesterol concentrations than normal women, even when matched for body weight [6]. Kissebah, in Chapter 31, reviews the evidence relating body fat topography, androgens and metabolism in nonhirsute women. In an independent investigation, we have found that the previously described changes in levels of triglycerides and HDL-cholesterol were independently related to levels of androgens and insulin [7]. We have hypothesized that, in contrast to the more gynoid (feminine) distribution of fat, women with PCO (either as a result of different genetic endowment or through modulation of programmed genetic expression by sex steroids at a critical time in either prenatal, neonatal or adolescent

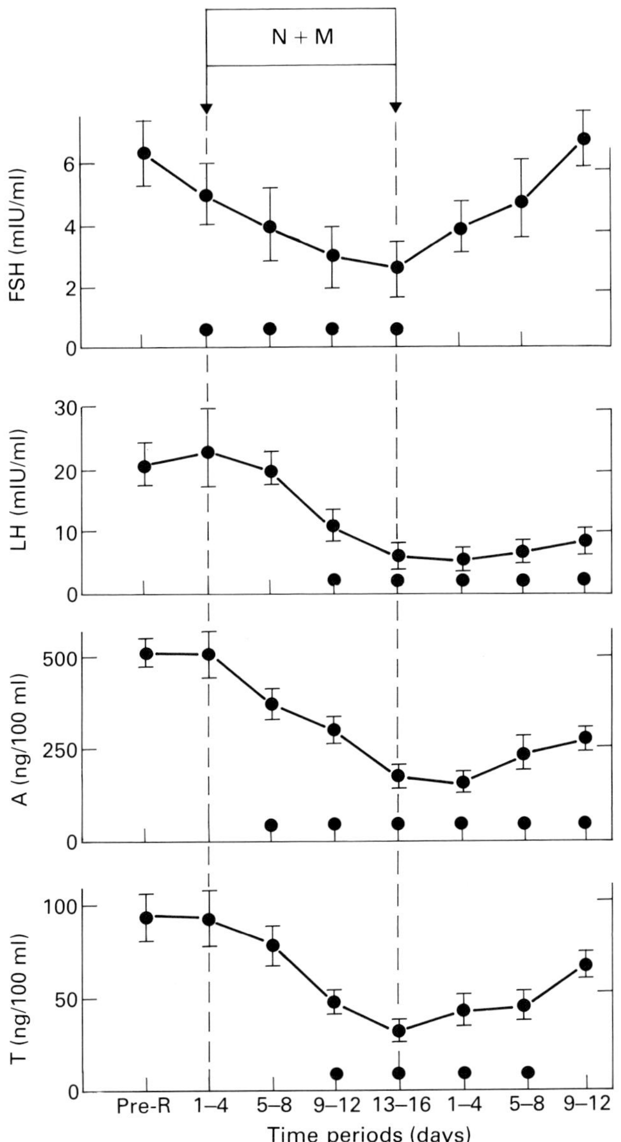

Fig. 26.3 Gonadotropin and androgen suppression with a combination sex-steroid in patients with PCO. (Reprinted, with permission, from Givens *et al.* [2], © by The Edocrine Society.)

development), who have significant metabolic aberrations, frequently have an android distribution of fat. It is possible that a critical threshold effect exists. Kirschner has recently demonstrated that the rate of testosterone production is greater in android than in gynoid obesity [8]. He recently made the observation that he does not recall ever seeing a

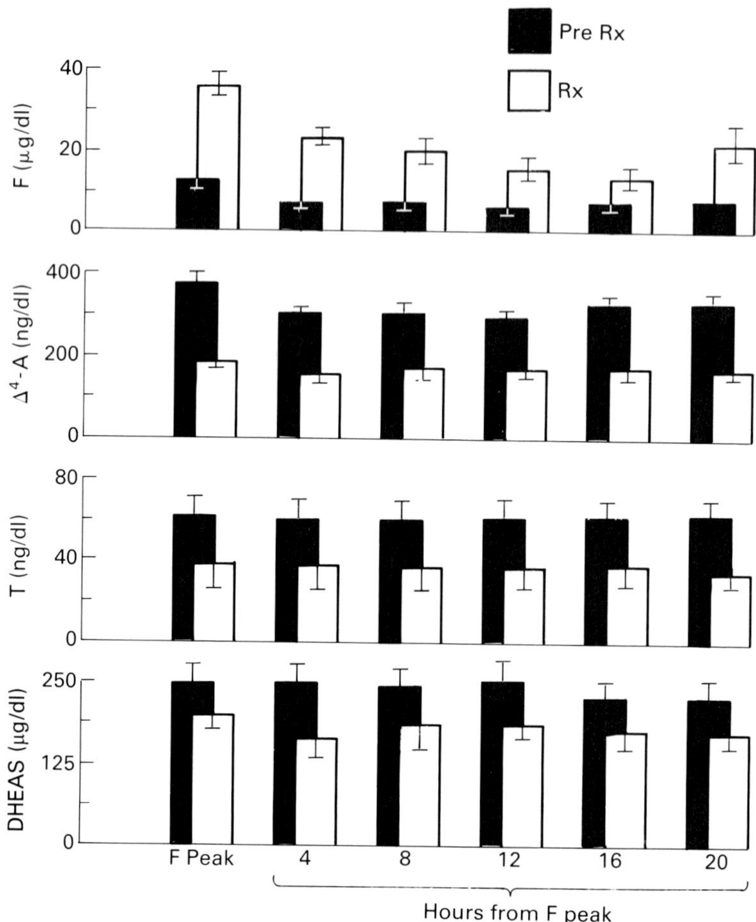

Fig. 26.4 Diurnal inhibition of adrenal androgens with combination sex-steroid suppression in patients with PCO. (Reprinted, with permission, from Wild *et al.* [3], © by The Endocrine Society.)

woman with a purely gynoid distribution of fat who was hirsute (unpublished observation). On the contrary, when the distribution of body fat is more android in character, hirsutism is more likely. Because women with PCO are heterogeneous with respect to sources of hyperandrogenism, it is our belief that their lipoprotein lipid alterations and probably their risk of CVD is likewise heterogeneous [9]. It is also our belief that clinical signs of androgen excess are risk factors for CVD [10].

There are thus a number of reasons why we believe that the consequences of PCO should alter our concepts of treatment. Chang and Cragun, in Chapter 28, review both medical and surgical therapies for PCO. It is our contention that improvement in metabolic parameters and reduction of long-term consequences of the disorder should be important principles in guiding the choice of therapy. The challenge before us is to move toward prevention of the now well-described consequences of the disorder and to develop newer treatment strategies that mitigate against risks associated with this disorder.

References

1 Givens JR, Wiser WL, Coleman SA, Wilroy RS, Anderson RN, Fish SA. Familial ovarian hyperthecosis: a study of two families. Am J Obstet Gynecol 1971; 110:959–72.

2 Givens JR, Anderson RN, Wiser WL, Fish SA. Dynamics of suppression and recovery of plasma FSH, LH, androstenedione and testosterone in polycystic ovarian disease using an oral contraceptive. J Clin Endocrinol Metab 1974; 38:727–32.

3 Wild RA, Umstot ES, Andersen RN, Givens JR. Adrenal function in hirsutism. II. Effect of an oral contraceptive. J Clin Endocrinol Metab 1982; 54:676–81.

4 Burghen GA, Givens JR, Kitabchi AE. Correlation of hyperandrogenism with hyperinsulinism in polycystic ovarian disease. J Clin Endocrinol Metab 1980; 50:113–16.

5 Wild RA, Painter PC, Coulson PC, Carruth KB, Rainey GB. Lipoprotein lipid concentrations and cardiovascular risk in women with polycystic ovary syndrome. J Clin Endocrinol Metab 1985; 61:946–51.

6 Wild RA, Bartholomew MJ. The influence of body weight on lipoprotein lipids in patients with polycystic ovary syndrome. Am J Obstet Gynecol 1988; 159:423–7.

7 Wild RA, Applebaum-Bowden D, Demers LM, Bartholomew M, Landis JR, Hazzard WR, Santen RJ. Lipoprotein lipids in women with androgen excess: independent associations with increased insulin and androgen. Clin Chem 1990; 36:283–9.

8 Kirschner MA, Samojlik E, Drijka M, Szmae E, Schneider G, Ertelin L. Androgen–estrogen metabolism in women with upper body versus lower body obesity. J Clin Endocrinol Metab 1990; 70:473–9.

9 Wild RA, Bartholomew M, Applebaum-Bowden D, Demers L, Hazzard W, Santen RJ. Evidence for heterogenous mechanisms of lipoprotein lipid alterations in hyperandrogenic women. Am J Obstet Gynecol 1990; 163: 1998–2005.

10 Wild RA, Grubb BG, Hartz A, VanNort JJ, Bachman W, Bartholomew M. Clinical signs of androgen excess as risk factors for coronary artery disease. Fertil Steril 1990; 54:255–9.

Chapter 27
Androgen Secretion in the Syndrome of Hyperandrogenic Chronic Anovulation

ROGERIO A. LOBO

Defining the syndrome

While it is difficult for most endocrinologists to agree on specific diagnostic criteria for polycystic ovary syndrome (PCO), there is general agreement that this is a heterogeneous group of disorders. Although heterogeneous, it appears clear that the features which most characterize these patients are the findings of chronic anovulation and hyperandrogenism. It is the latter finding that is the focus of this review. Because of the difficulty in defining and diagnosing PCO, we have preferred to use a more global term for these patients and have chosen to refer to them as having the syndrome of hyperandrogenic chronic anovulation (HCA). While in essence HCA includes "classic" PCO, the use of the term HCA allows for a more flexible and all-encompassing diagnosis appropriate for the majority of patients who have the two most important components of PCO: chronic anovulation and hyperandrogenism.

Ovarian morphologic focus in the diagnosis

Although early studies of PCO were entirely focused on ovarian morphology, there is evidence that such an exclusive emphasis is misplaced. Enlarged polycystic ovaries may occur in Cushing's syndrome, congenital adrenal hyperplasia, in association with some ovarian or adrenal tumors and, occasionally, in normal young children [1,2]. Furthermore, women with otherwise classic aspects of this syndrome may have ovaries of normal size. In Fig. 27.1 are the ovarian findings of a phenotypic male with 46,XX congenital hyperplasia due to incomplete 21-hydroxylase deficiency who was treated at our medical center. Similar findings have been reported by Erickson *et al.* [3].

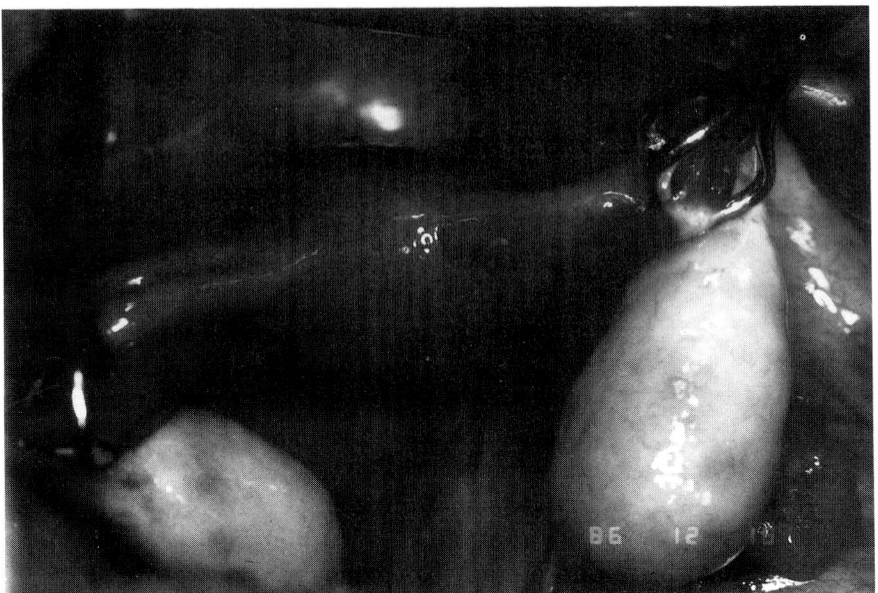

Fig. 27.1 Ovaries and uterus from a patient with 21-hydroxylase deficiency.

While ovarian size need not be a specific criterion for the diagnosis of PCO, certain characteristics described by ultrasound have popularized this technique for the diagnosis of PCO [4]. The current use of vaginal ultrasound has further enhanced our ability to detect ovarian morphologic changes. However, ovarian ultrasonographic changes cannot be taken in isolation to diagnose this syndrome. Indeed, the sonographic appearance need not be uniform and a spectrum of "PCO ovaries" is known to exist [5].

It has been proposed that up to 25% of "normal" women will have the ultrasound findings of PCO and that this figure increases to 76% if women are included who have some degree of menstrual irregularity [6]. However, the mere finding of cystic ovaries alone (without anovulation or hyperandrogenism) should not be confused with HCA, or PCO in particular.

While it is most common to have a characteristic ovarian picture of HCA, it is not essential for a firm diagnosis. On the contrary, women may have normal ovulatory cycles, no preexisting hyperandrogenism or infertility and ovaries that resemble PCO (Fig. 27.2). In understanding how normal ovaries may undergo cystic changes and hypothesizing that androgens may be implicated, it is arguable that, in such a normal patient as described above, subtle hyperandrogenism may exist and is difficult to rule out.

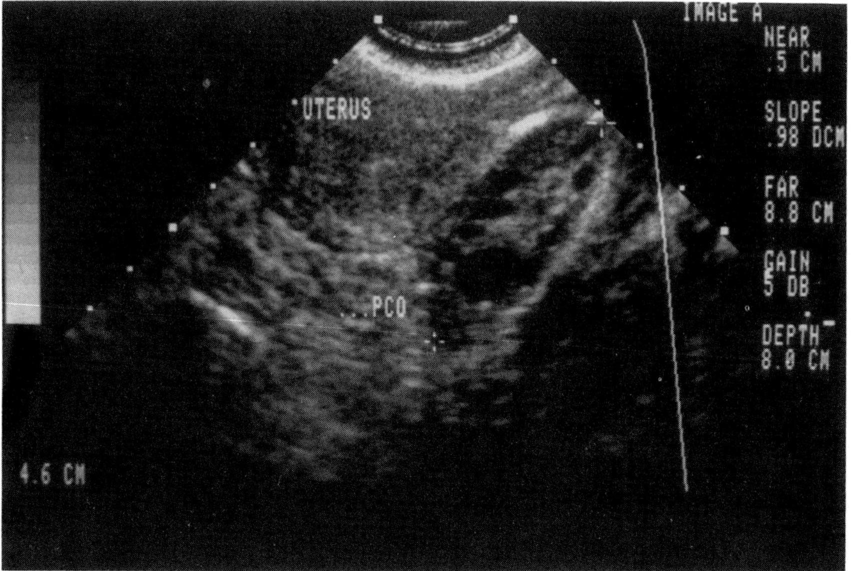

Fig. 27.2 Vaginal ultrasound of a normal ovulatory nonhirsute woman in the midfollicular phase.

That an increase in androgen may induce cystic or PCO-like changes in the ovaries is irrefutable. At least two studies where female to male transsexuals have been treated with androgen [7,8] have provided evidence for this evolution (Fig. 27.3). Indeed, any combination of chronic anovulation coupled with hyperandrogenism (either ovarian or adrenal) may be expected to result in cystic ovarian changes. In that these are the two salient, critical factors for the diagnosis of HCA, it is most characteristic for such patients to have cystic ovarian changes, but the latter are not requirements of the diagnosis.

Subgroups and mimics in the diagnosis of HCA

Diagnosing all women with chronic anovulation and hyperandrogenism as having HCA would include many other syndromes and disease states that should not be considered. Specifically excluded should be women with the diagnoses of congenital adrenal hyperplasia and Cushing's syndrome as well as those with ovarian or adrenal tumors. Since the specific diagnosis of stromal hyperthecosis requires histologic confirmation, HCA as a working clinical diagnosis may be appropriate. Other mimics of HCA may include patients with thyroid disease, simple obesity and women with significant hyperprolactinemia.

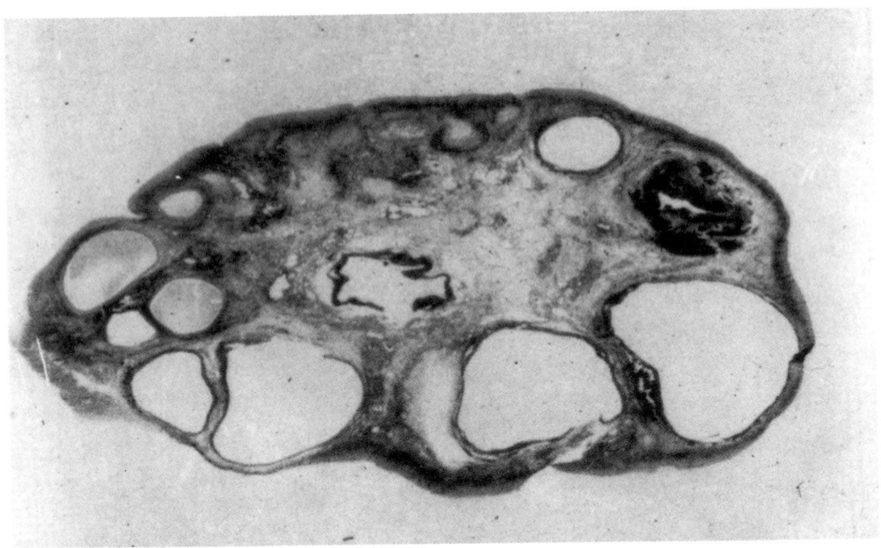

Fig. 27.3 Section of polycystic ovary in androgen-related patient showing multiple cystic follicles distributed beneath a thickened collagenized external ovarian cortex. Whole mount, ×2.5. (Reprinted, with permission, from Futterweit and Deligdisch [7], © by The Endocrine Society.)

Multicompartmental androgen production in HCA

In attempting to elucidate the source(s) of androgen production in women, we have stressed the existence of three compartments, each of which is not mutually exclusive. These are the ovary, adrenal and the periphery; the latter includes skin and more specifically the pilosebaceous units. In HCA, usually more than one compartment is involved and frequently all three.

Compared to other women with chronic anovulation or hypothalamic–pituitary dysfunction alone, patients with HCA have evidence for increased blood production of several androgens [9] (Fig. 27.4), whether or not hirsutism is present. Because the metabolic clearance of androgens may be increased in HCA, particularly with obesity, measurements in blood may not always reflect this increased production, yet with the measurement of several androgens one or more will usually be found to be elevated.

The ovarian compartment

Ovarian hyperandrogenism is perhaps most common and has been determined by elevated peripheral levels of total and unbound testos-

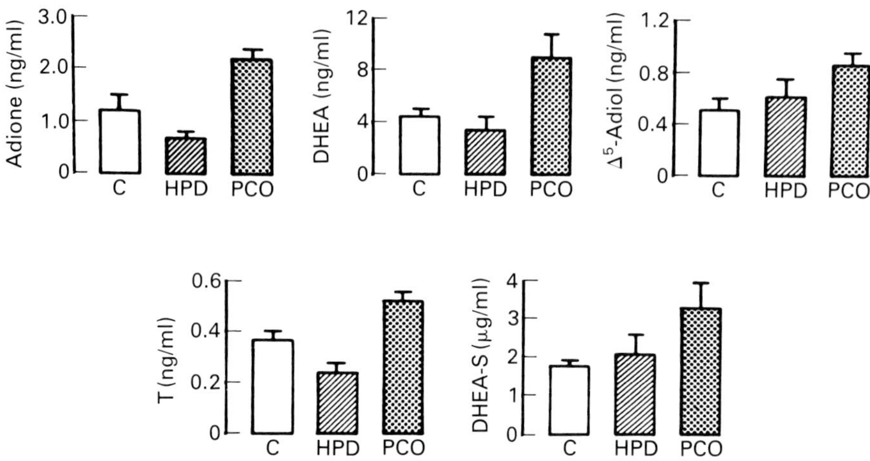

Fig. 27.4 Serum androstenedione (Adione), dehydroepiandrosterone (DHEA), Δ^5-androstenediol (Δ^5-Adiol), testosterone (T) and dehydroepiandrosterone sulfate (DHEA-S) in control subjects (C) and in women with hypothalamic–pituitary dysfunction (HPD) and those with polycystic ovary syndrome (PCO). (Reprinted, with permission, from Lobo *et al.* [9].)

terone as well as by direct ovarian vein catheterization studies, ovarian stimulation with gonadotropins, and ovarian down-regulation with the gonadotropin-releasing hormone (GnRH)-agonist [9–13]. Recent evidence has pointed to an enzymatic dysregulation in ovarian steroidogenesis. This hypothesis holds that ovarian and perhaps adrenal androgen production is enhanced in HCA because of cytochrome P-$450_{17\alpha}$ dysregulation resulting in increased 17α-hydroxylase and 17, 20-lyase activities [14] (see Chapter 9). Because ovarian hyperandrogenism is perhaps the least controversial of the findings in HCA, an in-depth discussion will not follow. However, Fig. 27.5 demonstrates the classic findings of the suppression of ovarian hyperandrogenism with the use of the GnRH-agonist [12]. While elevated levels of testosterone and androstenedione were significantly suppressed by gonadotropin and ovarian down-regulation, serum dehydroepiandrosterone (DHEA) and DHEA sulfate (DHEAS) elevated in baseline samples were not suppressed [12]. It has also been determined that GnRH-agonist down-regulation requires a larger dose of agonist for ovarian androgen suppression than for estradiol [13].

That ovarian hyperandrogenism is dependent, at least in part, on gonadotropin secretion is supported by the GnRH-agonist data but also by direct correlations of serum testosterone and unbound testosterone with serum immunoreactive and bioactive luteinizing hormone (LH) in patients considered to have PCO [15]. In concert with this, is the tropic influence of insulin and other growth factors on theca-stromal androgen production [16], which is the subject of other discussions in this volume (see Chapters 18 and 21). Finally, it must be appreciated that the ovaries of many patients with PCO, perhaps predominantly those with "classic" PCO, are more "sensitive" to gonadotropic stimulation. This trait, perhaps genetic, could in turn be related to cytochrome P-$450_{17\alpha}$ dysregulation [14]. This enhanced sensitivity is evident from the enhanced ovarian androgen response occurring from induction of ovulation, including the use of pulsatile GnRH [17] and with the use of exogenous human chorionic gonadotropin in particular.

For all practical purposes, serum total testosterone serves to signify ovarian hyperandrogenism in most patients. This is particularly true when levels of DHEAS are normal as this is a marker of adrenal androgen production. In patients with HCA, testosterone levels are usually no more than twice the upper normal range (20–70 ng/dl) and rarely above 150 ng/dl. In cases of stromal hyperthecosis, however, values may reach 200 ng/dl or more.

The adrenal compartment

While there has been some controversy about the role of the adrenal using the broader definition of this syndrome (HCA), patients with adrenal hyperandrogenism may be encountered frequently. However, in those studies where PCO was strictly defined and ovarian morphology was stressed, adrenal hyperandrogenism has been reported not to exist [18,19]. This, however, may be viewed as merely a selection bias. Adrenal uptake of iodomethylnorcholesterol has been found to be increased in patients considered to have PCO [20] and to overlap with the uptake of this tracer in patients with Cushing's syndrome.

In our medical center, adrenal hyperandrogenism is common. In patients with HCA, we have noted 50% of our patients to have elevations in serum DHEAS [21,22]. Further, these patients have been noted to have exaggerated responses of DHEAS to adrenocorticotropic hormone (ACTH) [21]. Another specific marker of adrenal androgen secretion is 11β-hydroxyandrostenedione. Measurements of this steroid have been reported to be normal in patients considered to have PCO [19]. However, DHEAS also may be normal in some patients with PCO. While not all patients with PCO or HCA will have an adrenal component, in our experience many patients have elevations in both DHEAS and 11β-hydroxyandrostenedione.

Recently, we have found increased responses of serum androgens

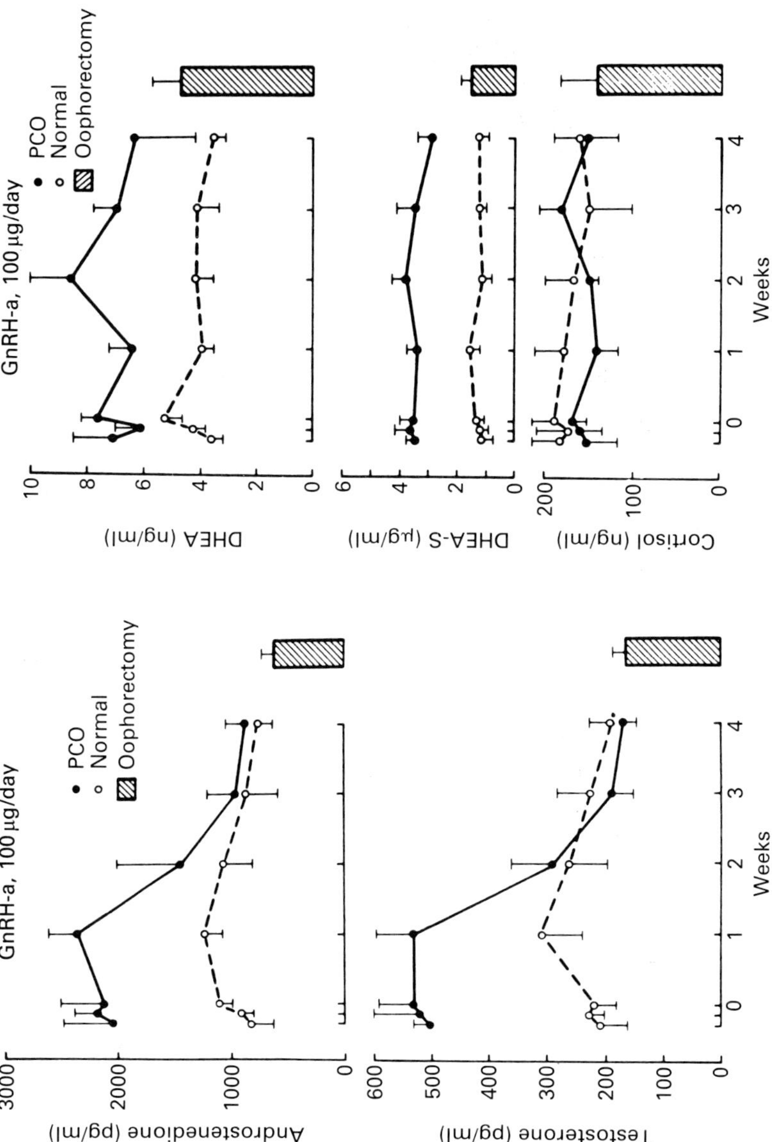

Fig. 27.5 Mean serum androstenedione, testosterone, dehydroepiandrosterone (DHEA), dehydroepiandrosterone sulfate (DHEA-S) and cortisol concentrations in polycystic ovary syndrome (PCO) and normal ovulatory subjects before and during gonadotropin-releasing hormone agonist (GnRH-a) treatment and in oophorectomized women. (Reprinted, with permission, from Chang *et al.* [12], © by The Endocrine Society.)

to corticotropin-releasing factor (CRF) stimulation [23] (Fig. 27.6) and this response was similar in patients with elevated LH levels as in "classic" PCO, as well as in those patients with normal gonadotropins considered to be "PCO-like." We have also found that many patients with HCA exhibit enhanced sensitivity to dexamethasone suppression (>60% reduction in levels of testosterone, unbound testosterone and androstenedione after 3 days of 2 mg/day suppression) [24]. In these these patients, however, basal levels were not helpful in predicting this dexamethasone sensitivity, including measurements of DHEAS, which were normal in some patients [24]. The dexamethasone sensitivity, however, was associated with a diminished response of ACTH to CRF stimulation, suggesting an increased adrenal sensitivity and an altered CRF–ACTH–adrenal axis in some patients (Fig. 27.7).

Androgen secretion and ovarian morphology

Is the appearance of the ovary associated with differences in the secretion of androgen from either ovary or adrenal? In studies of Moltz *et al.* [25], laparoscopic visualization of all hirsute hyperandrogenic patients was carried out prior to ovarian and adrenal venous catheterization studies. In those patients with and without ovaries considered to represent PCO, the pattern of androgen secretion and its severity did not differ [25]. Combined ovarian and adrenal hypersecretion was evident in 46% of "PCO cases," while in 21% and 12%, respectively, the hypersecretion was exclusively from the ovary or adrenal (Fig. 27.8). This pattern was similar in hyperandrogenic patients without the classic ovarian findings. From these data, we can draw the conclusion that in HCA there is evidence for both ovarian and adrenal androgenic hypersecretion and that the morphologic appearance of the ovary is not a valuable discriminating criterion.

Peripheral androgen secretion and the finding of hirsutism

In the retrospective series of Goldzieher and Axelrod [26], 30% of the patients described as having PCO were not hirsute. This figure may increase depending on the diagnostic criteria used for PCO or HCA and the ethnic origin of patients. In races where body hair is generally less (i.e. Orientals), it has been found that hirsutism is absent in over 80% of patients despite mixed hyperandrogenism and other "classic" criteria of PCO [27]. The concept that should be re-emphasized here is that it is skin 5α-reductase activity which largely determines the presence or

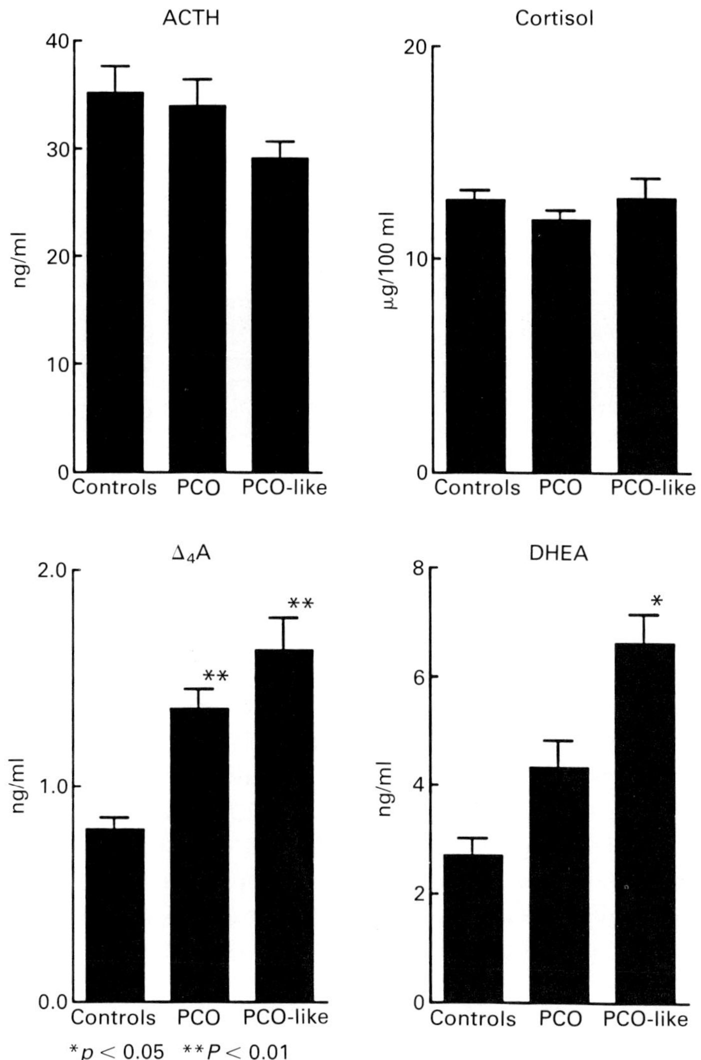

Fig. 27.6 Increase above baseline levels of ACTH and adrenal steroids after ovine corticotropin-releasing factor (1 μg/kg intravenously) in controls and patients. (Reprinted, with permission, from Carmina and Lobo [23].)

absence of hirsutism [28,29]. While patients with HCA and "classic" PCO are so diagnosed because of hyperandrogenemia, hirsutism need not be present. The hyperandrogenemia of adrenal or ovarian origin does not differentiate between patients with or without hirsutism.

In our previous work, patients who had strict criteria for the diagnosis of PCO with the exception of the presence or absence of hirsutism

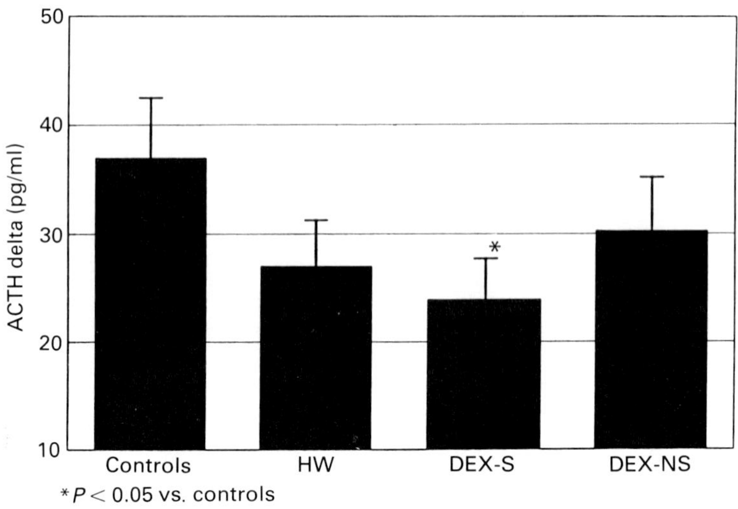

Fig. 27.7 Adrenocorticotropic hormone (ACTH) delta maximum responses of plasma ACTH (mean ± SE) after ovine corticotropin-releasing factor in controls, hirsute women (HW) and the dexamethasone-sensitive (DEX-S) and dexamethasone nonsensitive (DEX-NS) subgroups. (Reprinted, with permission of The American Fertility Society, from Carmina *et al.* [24].)

were divided into those with and without hirsutism [29]. While precursor androgens from the ovary or adrenal could not explain the presence or absence of hirsutism in these patients, a marker of peripheral androgen metabolism (serum 3α-diol G) and of 5α-reductase activity clearly made this distinction. Recent data have reconfirmed these findings and have included the measurement of several other markers of skin 5α-reductase activity [30] (Fig. 27.9).

The unifying concept to be recognized, therefore, is that, even though patients with HCA are hyperandrogenic, hirsutism is associated with the finding of enhanced 5α-reductase activity. This may be normal or elevated in patients and appears to be largely genetically or ethnically determined. Blood markers of 5α-reductase activity include primarily the glucuronide and sulfate conjugates of 3α-diol, but also the conjugates of androsterone. Our preliminary data suggest that 3α-diol G and androsterone glucuronide (Ao G) are most useful among these markers. These metabolites may be elevated even in the presence of normal 5α-reductase activity if precursor androgen levels are elevated and particularly if androstenedione is elevated, as the latter is the preferred substrate for 5α-reductase activity in women [31,32]. However, with only moderate elevations in androgens, high levels of 3α-diol G and Ao G signify enhanced 5α-reductase activity and correlate closely with the finding of hirsutism.

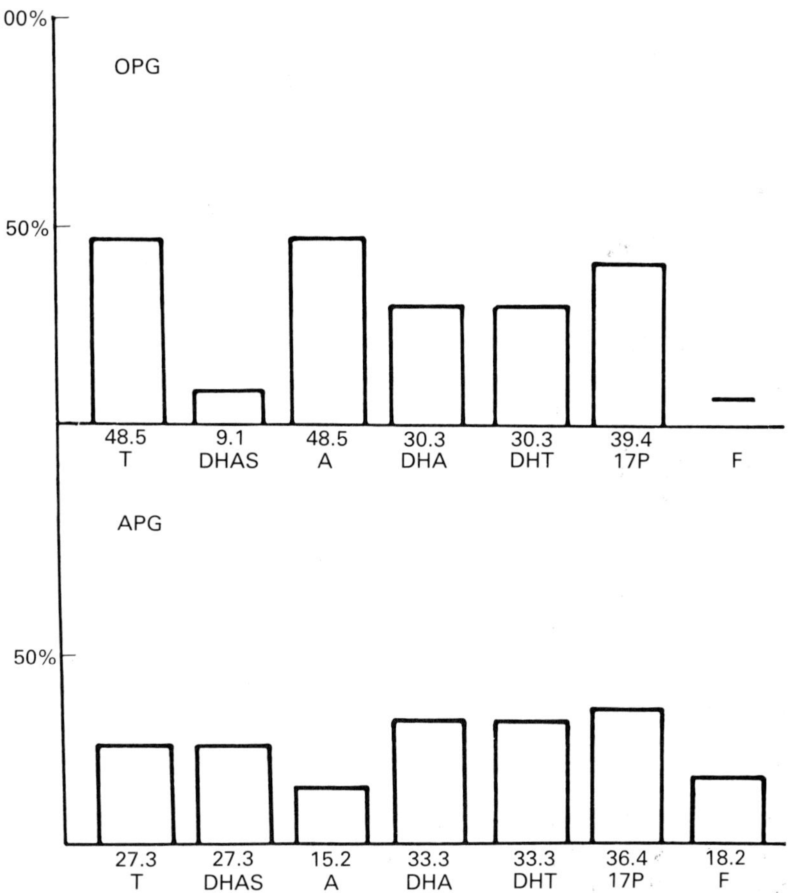

Fig. 27.8 Individual percentage increases of elevated ovarian- and adrenal-peripheral vein gradients (OPG, APG) in 33 patients with polycystic ovaries (> mean + two standard deviations of eight normal control subjects). (Reprinted, with permission, from Moltz *et al.* [25].)

Summary

Hyperandrogenism is one of the two hallmark features of HCA and distinguishes these patients from other patients with anovulation. Both ovarian and androgenic adrenal hyperfunction are present in the majority of patients and this is not influenced by ovarian morphologic findings. Since anovulation and hyperandrogenism may give rise to cystic ovarian changes, the latter finding, although not required for the diagnosis, is extremely prevalent. The causes for the mixed glandular androgenic hyperfunction in HCA include LH, insulin, growth factors and subtle

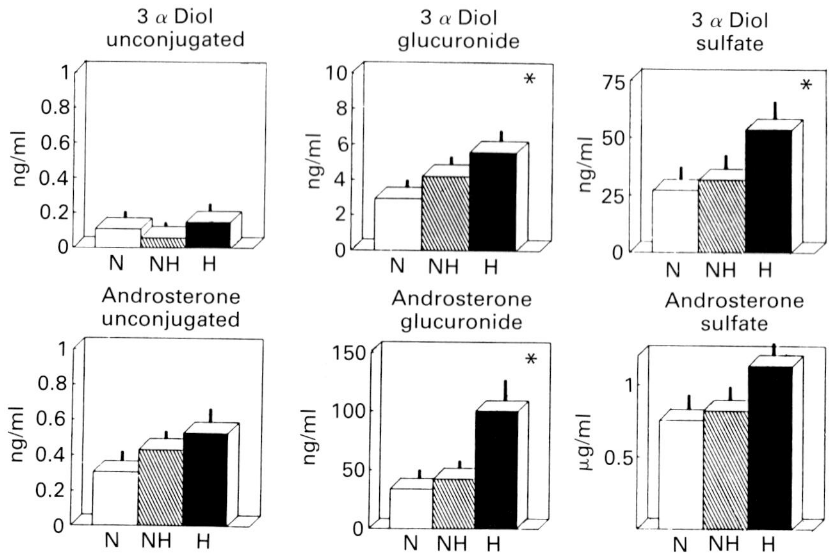

Fig. 27.9 Mean (±SE) of serum unconjugated 3α-diol and androsterone as well as their glucuronide and sulfate conjugates in normal women (N), nonhirsute women with polycystic ovary syndrome (NH) and hirsute women (H). *Significance of difference of H women compared with either N or NH women was $P < 0.05$. (Reprinted, with permission, from Matteri *et al.* [30].)

changes in adrenal sensitivity and the CRF–ACTH axis. Hyperandrogenism is not synonymous with hirsutism and the latter finding is highly associated with enhanced skin 5α-reductase activity. Specific blood markers of 5α-reductase activity may be helpful in determining the presence of enhanced 5α-reductase activity in hirsute patients with this heterogeneous clinical syndrome.

References

1 Vara P, Niemineva K. Small cystic degeneration of ovaries as incidental finding in gynecological laparotomies. Acta Obstet Gynecol Scand 1951; 31:94–107.
2 Givens JR. Polycystic ovaries—a sign, not a diagnosis. Semin Reprod Endocrinol 1984; 2:271–80.
3 Erickson GF, Magoffin DA, Jones KL. Theca function in polycystic ovaries of a patient with virilizing congenital adrenal hyperplasia. Fertil Steril 1989; 51:173–6.
4 Adams J, Polson DW, Franks S. Prevalence of polycystic ovaries in women with anovulation and idiopathic hirsutism. Br Med J 1986; 293:355–9.
5 Hann LE, Hall DA, McArdle CR, Seibel M. Polycystic ovarian disease: sonographic spectrum. Radiology 1984; 150:531–4.
6 Polson DW, Adams J, Wadsworth J, Franks S: Polycystic ovaries—a common finding in normal women. Lancet 1988; i:870–2.
7 Futterweit W, Deligdisch L. Histopathological effects of exogenously administered

testosterone in 19 female to male transsexuals. J Clin Endocrinol Metab 1986; 62: 16–21.
8 Spinder T, Spijkstra JJ, van den Tweel JG, Burger CW, van Kessel H, Hompes PGA, Gooren LJG. The effects of long term testosterone administration on pulsatile luteinizing hormone secretion and on ovarian histology in eugonadal female to male transsexual subjects. J Clin Endocrinol Metab 1989; 69:151–7.
9 Lobo RA, Granger LR, Paul WL, Goebelsmann U, Mishell DR Jr. Psychological stress and increases in urinary norepinephrine metabolites, platelet serotonin and adrenal androgens in women with polycystic ovary syndrome. Am J Obstet Gynecol 1983; 145:496–503.
10 DeVane GW, Czekala NM, Judd HL, Yen SSC. Circulating gonadotropins, estrogens, and androgens in polycystic ovarian disease. Am J Obstet Gynecol 1975; 121:496–500.
11 Moltz L, Schwartz U. Gonadal and adrenal androgen secretion in hirsute female. Clin Endocrinol Metab 1986; 15:229–45.
12 Chang RJ, Laufer LR, Meldrum DR, De Fazio J, Lu JKH, Vale WW, Rivier JE, Judd HC. Steriod secretion in polycystic ovarian disease after ovarian suppression by a long-acting gonadotropin-releasing hormone agonist. J Clin Endocrinol Metab 1983; 56: 897–903.
13 Rittmaster RS. Differential suppression of testosterone and estradiol in hirsute women with the superactive gonadotropin-releasing hormone agonist leuprolide. J Clin Endocrinol Metab 1988; 67:651–5.
14 Rosenfield RL, Barnes RB, Cara JF, Lucky AW. Dysregulation of cytochrome $P450_{C17\alpha}$ as the cause of polycystic ovarian syndrome. Fertil Steril 1990; 53:785–91.
15 Lobo RA, Kletzky OA, Campeau JD, diZerega GS. Elevated bioactive luteinizing hormone in women with the polycystic ovary syndrome. Fertil Steril 1983; 39:674–8.
16 Barbieri RL, Makris A, Randall RW, Daniels G, Kistner RW, Ryan KJ. Insulin stimulates androgen accumulation in incubations of ovarian stroma obtained from women with hyperandrogenism. J Clin Endocrinol Metab 1976; 62:904–10.
17 Filicori M, Campaniello E, Michelacci L, Pareschi A, Ferrari P, Bolelli G, Flamigni C. Gonadotropin-releasing hormone (GnRH) analog suppression renders polycystic ovarian disease patients more susceptible to ovulation induction with pulsatile GnRH. J Clin Endocrinol Metab 1988; 66:327–33.
18 Lachelin GCL, Barnett M, Hopper BR, Brink G, Yen SSC. Adrenal function in normal women and women with the polycystic ovary syndrome. J Clin Endocrinol Metab 1979; 49:892–8.
19 Polson DW, Reed MJ, Franks S, Scanlon MJ, James VHT. Serum 11β-hydroxyandrostenedione as an indicator of the source of excess androgen production in women with polycystic ovaries. J Clin Endocrinol Metab 1988; 66:946–50.
20 Gross MD, Wortsman J, Shapiro B, Meyers LC, Woodbury MC, Ayers JWT. Scintigraphic evidence of adrenal cortical dysfunction in the polycystic ovary syndrome. J Clin Endocrinol Metab 1986; 62:197–201.
21 Hoffman DI, Klove K, Lobo RA. The prevalence and significance of elevated dehydroepiandrosterone sulfate levels in anovulatory women. Fertil Steril 1984; 42:76–81.
22 Lobo RA. The role of the adrenal in polycystic ovary syndrome. Semin Reprod Endocrinol 1984; 2:251–62.
23 Carmina E, Lobo RA. Pituitary–adrenal responses to ovine corticotropin-releasing factor in polycystic ovary syndrome and in other hyperandrogenic patients. Gynecol Endocrinol 1990; 4:225–32.
24 Carmina E, Levin JH, Malizia G, Lobo RA. Ovine corticotropin-releasing factor and dexamethasone responses in hyperandrogenic women. Fertil Steril 1990; 54:245–50.
25 Moltz L, Sörensen R, Römmler A, Schwartz U, Hammerstein J. Polyzystische ovarien: Eigenständiges krankheitsbild oder unspezifisches symptom? Geburtshilfe und Frauenheilkunde 1985; 45:107–14.

26 Goldzieher JW, Axelrod LR. Clinical and biochemical features of polycystic ovarian disease. Fertil Steril 1963; 14:631–53.
27 Aono T, Miyazaki M, Miyake A, Kinugasa T, Kurachi K, Matsumoto K. Responses of serum gonadotropins to LH-releasing hormone and oestrogens in Japanese women with polycystic ovaries. Acta Endocrinol 1977; 85:840–9.
28 Serafini P, Alban F, Lobo RA. 5α-Reductase activity in the genital skin of hirsute women. J Clin Endocrinol Metab 1985; 60:349–55.
29 Lobo RA, Goebelsmann U, Horton R. Evidence for the importance of peripheral tissue events in the development of hirsutism in polycystic ovary syndrome. J Clin Endocrinol Metab 1983; 57:393–7.
30 Matteri RK, Stanczyk FZ, Gentzschein EE, Delgado C, Lobo RA. Androgen sulfate and glucuronide conjugates in nonhirsute and hirsute women with polycystic ovarian syndrome. Am J Obstet Gynecol 1989; 161:1704–9.
31 Silva PD, Gentzschein EEK, Lobo RA. Androstenedione may be a more important precursor of tissue dihydrotestosterone than testosterone in women. Fertil Steril 1987; 48:419–22.
32 Gompel A, Wright F, Kuttenn F, Mauvais-Jarvis P. Contribution of plasma androstenedione to 5α-androstanediol glucuronide in women with idiopathic hirsutism. J Clin Endocrinol Metab 1986; 62:441–4.

Chapter 28
Medical and Surgical Treatment of Polycystic Ovary Syndrome

R. JEFFREY CHANG & JEFFREY R. CRAGUN

Polycystic ovary syndrome (PCO) is a disorder of apparently heterogeneous etiology that is associated with widespread variation in clinical presentation. Despite the recognized diversity in the manifestation of this condition, there appear to be at least two major features that define PCO: chronic anovulation and evidence of hyperandrogenism, the latter usually being reflected by increased hair growth or, on occasion, virilization. In 50% of cases there is associated obesity and, to a lesser extent, acne [1]. The diagnosis generally can be made from a careful history of infrequent or absent menstruation and the gradual appearance of excessive hair growth. The distribution of hirsutism usually involves the face but may also involve the lower abdomen and chest. In the classical description of this disorder, the ovaries were bilaterally enlarged and occupied by cystic follicles in the area of the cortex [2]. In addition, a thick sclerotic coat encapsulated each ovary.

The endocrine profile usually demonstrates elevated levels of circulating androgens, of which the most biologically active originate from the ovaries. Adrenal androgens are increased in 50% of patients. The abnormally increased androgens are converted peripherally to estrogens, which are unopposed by progesterone as a result of the anovulatory state. This hormonal environment can lead to chronic endometrial stimulation and even to endometrial carcinoma. Thus, the clinical and hormonal features of PCO give rise to three major areas of therapeutic concern: an excess of hair growth and acne due to target organ stimulation by abnormal androgen production; chronic anovulation resulting in infertility; and the possibility of endometrial hyperplasia and, potentially, of endometrial cancer due to uninterrupted estrogen secretion.

Hirsutism

The occurrence of hirsutism and acne in PCO represents three interrelated functions. The first of these is abnormal androgen production by the ovary and the adrenal gland. It is evident that the most biologically active hormones, androstenedione and testosterone, are derived from the ovary [3]. The relatively weaker androgens, dehydroepiandrosterone (DHEA) and its sulfate (DHEAS), arise from the adrenal gland. This distinction is of clinical importance, since it impacts upon therapeutic considerations. The evaluation of hirsutism allows for this differentiation to be made. When total serum testosterone is elevated, hyperandrogenism is likely to be due to an ovarian source. An increase in levels of DHEAS would suggest an adrenal origin. If levels of both hormones are elevated in serum, then treatment is directed toward suppression of ovarian production of androgen. Adrenal suppression should only be considered if levels of DHEAS alone are increased. A careful pelvic examination should be performed to rule out the possibility of an ovarian neoplasm. If the androgen levels are high enough to suggest a neoplastic process, then imaging of the ovaries and the adrenal glands is imperative. The second aspect of hyperandrogenism involves the transport of androgens in the circulation. In the normal female, 99% of circulating testosterone is bound to sex hormone-binding globulin (SHBG). In the hyperandrogenic state SHBG is reduced and, as a result, circulating levels of free testosterone are elevated. The role of SHBG appears to be clinically relevant since the extent of excess free testosterone correlates best with the severity of hirsutism [4]. The third process in the development of hirsutism is target organ responsiveness to androgen. This responsiveness is dictated in part by ethnic background. In addition, some patients with hirsutism appear to exhibit increased rates of conversion of testosterone to dihydrotestosterone (DHT), which is the intracellular hormone that is primarily responsible for stimulation of the pilosebaceous unit. Thus, hair growth actually represents the combined effects of increased rates of intracellular conversion of testosterone to DHT, increased levels of free androgen in the circulation, and the relative biologic activity of differing types of androgen. A critical factor in the outcome of treatment for hirsutism is the fact that the life cycle of hair on the bearded area of the face is approximately 6 months. Thus, any treatment should be continued for at least this interval and, most likely, for one year. Treatment is directed toward arresting new growth of hair while hair that is present may enter the catagen stage and eventually be shed from the follicle. Another important consideration is the extent of hair growth at the time of initiation of treatment. Those individuals who have severe hirsutism are much less likely to obtain complete relief with any current modality of treatment. Thus, it is important to institute therapy as soon as possible in such patients.

Currently, the primary therapy for hirsutism in women with PCO is ovarian suppression, which is achieved by the administration of a combination of oral contraceptives. Suppression of gonadotropin secretion by combined estrogen and progestin leads to reduced ovarian steroidogenesis and decreased androgen production [5]. The estrogen content of the combined preparation increases levels of SHBG, which decrease serum levels of free testosterone. It is also likely that estrogen is antiandrogenic at the target organ. The progestin component has been shown to increase the clearance of testosterone, thereby contributing to an overall reduced androgen effect. It should be noted that synthetic progesterones are derived from 19-nortestosterone compounds. Therefore, those derivatives that have the highest androgenic potential should be avoided in the treatment of PCO (e.g. levonorgestrel).

Recently, marked suppression of ovarian steroidogenesis in PCO has been achieved by the administration of a long-acting agonist of gonadotropin-releasing hormone (GnRH) [3]. Studies in PCO patients and in women with regular ovulation and endometriosis revealed the total obliteration of ovarian steroid production. Not surprisingly, the arrest of ovarian steroid production was associated with postmenopausal symptomatology, such as hot flashes and vaginal dryness. Over a period of administration of 6 months hair growth was reduced in the majority of patients and skin oiliness was eliminated in all patients. Whether this therapeutic modality is practical remains unclear since circulating levels of estrogens are decreased to castrate levels. These low levels raise the possibility of bone loss and the risk of cardiovascular disease with prolonged administration. Long-term follow-up of patients who completed the study indicated a resumption of clinical symptomatology within approximately 3 months. The possible therapeutic utility of this compound is currently under investigation.

Excessive adrenal androgen production may be adequately treated by the administration of dexamethasone or similar glucocorticoid [6]. This treatment has been shown to benefit patients with PCO, particularly those with mild hirsutism. In theory, the effectiveness of this treatment may be limited since major reductions occur only in levels of the weak androgens DHEA and DHEAS and not in levels of the major bioactive steroids, androstenedione and testosterone. Combined ovarian and adrenal suppression has been utilized in the past. However, this form of therapy has not always been proven to be effective or tolerable.

The introduction of antiandrogen therapy in the USA has significantly influenced the treatment of hirsutism. Antiandrogens reduce hair growth primarily by blocking the action of testosterone at the target organ through competitive binding to its receptor. In the USA only spironolactone and cimetidine are available for use at this time. Spironolactone exerts an additional effect on androgen metabolism by interfering with cytochrome P-450. This interference results in defective steroidogenesis and a decrease in testosterone production [7]. The combination of an oral contraceptive with spironolactone has proven to be satisfactory for those patients who do not respond to either compound alone. As an aldosterone antagonist, spironolactone may also be associated with a mild reduction in blood pressure and a mild elevation in serum potassium levels. Cimetidine has been reported to decrease hair growth in hirsute individuals. The clinical benefit from this drug has been disappointing and it is not used frequently.

Local measures have been used by many patients to remove excessive hair. The most successful of these methods is electrolysis. Unfortunately, electrolysis can be painful and is expensive. Depilatory creams are available without prescription and may be used very successfully by some individuals. Some caution should be exercised by those women who tend to have sensitive facial skin. Waxing and plucking of hairs should be avoided since surrounding hair follicles are stimulated by these techniques.

Anovulation

Since approximately 1–4% of women in their childbearing years exhibit the syndrome of polycystic ovaries, the concern for anovulation and infertility is significant. The precise mechanism for the failure of ovulation in these women is unknown. Careful studies have demonstrated a pattern of diminished pituitary follicle-stimulating hormone (FSH) secretion that, presumably, results from the negative feedback effects of chronic estrogen secretion [8]. It is noteworthy that a significant characteristic of FSH secretion is an absence or diminution of pulse frequency. The impact of low-amplitude FSH pulses is underscored by the fact that the absolute concentration of circulating FSH is usually in the normal range (see Chapters 3 and 4). Another important consideration in the anovulatory process is the presence of high intraovarian androgen concentrations, which may, perhaps, inhibit folliculogenesis (see Chapter 10). It has been demonstrated in animal studies that elevated intraovarian concentrations of androgens are associated with decreased ovarian weight and an increase in the presence of atretic follicles, presumably as a result of androgen effect [9]. The question of oocyte health in relation to this hyperandrogenic environment has not been addressed. Another consideration is whether or not hyperprolactinemia plays a role in the anovulation associated with PCO. It has been reported that 25–30% of patients with PCO will exhibit increased levels of circulating prolactin levels [10]. Informative data are lacking in this area.

Induction of ovulation in women with PCO is most commonly attempted by the administration of clomiphene citrate. This drug is similar in molecular structure to diethylstilbestrol (DES) and may exhibit both estrogenic and antiestrogenic properties. While the mechanism is not totally understood, it is believed that clomiphene citrate interrupts the negative feedback effects of estrogen by binding to estrogen receptors in the hypothalamus and pituitary gland. This blockade of estrogen negative feedback allows for increased FSH secretion and follicle stimulation with eventual ovulation. The precise action of clomiphene citrate is unknown, although experimental evidence suggests that there are effects at the levels of the hypothalamus, the pituitary and the ovary [11]. The usual initial starting dose is 50 mg/day for 5 days, commencing on day 2 or 3 of spontaneous or progesterone-induced menses. Progesterone-induced menses may be achieved by either a 5-day course of Provera, 10 mg/day, or an injection of progesterone and oil, 100 mg. Subsequent vaginal bleeding provides a reference point for the commencement of therapy, assures adequate levels of estrogen, and safely confirms the absence of pregnancy. A rise in the basal body temperature (BBT) at approximately 12–14 days followed by spontaneous vaginal bleeding or a serum progesterone level above 10 ng/ml in the midluteal phase is indicative of a normal ovulatory response. The same dose of clomiphene citrate is repeated during the next cycle if pregnancy does not occur. In the absence of spontaneous menses, the dose is then increased by increments of 50 mg to a total daily dose of 150 mg for 5 days, or until an ovulatory response is achieved as indicated by a biphasic BBT or an elevated luteal level of progesterone. Higher doses of clomiphene citrate, up to 250 mg/day, have been employed in some patients but the success rate has been low. It may be more appropriate to modify the regimen by reducing the dose of clomiphene citrate to 100 mg/day and giving human chorionic gonadotropin (HCG) (10 000 IU) on day 13 of administration of clomiphene citrate. Extension of the duration of treatment or imposition of an incremental dose regimen has not proven highly successful.

In cases where there is evidence of concomitant adrenal hyperandrogenism, it is reasonable to combine clomiphene citrate therapy with administration of dexamethasone. Previous studies have demonstrated that patients with slightly increased levels of DHEAS exhibit higher rates of ovulation and pregnancy after administration of combined therapy than after therapy with clomiphene citrate alone [12]. The increase in levels of DHEAS need not necessarily exceed the upper normal range but should, rather, be higher than the mean concentration established by a given laboratory.

In the presence of coexistent hyperprolactinemia, it is unclear whether bromocriptine therapy results in a significantly increased rate of ovulation. Moreover, addition of bromocriptine to clomiphene citrate therapy has not been adequately studied. Until more convincing data are available, it is not recommended to use bromocriptine for ovulation induction in women with PCO.

Up to 30% of women with PCO will not ovulate in response to clomiphene citrate alone or in combination with other indicated drugs. This situation is best addressed by a consideration of gonadotropin therapy. Gonadotropins may be administered either as human menopausal gonadotropins (Pergonal) or as purified urinary FSH (Metrodin). These drugs stimulate the ovary directly to effect follicular development and require the use of HCG to trigger actual ovulation. Gonadotropin therapy is more complex than clomiphene citrate therapy and, because of potentially serious side effects, it requires careful monitoring. The use of ultrasound and techniques for the rapid determination of estrogen levels have proven to be highly beneficial in reducing the incidence of hyperstimulation. While mild degrees of hyperstimulation are quite common with the use of this drug regimen, severe cases, marked by proteinuria, ascites, hydrothorax, and hypovolemia, are uncommon. The dose of gonadotropins is adjusted according to the follicular response of each individual. Thus, there is a need for careful monitoring on an individual basis.

Some patients with PCO will not respond to any of the above therapies and, in such cases, consideration may be given to an ovarian wedge resection. The classical description of an ovarian wedge resection involved removal of a significant piece of ovarian tissue by sharp dissection. Early experiences with the procedure were associated with considerable pelvic adhesions, thereby increasing the problem of infertility. Recently, this procedure has been re-examined with the introduction of capsule penetration either by cautery or with laser therapy [13]. In some instances, direct aspiration of follicles has also resulted in a short-term ovulatory response. It is important to emphasize that the results of capsule penetration are usually short-lived and, commonly, the pretreatment condition of anovulation recurs. A second major consideration is the fact that with cautery and laser therapy there may be substantial incidence of pelvic adhesions, which again serve only to further impair fertility in these patients.

Endometrial hyperplasia

While their immediate concerns regarding hirsutism and anovulatory infertility are of great importance to patients with PCO, a far greater and more serious threat to life exists with respect to exposure to chronic unopposed estrogen. It is well known that continuous administration of high doses of estrogen in postmenopausal women leads to endometrial hyperplasia. This phenomenon is similar to the presence of long-term unopposed estrogen in women with chronic anovulation. In women with PCO there appears to be a greater incidence of endometrial hyperplasia than in normal women and, in some instances, endometrial carcinoma is encountered. The histologic pattern of disease usually involves well-differentiated or moderately well-differentiated endometrial adenocarcinoma. The importance of the recognition of these sequelae of chronic anovulation in PCO is underscored by the typical histories of young women who are found to have endometrial cancer [14]. This process is compounded in the presence of obestity. Thus, endometrial sampling should be mandatory in patients with a long history of chronic anovulation, in particular when it is associated with obesity.

Consideration of the development of endometrial hyperplasia or adenocarcinoma requires active therapeutic intervention to eliminate the unopposed estrogen state. Commonly, such intervention involves the introduction of progesterone either by exogenous administration or endogenously through ovulation induction. If prevention of endometrial hyperplasia is the primary therapeutic concern, then medroxyprogesterone acetate (Provera) should be administered at a dose of 10 mg/day for at least 10 days each month to induce menstrual bleeding. Other progestins, including derivatives of 19-nortestosterone, may be used but the known adverse side effects as they relate to lipid metabolism must be considered. Previous studies have demonstrated that the administration of GnRH agonists may cause a hyperplastic endometrium to revert to an atrophic or normal proliferative appearance [3]. Such agonist therapy remains an investigational protocol at this time. If the patient is seeking fertility, then successful ovulation induction by either clomiphene or gonadotropin therapy will be sufficient to counter the stimulatory effects of chronic estrogen secretion. These therapeutic modalities are designed to eliminate the risk of endometrial disease. However, it is likely that they do not entirely exclude the risk of endometrial cancer. Therefore, in the presence of abnormal bleeding, a sampling of the endometrium must be performed.

References

1 Goldzieher JW, Green JA. The polycystic ovary. I. Clinical and histologic features. J Clin Endocrinol Metab 1962; 22:325–37.

2 Stein IF, Leventhal ML. Amenorrhea associated with bilateral polycystic ovaries. Am J Obstet Gynecol 1935; 29:181–91.

3 Chang RJ, Laufer LR, Meldrum DR, De Fazio J, Lu JKH, Vale WW, Rivier JE, Judd HL. Steroid secretion in polycystic ovarian disease after ovarian suppression by a long-acting gonadotropin-releasing hormone agonist. J Clin Endocrinol Metab 1983; 56:897–903.

4 Rosenfield RL. Plasma testosterone-binding globulin and indexes of the concentration of unbound plasma androgens in normal and hirsute subjects. J Clin Endocrinol Metab 1971; 32:717–28.

5 Givens JR, Anderson RN, Wiser W, Umstot ES, Fish SA. The effectiveness of two oral contraceptives in suppressing plasma androstenedione, testosterone, LH, and FSH, and in stimulating plasma testosterone-binding capacity in hirsute women. Am J Obstet Gynecol 1976; 124:333–9.

6 Smith KD, Steinberger E, Perloff WH. Polycystic ovarian disease. A report of 301 patients. Am J Obstet Gynecol 1965; 93:994–1001.

7 Cummings DC, Young JC, Rebar RW, Yen SSC. Treatment of hirsutism with spironolactone. JAMA 1982; 247:1295–8.

8 Rebar RW, Judd HL, Yen SSC, Rakoff J, Van Den Berg G, Naftolin F. Characterization of the inappropriate gonadotropin secretion in polycystic ovary syndrome. J Clin Invest 1976; 57:1320–9.

9 Febres F, Gondos B, Siiteri P. Androgen-induced ovarian follicular atresia in the rat. Gynecol Invest 1976; 7:52.

10 Parkes D. Bromocriptine. N Engl J Med 1979; 301:893–898.

11 Adashi EY. Clomiphene citrate: mechanism(s) and site(s) of action—a hypothesis revisited. Fertil Steril 1984; 42:331–44.

12 Daly DC, Walter CA, Soto-Albors CE, Tohan N, Riddick DH. A randomized study of dexamethasone in ovulation induction with clomiphene citrate. Fertil Steril 1984; 41:844–8.

13 Greenblatt E, Casper RF. Endocrine changes after laparoscopic ovarian cautery in polycystic ovarian syndrome. Am J Obstet Gynecol 1987; 156:279–85.

14 Fechner RE, Kaufman RH. Endometrial adenocarcinoma in Stein–Leventhal syndrome. Cancer 1974; 34:444–52.

Chapter 29
Psychosocial Consequences of Androgen Effects

ANKE A. EHRHARDT

Gender identity

When patients experience problems of intersexuality from an early age, the various components of psychosexual differentiation and their determination by genetic, hormonal and social environmental factors must all be considered by the physician. Perhaps the most important aspect of behavioral development, as well as the most basic aspect of personality development, is gender identification. This is determined very early and usually remains constant throughout life, and is thus a critical consideration in the case of women who show excessive androgen effects in adulthood. While anecdotal clinical reports often imply that such patients frequently question their gender identification, this is, in fact, extremely rare. Rather, gender identification, once formed either as male or female, tends to remain firm despite the many incongruous physical symptoms that may occur.

Gender differences

In terms of hormones, research into gender differences of behavior is thus probably more fruitful than is research into gender identification. Indeed, there is a whole field of animal experimentation that has examined prenatal and neonatal sex hormones and their effects on the brain and behavior. The classic model in human development is congenital adrenal hyperpasia (CAH), which is described by Maria New in Chapter 13. We now have a considerable body of knowledge regarding childhood behavior as it may be influenced by high levels of prenatal androgens either naturally occurring, as in CAH, or via exogenous administration of androgen to the mother. Over the last 20 years, a number of studies have looked at the potential behavioral effects of high-level prenatal androgens in CAH [4]. Using various control groups and study designs, it has been fairly well established that prenatally androgenized girls tend to be higher in a cluster of behaviors having to do with physical energy, but tend to be lower than controls in those behaviors that relate to parenting interest and nurturance. Before one can assume, however, that prenatal androgens determine these behaviors, one must consider the overlap between boys and girls in sexually dimorphic behavior, or gender differences in behavior, among human beings. For example, while among preschoolers there is a mean difference and different distributions between the sexes in physical energy, resulting in more boys than girls having high levels, there is an enormous overlap. Thus, if we are considering sex differences that may be influenced by prenatal hormones (or for that matter, by postnatal hormones), we are talking about slight differences in the expression rather than the determination of a whole set of behaviors. And therefore, the behaviour, of course, is not truly sexually dimorphic. An additional difficulty is that all hormone actions interrelate to some extent with social environmental factors, so that direct hormonal effects will tend to be obscured.

Even less is known about the continuing effects of prenatal androgens on adult behavior. We do not have a body of data on adult behavior subsequent to high levels of prenatal androgens. We know a little more, however, about some of the exogenous hormones, notably diethylstilbestrol (DES). As is well known, DES is a peculiar substance because, in animal experiments, it is not bound like other estrogens either by α-fetoprotein or by the placental barrier, but to a large extent passes to the brain and thus acts like an aromatized androgen, binding with estrogen receptors. Recently, we examined [2] a sample of those young men and women whose mothers took DES to address the question whether there is any evidence that prenatal DES has a long-term effect on adult behavior.

After studying several hundred DES daughters, sons, mothers and siblings, and comparing them to various control groups, we have found that, as a group and in terms of psychosexual milestones, DES daughters do not differ from controls. However, they do differ in some of their sexual functioning, in terms of sexual desire and/or in aspects of their sexual behavior. We also found [3,4], somewhat unexpectedly, a significantly elevated level of bisexual behavior in DES females, particularly in the areas of arousal, interest and attraction. Further, compared to one control group, we found more general depression and slightly less feminine behavior. Compared to a second control group, the differences were not as strong, although they were in the same direction. These findings suggest that prenatal DES (an estrogen that acts in one way like an androgen) has an effect on some aspects of psychosexual differentiation.

Androgens and women

More specifically, what do we know about androgens and their effects on adult female behavior? Unfortunately, our understanding of how elevated androgens affect normal female behavior, whether as a result of treatment with exogenous androgens or of endogenous hyperandrogenism, remains far from perfect. Most studies that address such issues have been in the areas of sexual behavior, psychopathology (such as coping), body image, depression, and personality, including the areas of masculine and feminine behavior. John Bancroft, who perhaps has done the most in the area of behavior and androgen, recently reviewed what is known [1]. His findings indicate that, for women, the situation is little short of chaotic because so many studies are contradictory in what they suggest about the role androgens play in behavior. The root of this chaos probably lies in incorrect definition of the behavior entities involved and in the lack of appropriate hormonal studies, rather than in any inherent quality of the field.

Androgens and men

As Bancroft notes, much more is known about the role of androgens in men. For example, there is a whole body of studies concerning normal men and the correlation of plasma testosterone levels with sexual behavior. When studies in this field began, it was believed that men with higher androgen levels might evince some unusual features of sexual functioning. We are now aware that, within the normal range of androgen levels, there does not seem to be a correlation between higher androgen and higher sex drive. Instead, a kind of threshold effect has been assumed.

A number of studies has been conducted on men who present with either erectile dysfunctions or low sexual desire [1]. So far, it appears that therapy with exogenous androgens may increase sexual interest, but not necessarily erectile function. This is very important, because it points to the fact that different aspects of sexual behavior may very well be affected by different kinds of hormones. Therefore, it is incorrect to think in terms of a global measure of libido. Human sexual behavior needs to be divided into different components, similar to those applied by animal experimentalists, ranging from sexual desire to sexual attraction to actual sexual behavior. Of course, sexual behavior itself is enormously complex, being affected by availability of a partner and by that partner's reactions.

In Europe, and in Germany in particular, a large body of knowledge has been accumulated on cyproterone acetate (CPA) treatment for sex offenders [1]. It has been established over the past 15–20 years that both sexual interest and sexual behavior can be decreased by CPA. However, a peculiar finding remains that when sex offenders on CPA are provided with sexual stimuli, such as erotic films related to their particular sexual disorder, their erectile function is normal and not decreased. In contrast, in laboratory environments where male subjects are asked to produce their own sexual fantasies, CPA is shown to decrease erectile function. Thus, the findings indicate that CPA will not affect a male's sexual interest and desire in instances where there is a strong, external stimulus, but that it will negatively affect sexual interest and desire if there are no outside stimuli.

Menstrual cycle

Among women, research has focused on the normal variations of androgen over the menstrual cycle in addition to the various clinical syndromes of hyperandrogenism such as hirsutism, polycystic ovary syndrome (PCO), and the adrenogenital syndrome, and on the effects of treatment with androgens. In terms of menstrual cycle research alone, about 50 studies have looked at sexual behavior and mood [1]. They have produced conflicting evidence regarding androgen action. An obvious correlation to test was between the peak of androgen over the menstrual cycle and different sexual behavior parameters. Generally no such correlation has been established. If anything, it seems that the androgen peak coincides with low sexual interest, and there are a number of arguments as to why this should occur. It may have to do with the fact that the effect is delayed several days as is known from treatment studies, but this remains uncertain.

A number of studies have looked at women with relatively high levels of androgen that fall nonetheless within the normal range [1]. Results consistently suggest that relatively high androgen levels in women correlate with more masturbation, which suggests more sexual interest in the absence of partner stimulus. Further, some studies indicate that women with relatively high levels of androgen tend to be more bisexual or less heterosexual in their activities. Studies of androgen levels in lesbians are equivocal [5]. It has been suggested that about 30% of homosexual women tend to have higher levels of androgens than the average of heterosexual women. However, our own group did a very small, careful study of plasma testosterone and other hormone levels in lesbian women carefully matched to heterosexual women, and did not generally confirm these findings [6]. However, it appears that there is a subgroup of lesbian women who tend to have high androgen levels.

Hirsutism and PCO

Relatively little is known about women with hirsutism or PCO, and this is certainly an area where better studies are needed. Earlier clinical observations typically found that women with hirsutism presented with problems of self-worth and body image, and seemed to be more masculine psychologically. Before such cases were carefully examined, it was generally assumed that women who looked more masculine should be, or would be, more masculine. In fact, a couple of studies [1] that have carefully examined general behavior did not confirm these earlier assumptions.

Studies of the effects of hyperandrogenism and its control in women with hirsutism and PCO were performed in 61 women who were treated with CPA [7]. It was found that 44% reported reduction of sexual interest, desire, and capacity for orgasm. A subanalysis was then conducted of those women who had regular sexual partners and had reported normal sex lives before treatment. Among these women, 61% complained about reduction of sexual interest. Thus, the researchers strongly recommend that any treatment of this kind needs carefully to consider unwanted effects in terms of sexual behavior. Another study, which did not involve treatment [8], carefully compared hirsute women with a control group. The findings indicate that there were significant differences in history, menarche (which was delayed), body weight increase, mood disturbances, number of sexual partners (there were fewer), body image problems, and somatic complaints. However, when gender role was systematically examined, no difference was found.

Menopause

Another area where better studies are needed is treatment of menopausal symptoms, particularly after surgical menopause via bilateral oophorectomy. Sherwin and colleagues [9,10] looked very carefully at estrogen treatment in a crossover study with placebo, estrogen and androgen alone. There was convincing evidence that the most effective treatment is to give estrogen and androgens in combination. They documented that this combination increases energy and a sense of well-being. Clearly, estrogen is critical for vaginal lubrication and may be hot flushes, but it is androgens, in particular, that increase the motivational aspects of sexuality. Clearly, studies of this kind give us substantial evidence about the role of androgens in female behavior. But while it is important to define the syndrome clinically and behaviorally, it is equally critical to define the different subgroups and the behaviors that the various hormonal aspects may influence.

References

1 Bancroft J. Human Sexuality and its Problems, 2nd edn. Edinburgh: Churchill Livingstone, 1989.

2 Ehrhardt AA, Meyer-Bahlburg HFL, Rosen LR, Feldman JD, Veridiano NP, Elkin EJ, McEwen BS. The development of gender-related behavior in females following prenatal exposure to diethylstilbestrol (DES). Horm Behav 1989; 23:526–41.

3 Ehrhardt AA, Meyer-Bahlburg HFL, Rosen LR, *et al.* Sexual orientation after prenatal exposure to exogenous estrogen. Arch Sex Behav 1985; 14:57–77.

4 Ehrhardt AA, Meyer-Bahlburg HFL. Effects of prenatal sex hormones on gender-related behavior. Science 1981; 211:1312–18.

5 Meyer-Bahlburg HFL. Sex hormones and female homosexuality: a critical examination. Arch Sex Behav 1979; 8:101–19.

6 Downey J, Ehrhardt AA, Schiffman M, Dyrenfurth I, Becker J. Sex hormones in lesbian and heterosexual women. Horm Behav 1987; 3:347–57.

7 Appelt H, Strauss B. The effect of anti-androgen treatment on the sexuality of hirsute women. Psychother Psychosom 1984; 42:177–81.

8 Strauss B, Appelt H. Psychological effects on the evaluation of physical symptoms. Psychother Psychosom Med Psychol 1984; 34:179–85.

9 Sherwin BB. Estrogen and/or androgen replacement therapy and cognitive functioning in surgically menopausal women. Psychoneuroendocrinology 1988; 13:345–57.

10 Sherwin BB, Gelfand MM. Sex steroids and affect in the surgical menopause: a double-blind, cross-over study. Psychoneuroendocrinology 1985; 10:325–35.

Chapter 30
Diabetes Mellitus and Polycystic Ovary Syndrome

ANDREA DUNAIF

Background

The observation that diabetes mellitus is associated with hyperandrogenism is not new. Indeed, in 1921, the French scientists Achard and Thiers [1] named this phenomenon "le diabete des femmes à barbe" (the diabetes of bearded women). Although the association of diabetes with hyperandrogenism continued to be reported, it was not until the mid 1970s that Kahn and coworkers [2] described a distinct syndrome in adolescent girls of insulin-resistant diabetes mellitus and hyperandrogenism associated with the dermatologic lesion acanthosis nigricans (AN). They named this constellation the type A syndrome of insulin resistance and recent studies [3,4] have identified several mutations in the insulin receptor gene as causal of the insulin resistance in a few individuals affected with this rare disorder (see Chapter 20 for review).

Several rare syndromes of extreme insulin resistance and AN, often with hyperandrogenism, were identified [5] (e.g. type B, lipoatropic diabetes, Rabson–Mendenhall, leprechaunism). That a disorder of insulin action might be associated with the commonly encountered hyperandrogenic condition polycystic ovary syndrome (PCO) was initially recognized by Burghen, Givens and Kitabchi [6]. These investigators reported that women with PCO had basal and glucose-stimulated hyperinsulinemia compared to obese weight-matched normal women. Further, they noted significant positive linear correlations between insulin and androgens levels and suggested that this might have etiologic significance.

Flier and colleagues [7] as well as Dunaif and colleagues [8], noted that AN occurred more commonly than previously appreciated in hyperandrogenic women. These investigators determined that such women had a distinct disorder of insulin action compared to the rare syndromes of extreme insulin resistance. Indeed, these women had typical PCO, although on histologic examination of their ovaries there was an increase in stromal hyperthecosis suggesting that the insulin-resistant state modified ovarian function. Stuart's group also reported [9] a commonly encountered group of hirsute women with AN and insulin resistance. It is likely that these women also had typical PCO. At the same time, a number of investigators [10–12] were confirming and extending the original observation that women with PCO had hyperinsulinemia, independent of obestity, and secondary to some degree of insulin resistance. Thus, it was evident PCO represented a new uncharacterized disorder of insulin action.

Which groups of hyperandrogenic women are insulin resistant?

In order to determine whether hyperinsulinemia was a unique feature of PCO or a feature of hyperandrogenic states in general, we prospectively evaluated 62 hyperandrogenic women, stratified on the basis of weight and ovulatory status, for basal and glucose-stimulated insulin secretion and glucose tolerance [13]. The presence of AN on clinical examination was noted, and, since ~50% of the obese PCO women had this, it was also used to stratify this group. We found that only anovulatory hyperandrogenic women, whom we diagnosed as having PCO (since adrenal and pituitary disorders had been excluded) (see Chapter 32) had basal and/or glucose-stimulated hyperinsulinemia, independent of obesity (Fig. 30.1). Ovulatory hyperandrogenic women were not hyperinsulinemic. This finding was well supported in the nonobese women because a large sample of ovulatory hyperandrogenic women were studied but was less well supported in the obese women because only five such subjects were studied. It is noteworthy that the ovulatory hyperandrogenic women had higher dehydroepiandrosterone sulfate (DHEAS) levels than the ovulatory control women and the PCO women, consistent with the hypothesis that the androgen profile itself may have some impact on insulin sensitivity (see Chapter 24). These findings strongly suggested that hyperinsulinemia was a unique feature of PCO and not of hyperandrogenic states in general.

The PCO women with AN had significantly higher insulin responses than those without this skin change on clinical examination (Fig. 30.1). Otherwise, the sex hormone and gonadotropin levels were identical in these two subgroups of PCO women. Most importantly, 20% of the obese PCO women had previously undiagnosed frank diabetes mellitus

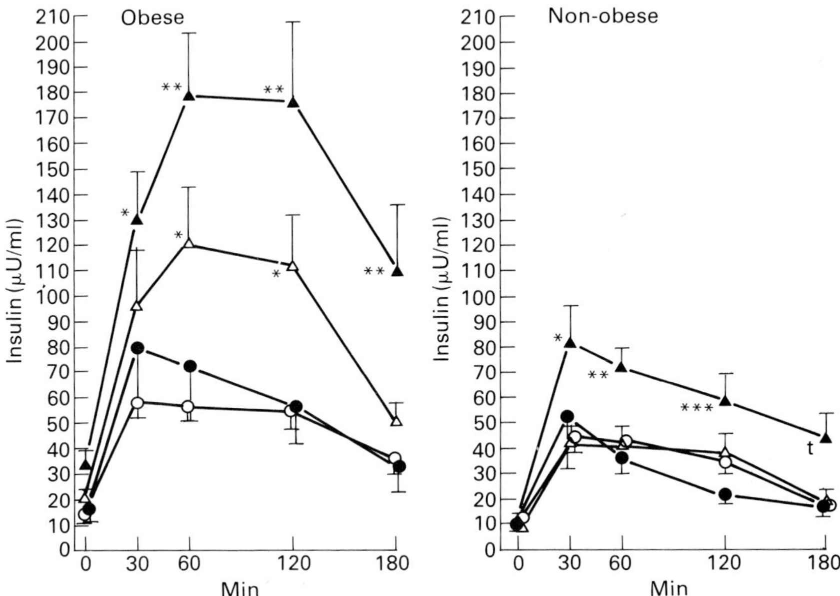

Fig. 30.1 Mean (±SM) serum insulin levels during an oral glucose tolerance test (40 g/m^2 glucose load) in obese (left panel) and nonobese (right panel) women. The obese PCO group is divided into two subgroups: one with AN (▲) and one without AN (△). The other groups are identified as follows. Left panel: ○, obese normal; ●, obese ovulatory hyperandrogenic; right panel: ▲, nonobese PCO; △, nonobese ovulatory hyperandrogenic; ○, nonobese normal; ●, nonobese anovulatory. *, Significantly greater than obese normal (left panel) or nonobese ovulatory hyperandrogenic and nonobese normal (right panel); **, significantly greater than obese PCO without AN, obese ovulatory hyperandrogenic and obese normal (left panel) or nonobese ovulatory hyperandrogenic, nonobese normal and nonobese anovulatory (right panel); ***, significantly greater than nonobese normal and nonobese anovulatory (right panel); t, significantly greater than nonobese normal (right panel). (Reprinted, with permission, from Dunaif *et al.* [13], © by The Endocrine Society.)

or impaired glucose tolerance, independent of the presence of AN (Fig. 30.2). The mean age of these women was 27 years. Thus, PCO represented a previously unappreciated risk factor for the development of noninsulin-dependent diabetes mellitus (NIDDM) at an extremely early age.

Insulin action in PCO

Hyperinsulinemia results from (except in rare instances of mutant insulins) target tissue insulin resistance [14]. In order to determine the magnitude of this defect in insulin action in PCO, we performed euglycemic glucose clamp studies in lean and obese women with PCO [15]. Muscle is the major site of insulin-mediated glucose disposal

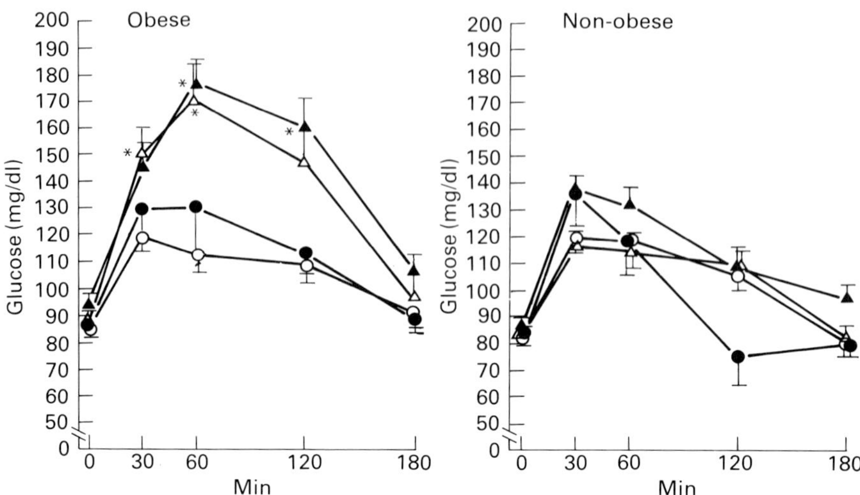

Fig. 30.2 Mean (±SM) plasma glucose levels during a 40 g/m² oral glucose tolerance test in obese (left panel) and nonobese (right panel) women. The groups are identified as in Fig. 30.1. *, Significantly greater than obese normal (left panel). (Reprinted, with permission, from Dunaif *et al.* [13], © by The Endocrine Society.)

[16,17], whereas fat mass independently decreases insulin-mediated glucose disposal [18]. There is an increased prevalence of obesity in women with PCO [19]. Indeed, it has been argued that insulin resistance in PCO is secondary to obesity [20], rather than an independent defect. It is also possible that PCO women might have increases in muscle mass because of their elevated plasma androgen levels [21]. To control for these potentially confounding factors, we matched lean and obese normal control women to the PCO women on the basis of fat and fat-free mass determined by hydrostatic weighing.

The euglycemic glucose clamp is the most accurate and widely accepted method for assessing insulin resistance *in vivo* [22]. This technique permits the measurement not only of peripheral (primarily muscle) insulin sensitivity but also the sensitivity of hepatic glucose production to insulin suppression (with the addition of an isotopically labeled glucose infusion) and of the metabolic clearance rate of insulin. A fixed dose of insulin is infused to produce the desired ambient insulin concentration. A variable infusion of glucose is administered to maintain euglycemia. The amount of glucose infused at steady state is equal to the peripheral glucose utilization (insulin-mediated glucose disposal) and is reported as the index of insulin action in these studies.

Despite the fact that none of the PCO women had a previous history of abnormalities in glucose tolerance, as a group the obese PCO women

Table 30.1 Glucose tolerance and basal hepatic glucose production (HGP) in PCO and normal women [15].

	Fasting glucose (mg/dl)	2-hour glucose (mg/dl)	Fasting insulin (μU/ml)	Basal HGP ($mg/m^2/min$)
Obese PCO ($n = 19$)	92 ± 2*	145 ± 8*	27 ± 5	66 ± 2*
Obese normal ($n = 11$)	84 ± 2	109 ± 6	15 ± 2	57 ± 2
Nonobese PCO ($n = 10$)	84 ± 2	107 ± 5	14 ± 3	63 ± 2
Nonobese normal ($n = 8$)	81 ± 4	84 ± 4	11 ± 2	65 ± 3
P ANOVA	<0.01	<0.001	NS	<0.01

* Mean ± SE, significantly different by least significant difference testing.

had significantly increased basal and 2-hour postglucose load glucose levels compared to the body composition-matched controls [15]. This was the result of significantly increased rates of basal hepatic glucose production (Table 30.1). There were significant statistical interactions between obesity and PCO on basal glucose levels and basal hepatic glucose production (Table 30.1). This suggested that PCO and obesity had a synergistic deleterious effect on glucose tolerance. Two obese PCO women had previously undiagnosed diabetes mellitus. Glucose tolerance and basal hepatic glucose production were completely normal in the lean PCO women (Table 30.1).

Peripheral insulin action was significantly and substantially decreased in lean and in obese PCO women compared to their body composition-matched control groups [15] (Fig. 30.3). The magnitude of the insulin resistance in PCO was similar in severity to that reported in NIDDM (Table 30.2) [22]. This is even more striking because PCO women are much younger (third and fourth decade) than individuals with NIDDM (sixth and seventh decade), since age independently decreases insulin action [25]. Insulin also failed to suppress hepatic glucose production in six PCO women, whereas it was completely suppressed in all normal subjects. This strongly suggests the presence of hepatic as well as peripheral insulin resistance, although the magnitude of this change did not achieve statistical significance. There was no significant difference in the metabolic clearance rate of insulin in PCO suggesting that decreased insulin clearance did not contribute to the hyperinsulinemia. Thus, this study [15] documented that women with PCO had a unique disorder of insulin action independent of obesity and impairment of glucose tolerance.

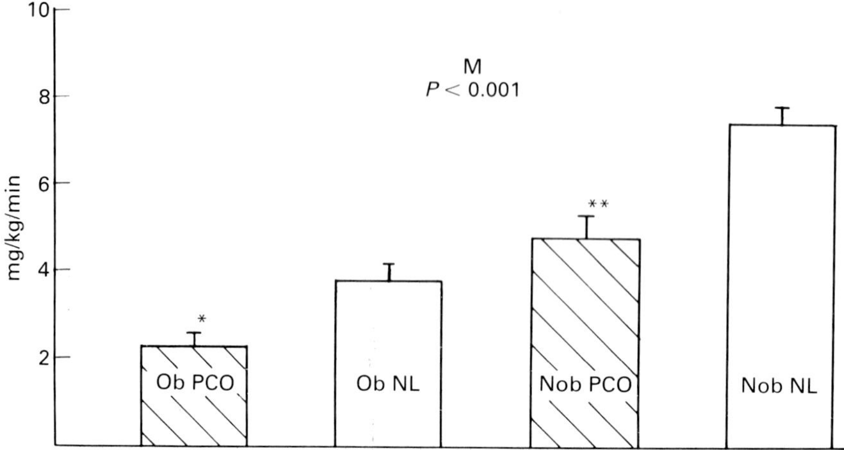

Fig. 30.3 Insulin-mediated glucose disposal (M) at 100 μU/ml insulin level in obese (Ob) and in nonobese (Nob) PCO women as compared to age- and body composition-matched normal (NL) women. Insulin-mediated glucose disposal is significantly decreased in the PCO women compared to controls.

Table 30.2 Comparison of insulin-mediated glucose disposal (M) at 100 μU/ml steady-state insulin level (values are mean ± SE).

	M (mg/kg/min)	Age (years)	Reference
Obese			
PCO	2.3 ± 0.2	26 ± 1	15
NIDDM	2.8 ± 0.2	55 ± 3	23
Nonobese			
PCO	4.8 ± 0.5	27 ± 2	15
NIDDM	5.6 ± 0.4	53 ± 2	24

Our studies have suggested that hyperinsulinemia is not a feature of non-PCO hyperandrogenic states. To our knowledge insulin action has been assessed in more detail in only one study in hyperandrogenic women. This study [26] reported that insulin action determined by the euglycemic glucose clamp was significantly decreased in hyperandrogenic women. The validity of these findings is arguable because the hyperandrogenic women were significantly more obese than the control group and PCO as a cause of the hyperandrogenism was not specifically excluded. This important question merits further study and could be optimally addressed by examining insulin action in women with non-classical 21-hydroxylase deficiency compared to body composition-matched controls.

Acanthosis nigricans and insulin action

There has been a tendency in the field to use the presence of the lesion AN on clinical examination to subgroup hyperandrogenic women [7–9,13]. The only reported biochemical difference is that acanthotic women have higher insulin levels than women lacking this skin change [9,13]. We found no differences in sex hormone levels or the pattern of pulsatile gonadotropin release in PCO women with and without this lesion [13,27].

Acanthosis nigricans is diagnosed by pathognomonic histologic changes: dermal thickening and papillomatosis, hyperkeratosis, and, at times, increased melanin [28]. In order to determine the sensitivity of clinical skin examination for diagnosing AN as well as the best biochemical correlates of this lesion, we prospectively performed skin biopsies in unselected PCO women and in age- and weight-matched normal women [29]. These biopsies were taken from the neck or the axilla and were evaluated blind by a dermatopathologist. Acanthosis nigricans was present on clinical examination in 11/13 obese PCO (Figs 30.4 and 30.5), 3/6 lean PCO, 4/14 obese normal, and 0/4 lean normal

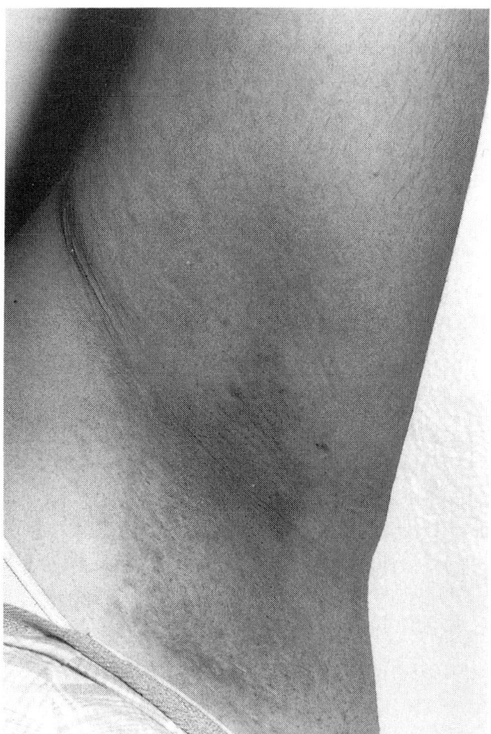

Fig. 30.4 Axilla of a PCO woman with clinically evident severe AN. Note the papillomatous hyperpigmented areas in the axilla.

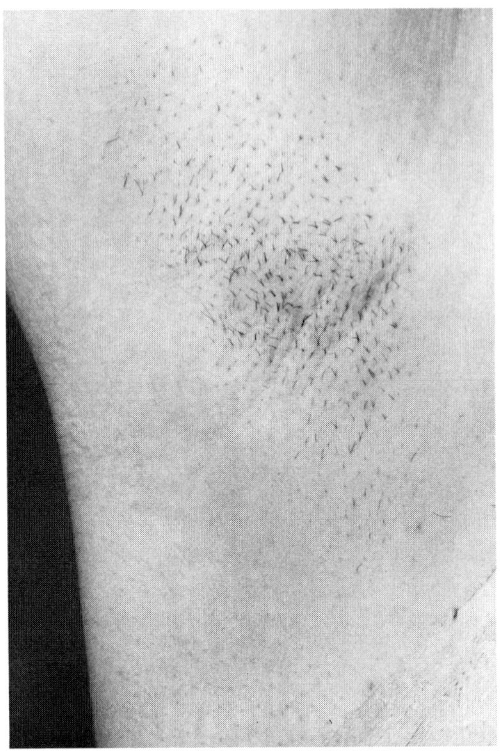

Fig. 30.5 Axilla from a PCO woman with no clinically evident AN. Histologic examination of a skin biopsy from this axilla showed the pathognomonic changes of AN.

women. Acanthosis nigricans was present on histologic examination (Fig. 30.6) in 13/13 obese PCO, 5/6 lean PCO, 13/14 obese normal, and 1/4 lean normal women. Acanthosis nigricans was present in women of all ethnic groups and skin types.

The severity of AN was most highly correlated with insulin-mediated glucose disposal ($r^2 = -0.37$, $P < 0.001$) rather than fasting ($r^2 = 0.21$, $P < 0.05$) or with glucose-stimulated insulin levels ($r^2 = 0.23$, $P < 0.01$). After statistical adjustment for insulin levels, only DHEAS levels were significantly correlated ($r^2 = 0.21$, $P < 0.01$) with AN.

Clinical examination of the skin proved to be quite insensitive for detecting AN. Thus, we found that AN was much more prevalent on microscopic examination of skin biopsies than clinically. The presence of this dermatologic change was most highly correlated with the magnitude of peripheral insulin resistance (i.e. decreased insulin-mediated glucose disposal) rather than basal or glucose challenge-induced hyperinsulinemia. The only sex steroid associated with AN was DHEAS. Acanthosis nigricans was present in normal as well as PCO women. This study indicates that AN is an epiphenomenon of insulin resistance and

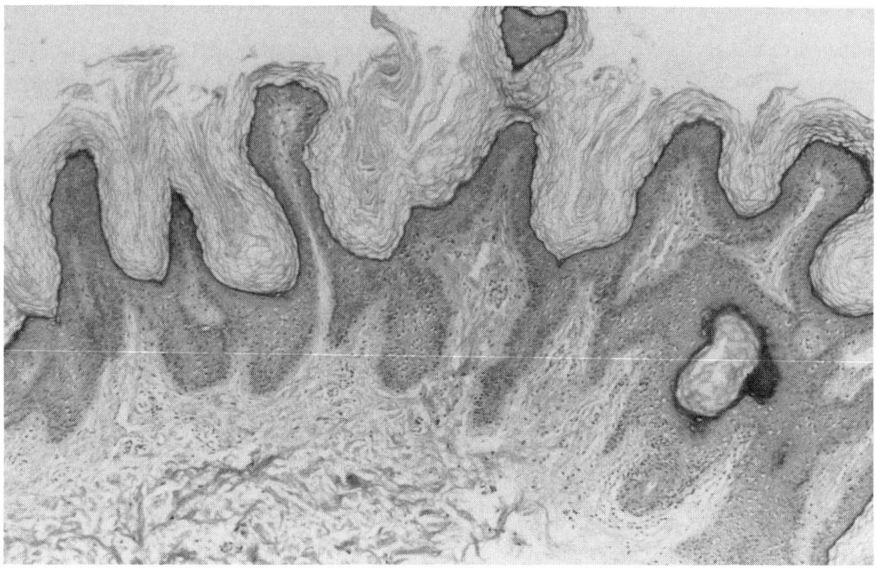

Fig. 30.6 Photomicrograph of a skin sample showing severe AN. Note the pronounced hyperkeratosis and the numerous dermal papillae.

that it is not valid to subgroup subjects on the basis of its presence on clinical examination (e.g. HAIR-AN, see Chapter 21).

Androgens and insulin resistance

Because of the significant positive correlations noted between androgen and insulin levels in PCO, it has been postulated that androgens may directly decrease insulin action [6]. Evidence to support this hypothesis comes from studies demonstrating that persons receiving anabolic steroids become hyperinsulinemic [30,31]. Conversely, natural androgen administration to men [32] and to female nonhuman primates [33] has not altered insulin levels or glucose tolerance. Studies altering androgen levels in PCO have been conflicting [34,35] and have been constrained by small sample size.

To investigate the causal role of endogenous hyperandrogenism in the insulin resistance of PCO, we suppressed gonadal steroid production for 12 weeks with a long-acting analog of gonadotropin-releasing hormone (GnRHa) [36]. Nine insulin-resistant women with PCO were studied. Despite suppressing androgen levels into the normal range for 10 weeks, there was no significant change in plasma insulin levels, hepatic glucose production, or in insulin-meditated glucose disposal determined by the euglycemic clamp technique. The sample size was adequate to detect a clinically significant change in insulin action (i.e. an improvement of insulin-mediated glucose disposal of $\geq 0.6\,mg/kg/min$).

This study indicated that plasma androgen elevations do not actively sustain insulin resistance in PCO. We cannot exclude, however, that the hyperandrogenic state caused an irreversible change in target tissue insulin sensitivity. If this were the case, then altering androgen levels would not have an effect on insulin action. The previous studies that suggested a direct action of androgens on insulin action [30,31] used orally active 17-alkylated synthetic androgens and these compounds may have different effects on glucose tolerance than natural androgens. Finally, suppressing androgen levels cannot be used as a therapeutic modality to improve insulin sensitivity and thereby decrease the risk of NIDDM in PCO.

Summary

Women with PCO have a unique disorder of insulin action. The magnitude of insulin resistance is similar to that seen in NIDDM. Indeed, obesity and PCO have a synergistic deleterious effect on glucose tolerance such that 20% of obese PCO women have impaired glucose tolerance or frank diabetes mellitus by their third decade. Acanthosis nigricans is not a specific marker for insulin resistance in PCO and its presence frequently escapes detection on clinical examination. It should therefore not be used as a criterion to subgroup hyperandrogenic women. Androgen excess does not sustain the insulin resistance in PCO and thus suppression of hyperandrogenism cannot be used for a therapeutic modality to improve insulin action.

References

1 Achard C, Thiers J. Le virilisme pilaire et son association à l'insuffisance glycolytique (diabete des femmes à barbe). Bull Acad Natl Med (Paris) 1921; 86:51–64.
2 Kahn CR, Flier JS, Bar RS, *et al.* The syndromes of insulin resistance and acanthosis nigricans. N Engl J Med 1976; 294:739–45.
3 Yoshimosa Y, Seino S, Whittaker J, *et al.* Insulin-resistant diabetes due to a point mutation that prevents insulin proreceptor processing. Science 1988; 240:784–7.
4 Kadowaki T, Kadowaki H, Rechler MM, *et al.* Five mutant alleles of the insulin receptor gene in patients with genetic forms of insulin resistance. J Clin Invest 1990; 86:254–64.
5 Dunaif A, Hoffman AR. Insulin resistance and hyperandrogenism: clinical syndromes and possible mechanisms. In: Pancheri P, Zichella L, eds. Biorhythms and Stress in the Physiopathology of Reproduction. Hemisphere Publishing Corp, 1988.
6 Burghen GA, Givens JR, Kitabchi AE. Correlations of hyperandrogenism with hyperinsulinism in polycystic ovarian disease. J Clin Endocrinol Metab 1980; 50:113–16.

7 Flier JS, Eastman RC, Minaker KL, Matteson D, Rowe JW. Acanthosis nigricans in obese women with hyperandrogenism: characterization of an insulin-resistant state distinct from the type A and B syndromes. Diabetes 1985; 34:101–7.
8 Dunaif A, Hoffman AR, Scully RE, Flier JS, *et al.* Clinical, biochemical, and ovarian morphologic features in women with acanthosis nigricans and masculinization. Obstet Gynecol 1985; 66:545–52.
9 Stuart CA, Peters JE, Prince MJ, Richards G, Cavallo A, Meyer WJ. Insulin resistance with acanthosis nigricans: the roles of obesity and androgen excess. Metabolism 1986; 35:197–205.
10 Pasquali R, Venturoli S, Paradis R, Capelli M, Parenti N, Melchionda N. Insulin and C-peptide levels in obese patients with polycystic ovaries. Horm Metab Res 1982; 14:284–7.
11 Chang RJ, Nakamura RM, Judd HL, Kaplan SA. Insulin resistance in nonobese patients with polycystic ovarian disease. J Clin Endocrinol Metab 1983; 57:356–9.
12 Shoupe D, Kumar D, Lobo RA. Insulin resistance in polycystic ovary syndrome. Am J Obstet Gynecol 1983; 147:588–92.
13 Dunaif A, Graf M, Mandeli J, Laumas V, Dobrjansky A. Characterization of groups of hyperandrogenic women with acanthosis nigricans, impaired glucose tolerance, and/or hyperinsulinemia. J Clin Endocrinol Metab. 1987; 65:499–507.
14 Defronzo RA. The triumvirate: beta-cell, muscle, liver. A collusion responsible for NIDDM. Diabetes 1988; 37:667–87.
15 Dunaif A, Segal KR, Futterweit W, Dobrjansky A. Profound peripheral insulin resistance, independent of obesity, in the polycystic ovary syndrome. Diabetes 1989; 38:1165–74.
16 Yki-Jarvinen H, Koivisto VA. Effects of body composition on insulin sensitivity. Diabetes 1983; 32:965–9.
17 DeFronzo RA, Jacot E, Jequier E, Maeder E, Wahren J, Felber JP. The effect of insulin on the disposal of intravenous glucose. Diabetes 1981; 30:1000–7.
18 Bogardus C, Lillioja S, Mott DM, Hollenbeck C, Reaven G. Relationship between degree of obesity and *in vivo* insulin action in man. Am J Physiol 1985; 248:E286–E291.
19 Goldzieher JW, Green JA. The polycystic ovary. I. Clinical and histologic features. J Clin Endocrinol Metab 1962; 22:325–38.
20 Sathanadan M, Mortola J, Kolterman OG, Yen SSC. Characterization of insulin resistance in polycystic ovary syndrome using hyperinsulinemic euglycemic clamp. 43rd Annual Meeting American Fertility Society, Reno, Nevada, 1987, p. 71, Abstract 176.
21 Wade GN, Gray JM. Gonadal effects on food intake and adiposity: a metabolic hypothesis. Physiol Behav 1979; 22:583–93.
22 Bergman RN, Finegood DT, Ader M. Assessment of insulin sensitivity *in vivo*. Endocr Rev 1985; 6:45–86.
23 Reaven GM, Doberne H, Greenfield MS. Comparison of insulin secretion and *in vivo* insulin action in nonobese and moderately obese individuals with non-insulin-dependent diabetes mellitus. Diabetes 1982; 31:382–4.
24 Rizza RA, Mandarino LJ, Gerich JE. Mechanism and significance of insulin resistance in non-insulin-dependent diabetes mellitus. Diabetes 1981; 30:990–5.
25 Rowe JW, Minaker KL, Pallota JA, Flier JS. Characterization of the insulin resistance of aging. J Clin Invest 1983; 71:1581–7.
26 Peiris AN, Aiman EJ, Drucker WD, Kissebah AH. The relative contributions of hepatic and peripheral tissues to insulin resistance in hyperandrogenic women. J Clin Endocrinol Metab 1989; 68:715–20.
27 Dunaif A, Mandeli J, Fluhr H, Dobrjansky A. The impact of obesity and chronic hyperinsulinemia on gonadotropin release and gonadal steroid secretion in the polycystic ovary syndrome. J Clin Endocrinol Metab 1988; 66:131–9.

28 Brown J, Winklemann RK. Acanthosis nigricans: a study of 90 cases. Medicine 1968; 47:33–51.
29 Dunaif A, Green G, Phelps RG, Lebwohl M, Futterweit W, Levy L. Acanthosis nigricans, insulin action, and hyperandrogenism: clinical, histologic and biochemical findings. J Clin Endocrinol Metab (in press).
30 Woodard TL, Burghen GA, Kitabchi AE, Williams JA. Glucose intolerance and insulin resistance in aplastic anemia treated with oxymetholone. J Clin Endocrinol Metab 1981; 53:905–8.
31 Cohen JC, Hickman R. Insulin resistance and diminished glucose tolerance in powerlifters ingesting anabolic steroids. J Clin Endocrinol Metab 1987; 64:960–3.
32 Friedl KE, Jones RE, Hannan CJ Jr, Plymate SR. The administration of pharmacological doses of testosterone or 19-nortestosterone to normal men is not associated with increased insulin secretion or impaired glucose tolerance. J Clin Endocrinol Metab 1989; 68:971–5.
33 Billiar RB, Richardson D, Schwartz R, Posner B, Little B. Effect of chronically elevated androgen or estrogen on the glucose tolerance test and insulin response in female rhesus monkeys. Am J Obstet Gynecol 1987; 157:1297–302.
34 Shoupe D, Lobo RA. The influence of androgens on insulin resistance. Fertil Steril 1984; 41:385–8.
35 Geffner ME, Kaplan SA, Bersch N, Golde DW, Landaw EM, Chang RJ. Persistence of insulin resistance in polycystic ovarian disease after inhibition of ovarian steroid secretion. Fertil Steril 1986; 45:327–33.
36 Dunaif A, Green G, Futterweit W, Dobrjansky A. Suppression of hyperandrogenism does not improve peripheral or hepatic insulin resistance in the polycystic ovary syndrome. J Clin Endocrinol Metab 1990; 70:699–704.

Chapter 31

Upper Body Obesity: Abnormalities in the Metabolic Profile and the Androgenic/Estrogenic Balance

AHMED H. KISSEBAH

Regional body fat patterning has emerged as an independent risk factor predisposing to a variety of metabolic disorders, including marked peripheral insulin resistance and abnormal insulin removal dynamics, disturbances in lipoprotein metabolism, and hypertension [1,2]. We have studied healthy premenopausal women to determine whether body fat distribution detects abnormalities in the metabolic profile that predict these disorders [2–4]. Increasing waist-to-hip ratio (WHR) is accompanied by progressively increasing fasting plasma glucose and insulin levels, and by higher insulin and glucose responses to oral glucose challenge. Fasting plasma triglyceride levels are increased and high-density lipoprotein (HDL)-cholesterol is decreased with increasing WHR. The effects of body fat topography are independent of and additive to those of obesity. Although WHR also correlates with the plasma cholesterol level, this association is dependent upon its correlation with increasing relative body weight. Body fat distribution and the degree of obesity are also independently and additively correlated with systolic and diastolic blood pressure. Similar findings have been reported in men [5].

Abdominal obesity in women is correlated with increased free testosterone and decreased sex hormone-binding globulin (SHBG) levels. Increased androgenicity is also associated with abnormalities in the metabolic profile. Thus, androgenicity may play an important part in the association between body fat distribution and metabolic health risks. This article summarizes research efforts to evaluate these associations and attempts to define areas for future research.

The metabolic profile

Glucose–insulin homeostasis

The coexistence of hyperinsulinemia and impaired glucose tolerance in upper body obesity suggests that diminished insulin sensitivity is the underlying abnormality [3,6,7]. Using the insulin impedance test and the insulin euglycemic clamp procedure, we have found that the glucose intolerance of upper body obesity is partially due to diminished sensitivity of insulin-mediated glucose disposal. A significant decline in muscle glycogen synthase-I activity suggests that the defect in skeletal muscle insulin sensitivity contributes to the impairment in overall glucose disposal. Although monocytes show diminished insulin binding with increasing WHR, these results suggest the presence of an additional postreceptor defect(s) in glucose metabolism. The significant intercorrelation between the metabolic variables measured is compatible with the complex glucose–insulin regulatory system in which a perturbation at one point evokes numerous secondary changes.

Compared with the nonobese, obese women have greater prehepatic insulin production and portal vein insulin levels basally and following oral glucose stimulation. These studies suggest that insulin hypersecretion is primarily related to total body fat mass but is uninfluenced by the distribution of body fat or the degree of insulin resistance. In addition, the upper body obese subjects demonstrate a significant decrease in hepatic insulin extraction both basally and during i.v. or oral glucose stimulation relative to the nonobese or the lower body obese. Consequently, posthepatic insulin delivery is progressively increased and correlates well with the degree of peripheral hyperinsulinemia. The diminished hepatic insulin extraction in these subjects is proportional to the magnitude of the decline in peripheral insulin sensitivity.

Lipoprotein metabolism

Abdominal obesity is also closely associated with noninsulin-dependent diabetes mellitus (NIDDM), and both disorders are associated with increased coronary heart disease risk. The results of these investigations have been reviewed in detail elsewhere [8–10]. Generally, plasma triglycerides (TG) and very-low-density lipoproteins (VLDL) are increased in NIDDM, while high-density lipoproteins (HDL) is often decreased. The lipoprotein kinetic pattern is characterized by increased VLDL turnover, which may be associated with hypertriglyceridemia, especially when the VLDL catabolic pathways cannot keep pace with the increased production. With the development of severe hyperglycemia and hypoinsulinemia, the efficiency of VLDL delipidation decreases, and a large fraction of VLDL is channeled into VLDL remnants. Derangements in low-density lipoprotein (LDL) metabolism that are consistent with increased LDL apolipoprotein B (apo-B) turnover have also been observed in NIDDM. An additive decrease in LDL catabolism is observed with worsening of the glycemic state and more marked insulin deficiency.

In nondiabetic subjects with upper body obesity, WHR and the size of the visceral fat mass strongly correlate with plasma TG and negatively with HDL concentrations [11]. Plasma levels of dense LDL are increased, and the larger LDL are decreased. Apolipoprotein B levels in plasma are also elevated with increasing WHR [8]. These abnormalities are similar to those found in NIDDM patients, particularly those with mild hyperglycemia.

Obese subjects often demonstrate abnormalities in lipoprotein metabolism that may not be associated with overt hyperlipidemia [8]. Increased VLDL-TG and apo-B synthesis is found in most obese subjects. These increases are proportional, resulting in increased secretion of VLDL particles. In the normolipemic obese individuals, the increased VLDL production is compensated by a comparable increase in its removal. As the efficiency of VLDL conversion to LDL is unimpaired, increased LDL is formed, which is compensated by increased LDL catabolic rate. The increase in VLDL and LDL apo-B flux rates is most apparent in individuals with severe diminution in insulin sensitivity and greater elevation in plasma insulin, who are likely to be upper body obese.

We have noted a close relationship between plasma free fatty acid (FFA) flux and VLDL-TG and apo-B production rates [12–14]. An increase of FFA flux might thus be important in the pathogenesis of the lipoprotein disorder in upper body obesity. The anatomic location of visceral fat facilitates a high exposure of the liver to FFA. The pronounced hyperinsulinemia of the upper body obese supports the overproduction of VLDL and the increased LDL turnover.

The precise mechanisms responsible for the decrease in HDL cholesterol (HDL-chol) concentration in upper body obese individuals are uncertain. The association between WHR and decreased HDL-chol is partially dependent upon the effect of body fat distribution on plasma TG concentrations. The WHR is also correlated positively with the plasma level of HDL_3 and negatively with HDL_2. Subjects with abdominal obesity have endogenous hyperinsulinemia and peripheral insulin resistance. This may result in decreased activity of adipose tissue lipoprotein lipase (LPL) and increased hepatic TG lipase, causing reductions in the conversion of HDL_3 to HDL_2 and in total HDL-chol. The inverse relationship between the degree of hyperinsulinemia and HDL concentrations observed in these individuals supports this hypothesis.

Blood pressure regulation

Upper body fat localization and increased visceral fat mass are associated with increased systolic and diastolic blood pressure. These associations are independent of the degree of overweight or total body fat mass. The frequency of hypertension is increased in individuals with upper or central body fat patterns [15,16]. Increasing evidence implicating insulin as an important determinant of blood pressure has been presented in human and animal studies [2]. Several mechanisms by which this may occur have been postulated, including insulin-mediated sodium retention [17], direct stimulation of the sympathetic drive [18], or through norepinephrine-mediated responses [19,20]. The relationship between fat distribution and blood pressure may not be entirely accounted for by insulin, however [21]. Visceral fat mass is significantly correlated with the blood pressure profile, but the subscapular/triceps ratio and the subscapular skinfold thickness are not significantly correlated, suggesting the possible existence of alternate mechanisms associating this fat depot with blood pressure levels.

Our studies thus suggest that abdominal and/or visceral adiposity accounts for a number of abnormal metabolic pathways, including marked peripheral insulin resistance, abnormal insulin removal dynamics, and disorders in lipoprotein and blood pressure regulation. Total body fat mass exerts synergistic effects via a mild decline in insulin sensitivity and increased pancreatic insulin production. Possible mechanisms for these aberrations are discussed below.

Androgenic/estrogenic balance

In healthy premenopausal women without significant history of hirsutism, amenorrhea, or clinical evidence of endocrine disorders, we observed a highly significant trend toward a decrease in the plasma level of SHBG and an increase in percent free testosterone (%FT) with increasing WHR [3,22]. A decrease in SHBG level with increasing WHR has also been observed by others [23]. Since the plasma SHBG level is determined largely by the androgen/estrogen balance, the decrease in SHBG and the increase in %FT thus indicates a relative increase in androgenic activity. In our study neither WHR nor obesity level correlated with total plasma androgen levels, suggesting that the decrease in SHBG signifies a relative increase in the proportion of unbound hormone. Indeed %FT rose proportionally as WHR increased. Since other androgenic 17β-hydroxysteroids, such as androstenedione, also bind to SHBG with high affinity, the decrease in SHBG may also result in an increase in the unbound concentrations of these steroids, further increasing total androgenicity.

That obesity and upper body fat predominance may contribute to the decrease in SHBG independently of changes in androgenic activity must also be considered. Decreased SHBG and increased %FT levels have been observed in obese men who, unlike obese women, also demonstrate decreased total testosterone (T) levels [2]. The calculated serum FT levels in these men is normal or slightly decreased, however, and there is no clinical evidence of diminished androgenic activity. Dihydrotestosterone (DHT) levels are normal [24], and the possibility that the levels of other androgens are increased has not yet been investigated. No studies, however, have examined in detail the relationship between body fat distribution and sex hormone metabolism in men.

In some studies the diminished SHBG levels associated with obesity have been observed to increase after weight reduction [25,26]. These studies, however, have included women with overt hyperandrogenism or massive obesity in whom additional defects may be involved and/or have been performed after jejunoileal bypass or during severe caloric restriction, the effects of which on the metabolism of SHBG and sex steroids are unknown. A study of premenopausal women with no gynecological abnormalities or elevated total androgen levels indicated no changes in plasma SHBG, %FT, or total T following long-term weight loss and dietary restabilization [22].

Regardless of whether the decrease in SHBG results from increased androgen production, some other undetermined mechanism associated with both obesity and upper body fat predominance, or a combination of the two, the decline in SHBG would result in a much greater change in unbound T than in unbound estradiol (E_2), and hence perpetuates a further increase in androgenic/estrogenic activity. Diminished SHBG also results in increased metabolic clearance rates of T and other androgens for which it has a high-binding affinity and may lead to enhanced turnover and tissue exposure to androgens despite normal plasma levels. Indeed Kirschner *et al.* in a preliminary study reported increase T production in a group of overweight upper body obese women [27]. Lower body obese women, on the other hand, demonstrated increased conversion of androstenedione to estrone. Androstenedione production was similar in the two obese groups.

Relationship of androgenic activity to regional body fat patterning

The importance of sex hormone activity in influencing body fat distribution is supported by the following observations.

1 The onset of androgen secretion in the pubertal male or administration of exogenous T to the hypogonadal male is accompanied by localization of fat in the upper body and a decrease in SHBG levels [28].

2 In individuals undergoing sexual transformation, T treatment in females increases upper body adipocyte cell volumes, whereas estrogen therapy in men increases fat cell number in the thigh [29].

3 In women with polycystic ovary syndrome (PCO), obesity and excess plasma androgens are frequently associated with the increases in fat deposition, which coincides with increased androgen production [30]. Many of these women exhibit a predominance of upper body fat, male-type obesity. Conversely, men with lower body fat (female-type obesity) have increased levels of estrogen [31].

4 In experimental animals androgens increase and estrogens decrease the activity of adipocyte LPL and, in turn, adipocyte and adipose tissue size [32–34]. An increase in LPL is the first abnormality to appear after administration of exogenous sex steroids and precedes changes in food intake, adipocyte volume, and body weight.

The strong correlation between the increases in androgenic activity and WHR suggests that body fat distribution might be a manifestation of the increased body exposure to unbound androgens [3]. The degree of androgenic activity (SHBG and %FT) correlates with the increased adipocyte volumes in the abdomen but not in the thigh, suggesting that hypertrophy of the abdominal adipocytes in upper body obesity might also be a manifestation of hyperandrogenicity. Like men, upper body obese women preferentially deposit fat intra-abdominally; the increase in the intra-abdominal/extra-abdominal fat mass ratio correlates highly with the increase in androgenic activity. Furthermore, in nonobese women, despite similar degrees of lean body mass, increasing plasma androgen levels, as in women with idiopathic hirsutism or PCO, are associated with increasing WHR [22]. Finally, Rebuffe-Scrive has proposed a regional specialization of adipose tissue depots that is governed by the sex hormone balance. Whereas the femoral–gluteal depot is primarily a storage organ dedicated to such female stresses as pregnancy and lactation, the abdominal–visceral depot is dedicated primarily to storage of easily and rapidly mobilizable energy reserves [35].

This well-documented occurrence of intersexual differences in the regional distribution of body fat suggests that the sex steroids may be involved in establishing topographical variations in tissue storage and fat mobilization. In order to examine the importance of ovarian factors in influencing regional differences in precursor cell development, we utilized a flow cytometric procedure (specifically labeling rat adipose tissue LPL, a putative marker for cells committed to becoming adipocytes) to quantify the differentiated and undifferentiated preadipocyte pools present in vascular adipose tissue stroma of visceral (perirenal and parametrial) and subcutaneous (dorsal and femoral) regions of female rats [36,37]. We then evaluated the possible role of ovarian factors in establishing regional disparity in preadipocyte recruitment and differentiation and their eventual transformation to mature adipocytes.

Sexual maturation of the female rat is associated with significant increases in the differentiated preadipocytes and fat cell number in all regions. This increase is accompanied by a significant decrease in the undifferentiated pool of preadipocytes in all depots except the femoral. In contrast to other regions, the femoral depot possesses an infinite capacity to provide precursor cells capable of rapid differentiation and transformation into mature adipocytes. This characteristic appears to be maintained by ovarian factors. Interestingly, the visceral depot in male rats contains an infinite pool of preadipocytes with an enhanced capacity for replication. Our observations thus raise the interesting question of whether variations in regional distribution of adipocyte precursors are dependent upon sex hormones.

Relationship of androgenic activity to the metabolic events

Androgenic activity may initiate abnormalities in the metabolic profile via two additive mechanisms. First, by influencing the deposition of adipocytes in areas around the waist (visceral and subcutaneous), which are morphologically and metabolically different from those deposited in the gluteofemoral region, androgens could increase plasma FFA flux and thus expose hepatic and extrahepatic tissues to excess levels of FFA. This mechanism is suggested by the following observations.

1 Upper body adipocytes are large and exhibit high rates of basal and catecholamine-stimulated lipolysis, presumably due to both increased β-to-α adrenergic activities and to diminished sensitivity to the anti-lipolytic action of insulin [3,35].

2 Upper body obese women demonstrate higher nocturnal levels of plasma FFA [38] and increased FFA flux [39], despite higher plasma insulin levels.

3 Feeding a high fat diet to rats increases portal vein plasma FFA levels and hepatic TG content, which correlates with a decline in hepatic insulin extraction [40].

4 Animal and human studies suggest that FFA could inhibit insulin stimulation of peripheral glucose metabolism and insulin suppression of hepatic glucose production [41,42]. Therefore, if similar mechanisms operate in upper body obesity, an increase in hepatic exposure to FFA could lead to increased posthepatic insulin delivery and to hyperinsulinemia. Increased FFA could also diminish hepatic and peripheral insulin sensitivity.

The second mechanism assumes that androgenic activity might be directly responsible for the abnormalities in insulin dynamics and in hepatic and extrahepatic insulin actions. The influence of increased androgen activity on carbohydrate metabolism is supported by the following observations.

1 Diabetes is more common in males than in age-matched and relative weight-matched females [43]. When expressed per kilogram lean body weight, insulin-mediated glucose disposal measured during the euglycemic clamp is 45% lower in healthy men relative to women of similar age and body weight [44].

2 Administration of T derivatives to women results in impaired glucose tolerance and hyperinsulinemia [45,46].

3 Hyperandrogenism and insulin resistance in women are associated with PCO and acanthosis nigricans and may abate with estrogen therapy [47,48]

4 Experimental exposure of animals to the encephalomyocarditis virus, streptozoticin, or to subtotal pancreatectomy results in a higher frequency of diabetes in male and female animals [49].

5 Estrogen administration reduces the activities of rat liver gluconeogenic enzymes, alters the glucagon response, and promotes a decrease in plasma glucose [50].

In premenopausal women increasing androgenic activity correlates significantly with plasma glucose and insulin levels, decreasing peripheral insulin sensitivity and a decline in hepatic insulin extraction [51]. We have also demonstrated a significantly impaired peripheral insulin sensitivity in nonobese hyperandrogenized hirsute women [52]. Thus our findings suggest that the association between upper body fat localization and the aberrations in hepatic insulin extraction and peripheral insulin sensitivity, and the resultant changes in the metabolic profile might be mediated by a common mechanism involving the increase in androgenic activity.

Support for the influence of androgens on hepatic removal of insulin comes from the elevation of plasma insulin, but not C-peptide levels, in men compared with age- and weight-matched women. Testosterone and insulin have similar clearance rates, with approximately 50% of each being removed from the splanchnic circulation via the liver. Androgen receptors have been demonstrated in the hepatic parenchymal cells of both rats and humans [53]. Studies in sexually mature rats demonstrate that hepatic insulin extraction is lower in males than in age- and weight-matched females [54]. Furthermore, in the SHR/N:Mcc-cp corpulent rat, male gender augments the reduction of hepatic insulin extraction induced by obesity [55]. This increase is accompanied by a decline in hepatocyte insulin receptor number and diminished receptor-mediated insulin degradation. The aberrations in hepatic insulin dynamics, most marked in the obese males, are associated with severe hyperinsulinemia, insulin resistance, and a high frequency of diabetes.

We have examined the relationship of sex hormones to hepatic insulin dynamics [56]. Insulin binding and receptor-mediated insulin processing were investigated in isolated hepatocytes from sexually maturing female rats and from age-matched animals that had undergone prepubertal ovariectomy. Insulin binding at tracer concentrations increases 50% from sexual immaturity at 3–4 weeks through pubescence at 6–8 weeks. Scatchard analysis indicates that the altered binding is due primarily to an increase in receptor number. Increased binding with sexual maturation results in correspondingly higher levels of insulin in each of the four compartments of processing (cell surface-bound, internalized, degraded, and released). A corresponding increase in receptor-mediated insulin degradation is also observed. The pubescence-related increase in insulin binding and degradation is abolished by prepubertal ovariectomy. More recent studies have shown that this increase can be reproduced in ovariectomized rats that received E_2 implants [57]. Thus, ovarian factors appear to be involved in the pubescence-associated regulation of hepatic insulin degradation in female rats, probably at the level of insulin binding.

Upper body obese women, like men, have a high preponderance of fast-twitch fibers, whereas the lower body obese resemble normal women, having a preponderance of slow-twitch fibers in their quadriceps muscle [58]. The degree of aberration of plasma insulin and glucose levels correlates highly with the relative abundance of fast-twitch b fibers. Differences in insulin receptor number, substrate processing, and insulin sensitivity between muscle fiber types are well recognized [59,60]. Whether the characteristic muscle fiber composition of upper body obesity is also part of an aberrant sexual dimorphism, and if so to what extent this could account for the accompanying decline in peripheral insulin sensitivity, is unknown.

Role of sexual dimorphism

We have suggested that abdominal and/or visceral adiposity is strongly associated with such abnormal metabolic pathways as marked peripheral insulin resistance, abnormal insulin removal dynamics, and disturbances in lipoprotein and blood pressure regulation. The mechanisms associating regional adiposity to the metabolic sequences are uncertain. Body fat distribution appears, in part, to be genetically determined [61], and each of the metabolic complications associated with it, including NIDDM, hyperlipidemia, hypertension, and coronary heart disease, has a genetic component in its pathogenesis. Upper body obese individuals also demonstrate a multitude of behavioral and psychological maladjustments to stress, and they also suffer from menstrual irregularities and other neuroendocrine dysfunctions. Abdominal obesity and its metabolic complications might thus result from a neuroendocrine aberration secondary to poor coping with environmental stresses [62]. Finally, body fat distribution and the accompanying metabolic abnormalities could be manifestations of a global disorder initiated by variability in an androgenic/estrogenic balance and in degree of sexual dimorphism. This last hypothesis has been extensively researched by our group and is detailed below.

The reasons for suggesting that the association between sex hormone balance, body fat distribution, and the abnormalities in the metabolic profile might be induced or exacerbated by an early developmental aberration in sexual dimorphism are as follows.

1 The association between body fat distribution and abnormalities in hepatic insulin extraction or peripheral insulin sensitivity, when adjusted for the effects of SHBG and %FT, although markedly reduced, are still detectable, suggesting that the androgen balance is not the sole determinant of these relationships [51].

2 In studies of nonobese hirsute women, plasma androgen levels are higher than in upper body obese nonhirsute women, but the impairments in insulin-mediated glucose metabolism are less pronounced [52].

3 Treatment of hirsute women with the antiandrogen spironolactone normalizes androgen levels and improves peripheral insulin sensitivity but does not consequently normalize insulin–glucose homeostasis [22].

4 Although moderately obese men have larger visceral fat depots (as determined by computed tomography), there is a marked intersexual overlap in the fat distribution ratio between visceral and subcutaneous fat, suggesting that the level of circulating androgens is not the sole determinant of fat deposition site [2,63].

5 Animal studies in the female liver have indicated higher levels of 5α-reductase activity, which converts T to its active metabolite, DHT [53]. The relative abundance of hepatic androgen receptors is also sex dependent. These sex differences in hepatic activities appear to be imprinted by prenatal and neonatal exposure to sex steroids [64,65].

Alterations in the prenatal hormonal environment appear important for proper postnatal development [66]. Much of this understanding has derived from metabolic diseases which influence sexual development. One such syndrome is the 5α-reductase deficiency [67], whereby genetic males cannot reduce testosterone to DHT and thus lack genital masculinization. Many of the female infants with the congenital adrenal genital syndrome lack 21-hydroxylase activity, which is responsible for the production of cortisol. With no or reduced negative feedback, the adrenals are exposed to high levels of adrenocorticotropic hormone (ACTH) and respond to this tropic stimulation with the release of adrenal androgens sufficient to masculinize the genitalia. Deficiency of this enzyme is inherited as an autosomal recessive trait closely linked to the HLA major histocompatibility complex [68], and there are specific associations between HLA haplotypes and different forms of 21-hydroxylase deficiency. 21-Hydroxylase deficiency appears to be due to deletions or other abnormalities of genes closely linked to the HLA markers, however, rather than being directly due to a genetic variation in an HLA molecule [69].

Experimental disruption of sexual dimorphism can be achieved in female rat pups by the perinatal injection of testosterone propionate. Relative to undisrupted animals, the inguinal fat pad of disrupted rats demonstrated a significant decrease in fat cell number and in undifferentiated preadipocytes, while neither event was affected in the femoral depot, nor did disruption influence the percentage of differentiated preadipocytes in the two regions [37]. Thus, preadipocyte differentiation capacity and the adipocyte number of the femoral, but not the visceral, depot are highly influenced by normal sexual dimorphism. An aberration in sexual dimorphism may result in diminished growth potential of the femoral region and a greater susceptibility for visceral adiposity in the female.

We have also examined the effects of disrupting the sexual dimorphism of female rat pups on hepatic insulin dynamics [56,57]. Perinatal androgen treatment reduces insulin binding by the liver cells from animals age-matched to sexually mature rats, but receptor-mediated insulin degradation is not similarly diminished. Both insulin receptor binding and receptor-mediated insulin processing appear to be sexually dimorphic phenomena. The complex interactions between sexual dimorphism and pubertal sex hormone development are currently under investigation.

We have proposed that body fat distribution with its adipocyte morphologic and metabolic characteristics and the accompanying abnormalities in insulin–glucose homeostasis are linked via an aberration in androgenic/estrogenic activity. A genetic and/or early developmental aberration occurring at the time of sexual dimorphism may thus induce or exacerbate the sensitivity to the androgenic milieu.

Summary

Increasing abdominal and/or visceral body fat is accompanied by progressively increasing plasma glucose and insulin levels in a manner that is independent of and additive to those due to total body fat mass. Increasing abdominal and/or visceral adiposity accounts for most of the abnormal metabolic pathways predisposing to NIDDM, including the marked peripheral insulin resistance and the abnormal insulin removal dynamics. Since perinatal exposure to androgens is known to influence behavior and maturation of the hypothalamic–hypophyseal–gonadal axis, it is possible that the psychological maladjustments to stress and the neuroendocrine disorders accompanying this form of obesity could be part of an aberrant sexual dimorphism. Furthermore, perinatal overexposure to androgens might result from a genetic disorder, and the possible occurrence of genetic linkages associating sex hormone balance, body fat distribution, and the metabolic sequelae has to be considered. These exciting possibilities deserve further examination, and they can be addressed more systematically now that the major metabolic pathways are known.

Acknowledgments

Studies from this laboratory were supported, in part, by grant No. HL34989 and General Clinical Research Center Grant No. RR00058 from the National Institutes of Health. Other major contributors to studies from this group include David J. Evans, Glenn R. Krakower,

Roland James, Robert A. Mueller, and Magda M. Hennes. The critical comments of Gabriele E. Sonnenberg are also greatly appreciated.

References

1 Kissebah AH, Peiris A, Evans DJ. Regional body fat distribution and morbidity: biologic connection to NIDDM. In: Lardy H, Stratman F, eds. Hormones, Thermogenesis, and Obesity. Elsevier Science Publishing, New York, 1989, pp. 77–91.

2 Kissebah AH, Peiris AN. Biology of regional body fat distribution: relationship to non-insulin-dependent diabetes mellitus. Diabetes Metab Rev 1989; 5:83–109.

3 Evans DJ, Hoffmann RG, Kalkhoff RK, Kissebah AH. Relationship of androgenic activity to body fat topography, fat cell morphology, and metabolic aberrations in premenopausal women. J Clin Endocrinol Metab 1983; 57:304–10.

4 Freedman DS, Jacobsen SJ, Barboriak JJ, Sobocinski KA, Anderson AJ, Kissebah AH, Sasse EA, Gruchow HW. Body fat distribution and male/female differences in lipids and lipoproteins. Circulation 1990; 81:1498–1506.

5 Krotkiewski M, Bjorntorp P, Sjostrom L, Smith U. Impact of obesity on metabolism in men and women. Importance of regional adipose tissue distribution. J Clin Invest 1983; 72:1150–62.

6 Evans DJ, Murray R, Kissebah AH. Relationship between skeletal muscle insulin resistance, insulin-mediated glucose disposal, and insulin binding; effects of obesity and body fat topography. J Clin Invest 1984; 74:1515–25.

7 Peiris AN, Mueller RA, Smith GA, Struve MF, Kissebah AH. Splanchnic insulin metabolism in obesity: influence of body fat distribution. J Clin Invest 1986; 78:1648–57.

8 Kissebah AH. Low density lipoprotein metabolism in non-insulin-dependent diabetes mellitus. Diabetes Metab Rev 1987; 3:619–51.

9 Kissebah AH, Schectman G. Polyunsaturated and saturated fat, cholesterol, and fatty acid supplementation. Diabetes Care 1988; 11:129–42.

10 Kissebah AH, Schectman G. Hormones and lipoprotein metabolism. In: Shepherd J, ed. Bailliere's Clinical Endocrinology and Metabolism, Vol. 1. London: WB Saunders, 1987, pp. 699–725.

11 Despres JP, Allard C, Tremblay A, Talbot J, Bouchard C. Evidence for a regional component of body fatness in the association with serum lipids in men and women. Metabolism 1985; 34:967–73.

12 Kissebah AH, Adams PW, Wynn V. Plasma free fatty acid and triglyceride transport kinetics in man. Clin Sci Mol Med 1974; 47:259–78.

13 Kissebah AH, Alfarsi S, Adams PW, Seed M, Folkard J, Wynn V. Transport kinetics of plasma free fatty acid, very low density lipoprotein, triglycerides and apolipoprotein in patients with endogenous hypertriglyceridemia: effects of 2,2-dimethyl (2,5-xylyloxy) valeric acid therapy. Atherosclerosis 1976; 24:199–218.

14 Kissebah AH, Alfarsi S, Adams PW, Wynn V. Role of insulin resistance in adipose tissue and liver in the pathogenesis of endogenous hypertriglyceridemia in man. Diabetologia 1976; 12:563–71.

15 Haffner SM, Stern MP, Hazuda HP, Rosenthal M, Knapp JA, Malina RW. Role of obesity and fat distribution in non-insulin dependent diabetes mellitus in Mexican Americans and non-Hispanic whites. Diabetes Care 1986; 9:153–61.

16 Blair D, Habicht JP, Sims EAH, Sylwester D, Abraham S. Evidence for an increased risk for hypertension with centrally located body fat and the effect of race and sex on this risk. Am J Epidemiol 1984; 119:526–40.

17 DeFronzo RA. Insulin and renal sodium handling: clinical implications. Int J Obes 1981; 5:93–104.

18 Rowe JW, Young JB, Minaker KL, Stevens AL, Pallotta J, Landsberg L. Effect of insulin and glucose infusions on sympathetic nervous system activity in normal man. Diabetes 1981; 30:219–25.
19 Owen NE. Regulation of Na/K/Cl co-transport in vascular smooth muscle cells. Biochem Biophys Res Commun 1984; 125:500–508.
20 Chipperfield AR. The (Na^+-K^+-Cl^-) co-transport system. Clin Sci 1986; 71:465–76.
21 Weinsier RL, Norris DJ, Birch R, Bernstein RS, Pi-Sunyer FX, Yang M-U, Wang J, Pierson RN, Van Itallie TB. Serum insulin and blood pressure in an obese population. Int J Obes 1986; 10:11–17.
22 Evans DJ. Body fat distribution and metabolic complications. MD Thesis, Univ. of Cardiff, UK, 1986.
23 Haffner SM, Katz MS, Dunn JF, Stern MP. Decreased sex hormone binding globulin (SHBG) is associated with hyperinsulinemia in premenopausal Mexican American (MA) women. Clin Res 1988; 36:482A.
24 Strain GW, Zumoff B, Kream J, Strain JJ, Deucher R, Rosenfeld RS, Levin J, Fukushima DK. Mild hypogonadotropic hypogonadism in obese men. Metabolism 1982; 31:871–75.
25 Zorn EM, Wieland RG, Hallberg MC. 17β-ol androgens and free index in hirsute and nonhirsute obese women. Fertil Steril 1976; 27:916–20.
26 O'Dea JPK, Wieland RG, Hallberg MC, Llerena LA, Zorn EM, Genuth SM. Effect of dietary weight loss on sex steroid binding, sex steroids and gonadotropins in obese postmenopausal women. J Lab Clin Med 1979; 93:1004–1008.
27 Kirschner MA, Samojlik E, Ertel N, Schneider G, Szmal E. Androgen–estrogen metabolism in women with upper body obesity. Endocrinology 1988; 122(suppl.): 209.
28 Vermeulen A, Verdonck L, van der Straeten M, Orie N. Capacity of the testosterone-binding globulin in human plasma and influence of specific binding of testosterone on its metabolic clearance. J Clin Endocrinol Metab 1969; 29:1470–80.
29 Vague J, Meignen JM, Negrin JF. Effects of testosterone and estrogens on deltoid and trochanter adipocytes in two cases of transsexualism. Horm Metab Res 1984; 16:380–81.
30 Yen SSC. The polycystic ovary syndrome. Clin Endocrinol 1980; 12:177–207.
31 Sparrow D, Bosse R, Rowe JW. The influence of age, alcohol consumption, and body build on gonadal function in men. J Clin Endocrinol Metab 1980; 51:508–512.
32 Wade GN, Gray JM. Theoretical review. Gonadal effects on food intake and adiposity: a metabolic hypothesis. Physiol Behav 1979; 22:583–93.
33 Krotkiewski M, Kral JG, Karlsson J. Effects of castration and testosterone substitution on body composition and muscle metabolism in rats. Acta Physiol Scand 1980; 109:233–7.
34 Gruen R, Hietanen E, Greenwood MRC. Increased adipose tissue lipoprotein lipase activity during the development of the genetically obese rat (fa/fa). Metabolism 1978; 27 (suppl. II):1955–66.
35 Rebuffe-Scrive M. Regional adipose tissue metabolism in men and in women during menstrual cycle, pregnancy, lactation, and menopause. Int J Obes 1987; 11:347–55.
36 Krakower GR, James RG, Arnaud C, Etienne J, Keller RH, Kissebah AH. Regional adipocyte precursors in the female rat: influence of ovarian factors. J Clin Invest 1988; 81:641–8.
37 James RG, Kissebah AH. Influence of sexual dimorphism on regional preadipocyte differentiation and fat cell number in female rats. Int J Obes 1989; 13:558.
38 Kissebah AH, Evans DJ, Peiris A, Wilson CR. Endocrine characteristics in regional obesities: role of sex steroids. In: Vague J, Bjorntorp P, Guy-Grand B, Rebuffe-Scrive M, Vague P, eds. Metabolic Complications of Human Obesities. Amsterdam: Elsevier Science Publishing, 1985, pp. 115–130.

39 Peiris A, Kissebah AH. Body fat distribution and free fatty acid metabolism. Clin Res 1988; 36:488A.

40 Stromblad G, Bjorntorp P. Reduced hepatic insulin clearance in rats with dietary-induced obesity. Metabolism 1986; 35:323–7.

41 Randle P, Garland P, Hales C, Newsholme E. The glucose–fatty acid cycle. Its role in insulin sensitivity and the metabolic disturbances of diabetes mellitus. Lancet 1963; i:785–9.

42 Ferrannini E, Barrett EJ, Bevilacqua S, DeFronzo RA. Effect of fatty acids on glucose production and utilization in men. J Clin Invest 1983; 72:1737–47.

43 West KM. Epidemiology of Diabetes and its Vascular Complications. New York: Elsevier Science Publishing, 1978, p. 231.

44 Yki-Jarvinen H. Sex and insulin sensitivity. Metabolism 1984; 33:1011–15.

45 Landon J, Wynn V, Samols E. The effect of anabolic steroids on blood sugar and plasma insulin levels. Metabolism 1963; 12:924–35.

46 Beck P. Contraceptive steroids: modification of carbohydrate and lipid metabolism. Metabolism 1973; 22:841–55.

47 Burghen GA, Givens JR, Kitabchi AE. Correlation of hyperandrogenism with hyperinsulinism in polycystic ovarian disease. J Clin Endocrinol Metab 1980; 50: 113–16.

48 Kahn CR, Flier JS, Bar RS, Archer JA, Gordon P, Martin MM, Roth J. The syndromes of insulin resistance and acanthosis nigricans. Insulin receptor disorders in man. N Engl J Med 1976; 294:739–49.

49 Paik SG, Michaelis MA, Kim YT, Shin S. Induction of insulin-dependent diabetes by streptozoticin: inhibition by estrogens and potentiation by androgens. Diabetes 1982; 31:724–9.

50 Mandour T, Kissebah AH, Wynn V. Mechanisms of oestrogen and progesterone effects of lipid and carbohydrate metabolism: alterations in the insulin–glucagon molar ratio and hepatic enzyme activity. Eur J Clin Invest 1977; 7:181–7.

51 Peiris AN, Meuller RA, Struve MF, Smith GA, Kissebah AH. Relationship of androgenic activity to splanchnic insulin metabolism and peripheral glucose utilization in premenopausal women. J Clin Endocrinol Metab 1987; 64:162–9.

52 Peiris A, Aimen EJ, Drucker WD, Kissebah AH. Contribution of androgen to peripheral insulin resistance in upper body obesity. Endocrinology 1988; 122 (suppl.):203.

53 Roy AK, Chatterjee B. Sexual dimorphism in the liver. Ann Rev Physiol 1983; 45: 37–50.

54 McCarroll AM, Buchanan KD. Physiological factors influencing insulin clearance by the isolated perfused rat liver. Diabetologia 1973; 9:174–7.

55 Hennes MM, McCune S, Shrago E, Kissebah AH. Synergistic effects of male gender and obesity on hepatic insulin dynamics: studies in the SHR/Mcc-c rat. Diabetes 1990; 39:789–95.

56 Krakower GR, Kissebah AH. Pubescence-related changes in hepatocyte insulin dynamics in female rats. Am J Physiol 1989; 256:E780–E787.

57 Krakower GR, Kissebah AH. Relationship of sexual dimorphism to estradiol-mediated regulation of hepatic insulin dynamics. Int J Obes 1989; 13:561.

58 Krotkiewski M, Bjorntorp P. Muscle tissue in obesity with different distribution and adipose tissue. Effects of physical training. Int J Obes 1986; 10:331–41.

59 Hom FG, Goodner CJ. Insulin dose–response characteristics among individual muscle and adipose tissues measured in the rat *in vivo* with ^{3}(H)2-deoxyglucose. Diabetes 1984; 33:153–9.

60 Lefaucheur L, LePeuch C, Barenton B, Vigneron P. Characterization of insulin binding to slices of slow and fast twitch skeletal muscles in the rabbit. Horm Metab Res 1986; 18:725–9.

61 Bouchard C. Inheritance of human fat distribution. In: Bouchard C, Johnston FE, eds.

Current Topics in Nutrition and Disease: Fat Distribution during Growth and Later Health Outcomes. New York: Alan R. Liss, 1988, p. 103.

62 Bjorntorp P. Fat distribution and risk for death, myocardial infarction and stroke. In: Bouchard C, Johnston FE, eds. Current Topics in Nutrition and Disease: Fat Distribution during Growth and Later Health Outcomes. New York: Alan R. Liss, 1988, p. 175.

63 Enzi G, Gasparo M, Biondetti PF, Fiore D, Semisa M, Zurlo F. Subcutaneous and visceral fat distribution according to sex, age and overweight, evaluated by computed tomography. Am J Clin Nutr 1986; 44:739–46.

64 Gustafsson J-A, Mode A, Norstedt G, Eneroth P, Hokfelt T. Growth hormone: a regulator of the sexually differentiated steroid metabolism in rat liver. In: MacLeod MS, Oakley AB, Spielberg SP, eds. Developmental Pharmacology. New York: Alan R. Liss, 1983, pp. 37–59.

65 Bardin CW, Catterall JF. Testosterone: a major determinant of extragenital sexual dimorphism. Science 1981; 211:1285–94.

66 Ehrhardt A, Meyer-Bahlburg HFL. Effects of prenatal sex hormones on gender-related behavior. Science 1981; 211:1312–18.

67 Imperato-McGinley J, Peterson RE, Gautier T, Sturla E. Male pseudohermaphroditism secondary to 5α-reductase deficiency—a model for the role of androgens in both the development of the male phenotype and the evolution of a male gender identity. J Steroid Biochem 1979; 11:637–45.

68 New MI, White PC, Pang S, DuPont B, Speiser PW. The adrenal hyperplasias. In: Scriver CR, Beaudet AL, Sly WS, Valle D, eds. The Metabolic Basis of Inherited Disease, Vol. II. New York: McGraw-Hill Publishing, 1989, pp. 1881–1917.

69 Dostyu DD, Amos DB. The HLA complex: genetic polymorphism and disease susceptibility. In: Scriver CR, Beaudet AL, Sly WS, Valle D, eds. The Metabolic Basis of Inherited Disease, Vol. I. New York: McGraw-Hill Publishing, 1989, pp. 225–49.

Section 9
Diagnostic Criteria: Towards a Rational Approach

Chapter 32
Diagnostic Criteria for Polycystic Ovary Syndrome: Towards a Rational Approach

JOANNA K. ZAWADZKI & ANDREA DUNAIF

Although polycystic ovary syndrome (PCO) is a very common syndrome, ironically it is also poorly understood. At a preliminary National Institute of Child Health and Human Development (NICHD) conference regarding PCO in April 1989, in a written questionnaire many participants described PCO as a manifestation of a disease rather than a specific disease entity or a specific diagnosis, in analogy to congestive heart failure or jaundice. Clinically, such a description can be useful, since a specific aspect of the syndrome, e.g. hirsutism or infertility, may be the presenting complaint, the patient's symptoms may evolve over time, and physicians focus on the patient as a whole rather than on the presenting symptom or syndrome *per se*. From a research viewpoint, however, such a vague description is a limitation rather than an asset. The spectrum of characteristics of PCO can be very extensive. It becomes almost impossible to compile conclusions from research data from different centers if the specific characteristics of subjects are unknown or actually greatly differ. One of the goals of the NICHD Conference on PCO (April 16–18, 1990) was the possible establishment of rational diagnostic criteria of PCO for clinical research. In this chapter, we will discuss some of the goals and limitations of establishing more specific criteria for PCO, the historical perspective from other disease classification systems and the processes by which they evolved, and some of the controversies that were stimulated by the discussions during the conference.

The major goal for establishing more specific criteria for PCO is further understanding of the pathogenesis of this disorder. Thus far, the etiology of PCO has been attributed to the gonad [1] (see Chapter 9), pituitary [2] (see Chapters 3 and 4), or even outside the hypothalamic–pituitary axis, e.g. hyperinsulinemia [3] or insulin-like growth factors

[4] (see Chapters 21–23). The descriptions of patients with this condition have been similarly broad. For example, the original report of Stein and Leventhal [1] described large cystic ovaries as the characteristic ovarian change, and hirsutism, oligomenorrhea, infertility, and obesity as the characteristic clinical presentation. However, of the seven patients described, all were oligo-ovulatory, but only two were obese and four were hirsute. The diversity of clinical presentation has been well described with normal-weight fertile women presenting with apparently polycystic ovaries and obese, oligomenorrheic, hirsute women with apparently normal gonads. In order for criteria of PCO to be useful in meeting the goal of defining the pathogenesis (or pathogeneses) of this disorder(s), the criteria should be as precise as possible in specifying a phenotype. With our current understanding of molecular biology, a phenotype can then be studied to perhaps identify a specific genotype (see Chapter 6).

In general, a good classification system depends on a clear purpose. The purpose of diagnostic criteria for research in PCO, as noted above, sets the stage for further understanding of the pathogenesis. Such classification depends on clear and objective terminology and definitions for the symptoms and signs associated with PCO. Standard classification or diagnostic criteria for the diagnosis of PCO are essential to assure homogeneity in reporting studies of pathogenesis, epidemiology, natural history, and therapy of the specific disease as well as to assure accuracy of diagnosis in the individual patient. In order for a classification system to function well, it must be reproducible both by experts and nonexperts and evolve rationally. Thus, it is preferable if it is based upon biologic facts rather than on an artificial construct or theory. The classification system should be able to include simple and difficult cases, and the system should not be too complex. As much as possible, a classification system must be objective and relate measurable, rather than subjective, data. Any potentially subjective findings, e.g. hirsutism, need to be regarded objectively as much as possible by defining them in terms of standardized rules, e.g. the Ferriman–Gallwey scoring system of hirsutism [5].

After the purpose of the classification system and the classification system itself are defined, experts should convene to make a tentative agreement on the features of the system, and the system must be tested or verified in actual cases. Sensitivity (the proportion of people with the disease who have a positive result), specificity (the proportion of people without the disease who have a negative result), and positive predictive value (probability of disease in people with a positive result) of the criteria can be established. The criteria should be judged on suitability and reproducibility, and differences should be identified. Then, the redefined criteria should be tested again on real cases. Finally, the criteria should be published.

This potential process of evolving a classification system of PCO has evolved from the observation of the development of classification systems of diabetes mellitus [6], arthritic disorders such as rheumatoid arthritis [7–10], and mucosal dysplasia staging in ulcerative colitis [11–12]. From these experiences, it appears that it is easier to formulate a classification system if one already has specific research questions. Particularly from the experiences in the arthritic diseases, it became apparent that a classification system may need to change over time as the disease or the understanding of the disease changes.

The current classification of diabetes mellitus was established in 1979 by the National Diabetes Data Group both for research and clinical use. Many of the definitions published by this group had actually evolved over decades prior to 1979 and some had been previously published in research literature. For example, the distinction between insulin-dependent diabetes mellitus (IDDM) and noninsulin-dependent diabetes mellitits (NIDDM) had previously been noted, and the usefulness of the 2-hour post 75-g glucose load value of 200 mg/dl as a distinction between diabetic and nondiabetic had been noted by both the Pima [13] and Bedford [14] studies and no studies had refuted it.

The diagnosis of rheumatoid arthritis evolved more slowly, with committee meetings in 1948, 1956, 1960, and 1966 redefining the criteria. The diagnostic criteria for rheumatoid arthritis were largely based on symptoms and signs. With current technology it is quite likely that such a process would be faster. The classification or staging system for mucosal dysplasia in ulcerative colitis was intended for use in clinical research. Expert pathologists agreed upon a tentative set of criteria and pathologic slides were reviewed. The criteria were then tested for suitability, reproducibility, and disagreements were identified. Slides were re-reviewed and criteria redefined.

The diagnosis of PCO shares some of the types of characteristics of diabetes mellitus and rheumatoid arthritis, and to a lesser extent mucosal dysplasia in ulcerative colitis. The diagnosis of diabetes mellitus depends on a glucose concentration, a measurement that is easily and precisely (within 3%) reproducible. In contradistinction, the diagnostic criteria of PCO frequently include hyperandrogenemia, though the actual measurement of androgens, such as testosterone or dehydroepiandrosterone sulfate (DHEAS), may vary by as much as 15–20% between different assays. Like the diagnosis of rheumatoid arthritis, the current working diagnosis of PCO includes a constellation of signs and symptoms, including hyperandrogenism, chronic oligo-ovulation, and polycystic ovaries on ultrasound. Although the ovaries in PCO are thought to have a distinct pathologic appearance, in many clinical studies as many as 30% of the ovaries appear normal on ultrasound, and very few patients actually undergo surgery. Thus, it would be difficult to develop specific pathologic criteria as were developed for mucosal dysplasia in ulcerative colitis, though the latter process lends insight into the development of specific criteria.

In order to facilitate the initial evolution of diagnostic criteria for PCO, a written questionnaire was distributed at the very beginning of the April 16–18, 1990 NICHD Conference on PCO. The questionnaire is reproduced as Table 32.1. There were several general questions in this questionnaire:

1 What is a clinical matrix of characteristics of PCO that might be useful in clinical research studies? Specifically, which are classical (>95% agreement), definite, probable (associated with some doubt), possible (which may be discarded over time), and exclusionary criteria? In fact, classical was omitted as a category since both in the 1989 NICHD preliminary conference and in communications before this meeting, no one could identify any classical criteria.

2 How specific is the current nomenclature of PCO? For example, are idiopathic hirsutism and hyperthecosis distinctly separate diagnoses from PCO?

3 Would scoring of the clinical characteristics of PCO be as helpful, for example, as the scoring system used in endometriosis?

The 58 responses to the question of research diagnostic criteria for PCO are summarized in Table 32.2. Of note, there was no more than about two-thirds agreement for any single criterion. A criterion is listed only if at least 40% of the responders had chosen it. Interestingly, one can see some trends in these responses and borderline concordance for diagnostic criteria of PCO among these expert responders.

The responses to the nomenclature of PCO were also divided, though certain trends again evolved. Most (88%) agreed that PCO is a manifestation of disease rather than a disease entity or specific diagnosis, and many (60%) agreed that PCO is a diagnosis of exclusion. The opinion was almost equally divided whether lean and obese women with PCO have the same disease and whether PCO and idiopathic hirsutism are distinctly separate diagnoses. However, most (73%) did not consider PCO and hyperthecosis as distinctly separate diagnoses.

Perhaps the most useful, albeit negative, responses on this questionnaire were to the scoring of clinical characteristics in a specific case presentation. If one plots the total scores that each responder ascribed

Table 32.1 Questionnaire distributed at the NICHD polycystic ovary syndrome conference (April 16–18, 1990): session on diagnostic criteria.

PLEASE ANSWER THE FOLLOWING QUESTIONS (AND SUB-QUESTIONS) AND MAKE ANY ADDITIONAL COMMENTS. THANK YOU.

I *The following are diagnostic criteria of polycystic ovary syndrome:*

Please circle a for a definite or possible criterion; b for a possible criterion; c for any irrelevant criterion.

a b c 1 clinical signs of hyperandrogenism (e.g. hirsutism, alopecia, acne)
a b c 2 biochemical hyperandrogenism ("hyperandrogenemia"); [*circle* if applicable: increased concentrations of testosterone, free testosterone, androstenedione, DHEAS]
a b c 3 menstrual dysfunction; [*circle* if applicable: ≤6 menses/yr]
a b c 4 elevated LH/FSH ratio; [*circle* if applicable: ≥1.5, ≥2, ≥2.5]
a b c 5 polycystic ovaries by ultrasound
a b c 6 perimenarchal onset of symptoms
a b c 7 insulin resistance
a b c 8 exclusion of attenuated congenital adrenal hyperplasia; [*circle* if applicable: 21-hydroxylase deficiency, 3-beta-hydroxysteroid dehydrogenase deficiency, or both?]
a b c 9 exclusion of other etiologies; [*circle* if applicable: Cushing's syndrome, androgen-producing adrenal or ovarian tumor, hyperprolactinemia]
a b c 10 decreased 34-k IGF binding protein

II *Nomenclature*:

Please circle T (true) or F (false).

T F 1 Polycystic ovary syndrome is a manifestation of disease rather than a disease entity or specific diagnosis.
T F 2 Polycystic ovary syndrome is a diagnosis of exclusion.
T F 3 Lean and obese women with PCO have the same disease.
T F 4 PCO and idiopathic hirsutism are distinctly separate diagnoses.
T F 5 PCO and hyperthecosis are distinctly separate diagnoses.

III *Scoring of PCO*: Case Presentation

Hx: 19 yo WF with chief complaint of excess facial hair, onset age 16, treated with electrolysis, not progressive; menarche age 13, cycles q 30–45 days
PE: Ht 4′11″ [mother 5′2″], Wt 57.3 kg, BP 113/64; sparse terminal hair on chin and upper lip; no clitoromegaly
LAB: Testosterone 108, repeat 87 ng/dl (NORMAL 20–80); DHEAS 229 μg/dl (NORMAL 60–230); LH 20 mIU/ml; FSH 11 mIU/ml; 17-OH-progesterone: 153 ng/dl, 1-h ACTH-stimulated 396 ng/dl; normal prolactin, fasting insulin, fasting glucose

Please score this case presentation according to the following criteria, each on a scale of 0–5.

0 1 2 3 4 5 (a) clinical signs of hyperandrogenism
0 1 2 3 4 5 (b) biochemical evidence of hyperandrogenism
0 1 2 3 4 5 (c) menstrual dysfunction
0 1 2 3 4 5 (d) elevated LH/FSH ratio
0 1 2 3 4 5 (e) polycystic ovaries by ultrasound
0 1 2 3 4 5 (f) perimenarchal onset of symptoms
0 1 2 3 4 5 (g) insulin resistance
0 1 2 3 4 5 (h) exclusion of attenuated congenital adrenal hyperplasia
0 1 2 3 4 5 (i) exclusion of other etiologies

____________ Total score

Table 32.2 Polycystic ovary syndrome (PCO) research diagnostic criteria (NIH April 1990, $n = 58$). Numbers in parentheses indicate number of participants who listed this criterion in this category.

Definite or probable	Possible
Hyperandrogenemia (37) 64%	Insulin resistance (40) 69%
Exclusion of other etiologies (35) 60%	Perimenarchal onset (36) 62%
Exclusion of CAH (34) 59%	Elevated LH/FSH (32) 55%
Menstrual dysfunction (30) 52%	PCO by ultrasound (30) 52%
Clinical hyperandrogenism (28) 48%	Clinical hyperandrogenism (30) 52%
	Menstrual dysfunction (26) 45%

to the case presentation, a bell-shaped distribution curve is obtained. Although negative, this information is critical. As Simpson has pointed out elsewhere in this book (see Chapter 6), particularly from a genetic point of view, it would be more helpful to identify subsyndromes rather than to lump all cases together.

The discussion that followed the presentation of these results was similarly diverse. Perhaps, some of the most important comments identified the necessity to better understand the pathogenesis of PCO. Some questioned the appropriateness of the name PCO, as many patients with this diagnosis lack the pathognomonic ovarian ultrasonographic features, as described by Franks (Chapter 2), and few currently undergo surgery. Furthermore, there was much discussion whether an ultrasonographic evaluation of the ovaries should be done in each subject because of the differing equipment and technical skills at different centers and because 30% of the subjects who appeared to have PCO clinically lacked the ultrasonographic findings (see Chapter 2). Alternatively, it was pointed out that some women who ovulate normally and who lack the other criteria of PCO may have polycystic ovaries ultrasonographically. Though a consensus was not reached in the round table discussion, many suggested that detection of polycystic ovaries by ultrasound was not essential for the diagnosis of PCO.

Rather, many concurred that a new term for the syndrome—chronic oligo-ovulatory hyperandrogenism—may be more descriptive. This suggestion raised the issue whether the name should be changed now or whether such a change was premature, because the pathogenesis of PCO is poorly understood and because a name change may inappropriately bias future research.

Instead, some suggested that it is premature to include or exclude criteria and that it would be more helpful to precisely describe what is measured and what is not examined. Because of the complexity of this syndrome, it is not surprising that approaches to the study of this syndrome vary. For example, Rosenfield and his colleagues, as described previously in this book (Chapter 9), have described criteria for PCO that are largely based on tests routinely done by their research group but not elsewhere, specifically the dexamethasone suppression test and gonadotropin-releasing hormone (GnRH) agonist test. Thus, this group's criteria for PCO may be more sensitive and specific, but their patients are difficult to compare to those selected by only clinical criteria.

Thus, the problems of the diagnostic criteria of PCO are multifold: we do not know the sensitivity or specificity of any of the criteria previously cited and there are different approaches to the study of PCO. If the criteria are not sufficiently specific, the spectrum of disorders that is included may actually be too large and diseases may be included that actually have another underlying pathogenesis. Thus, one agreement among the conference attendees was the necessity to describe the phenotype one is studying as accurately as possible so that researchers can compare results. There was general agreement, although less emphatic, that the major research criteria of PCO should include (in order of importance) (i) hyperandrogenism and/or hyperandrogenemia, (ii) oligo-ovulation, (iii) exclusion of other known disorders such as Cushing's syndrome, hyperprolactinemia, or congenital adrenal hyperplasia, and possibly (iv) polycystic ovaries on ultrasound. The last criterion was, however, particularly controversial for the reasons cited previously.

What are the major benefits of classification and diagnostic criteria in PCO? First of all, diagnostic criteria would enable the recognition of other specific syndromes, just as the diagnostic criteria of rheumatoid arthritis enabled the subsequent diagnosis of Lyme disease. Secondly, better standardization of laboratory tests could result. Thirdly, molecular genetics technology has a specific incentive to be a splitter; conversely, if a more homogeneous group is established, there is greater likelihood of establishing a molecular basis; if there is a common molecular basis, then the group can be put together clinically. Lastly, with establishment of diagnostic criteria, more specific approaches to the therapy of PCO will evolve.

References

1 Stein IF, Leventhal ML. Amenorrhea associated with bilateral polycystic ovaries. Am J Obstet Gynecol 1935; 29:181–91.

2 Yen SSC, Vela P, Rankin J. Inappropriate secretion of follicle-stimulating hormone and luteinizing hormone in polycystic ovarian disease. J Clin Endocrinol Metab 1970; 30:435–42.

3 Burghen GA, Givens JR, Kitabchi AE. Correlation of hyperandrogenism with hyperinsulinemia in polycystic ovarian disease. J Clin Endocrinol Metab 1980; 50:113–16.

4 Adashi EY, Resnick CE, D'Ercole AJ, Svoboda ME, Van Wyk JJ. Insulin-like growth factors as intraovarian regulators of granulosa cell growth and function. Endocr Rev 1985; 6:400–20.

5 Ferriman D, Gallwey JD. Clinical assessment of body hair growth in woman. J Clin Endocrinol Metab 1961; 21:1440–7.

6 National Diabetes Data Group. Classification and diagnosis of diabetes mellitus and other categories of glucose intolerance. Diabetes 1979; 28:1039–57.

7 Dictionary of the Rheumatic Diseases. Volume 1, Signs and Symptoms: Volume 2, Diagnostic Testing prepared, by ARA glossary, American Rheumatism Association, 1985.

8 Medsger TA, Masi AT. Epidemiology of the rheumatic diseases. In: McCarty DJ, ed. Arthritis and Allied Conditions. Philadelphia: Lee and Febiger, 1985, pp. 9–39.

9 Altman RD, Meenman RF, Hochberg MC, Bole Jr GG, Brandt K, Derek T, Cooke V, Greenwald RA, Howell DS, Kaplan D, Koopman WJ, Mankin H, Mikkelsen WM, Moskowitz R, Sokoloff L. An approach to developing criteria for the clinical diagnosis and classification of osteoarthritis. J Rheumatol 1983; 10:180–3.

10 Subcommittee for scleroderma criteria of the American Rheumatism Association diagnostic and therapeutic criteria committee. Preliminary criteria for the classification of systemic sclerosis (scleroderma). Arthritis Rheum 1980; 23:581–90.

11 Riddell RH, Goldman H, Ransohoff DF, Appelman HD, Fenoglio CM, Haggitt RC, Ahren C, Correa P, Hamilton SR, Morson BC, Sommers SC, Yardley JH. Dysplasia in inflammatory bowel disease: standardized classification with provisional clinical applications. Hum Pathol 1983; 14:931–68.

12 Ransohoff DF, Riddell RH, Levine B. Ulcerative colitis in colonic cancer. Problems in assessing the diagnostic usefulness of mucosal dysplasia. Dis Colon Rectum 1985; 28:383–8.

13 Bennett PH, Rushforth NB, Miller M, LeCompte PM. Epidemiologic studies of diabetes in the Pima Indians. Recent Prog Horm Res 1976; 32:333–76.

14 Keen H, Jarrett RJ, McCartney P. The ten year followup of the Bedford survey. Diabetologia 1982; 22:73–8.

Index

Page numbers in **bold** refer to figures, those in *italic* refer to tables